Contents

Medical Masterclass third edition

Editor-in-Chief

Dr John D Firth DM FRCP
Consultant Physician and Nephrologist
Addenbrooke's Hospital
Cambridge
UK

Rheumatology and clinical immunology

Editor

Dr Siraj A Misbah MSc FRCP FRCPath
Consultant Clinical Immunologist and Honorary Senior Clinical Lecturer
in Immunology
Oxford University Hospitals NHS Foundation Trust and University
of Oxford
Oxford
UK

Third edition

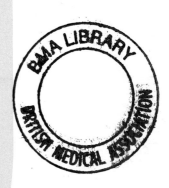

Disclaimer

Although every effort has been made to ensure that drug doses and other information are presented accurately in this publication, the ultimate responsibility rests with the prescribing physician. Neither the publishers nor the authors can be held responsible for any consequences arising from the use of information contained herein. Any product mentioned in this publication should be used in accordance with the prescribing information prepared by the manufacturers.

The information presented in this publication reflects the opinions of its contributors and should not be taken to represent the policy and views of the Royal College of Physicians of London, unless this is specifically stated.

Every effort has been made by the contributors to contact holders of copyright to obtain permission to reproduce copyrighted material. However, if any have been inadvertently overlooked, the publisher will be pleased to make the necessary arrangements at the first opportunity.

List of contributors

Dr Aamir Aslam DPhil MRCP
Consultant Rheumatologist and
Honorary Senior Lecturer
Leeds Teaching Hospitals
Leeds
UK

Dr Hilary J Longhurst MA PhD FRCP
FRCPath
Consultant Immunologist
Barts Health NHS Trust
London
UK

Dr Siraj A Misbah MSc FRCP FRCPath
Consultant Clinical Immunologist and
Honorary Senior Clinical Lecturer in
Immunology
Oxford University Hospitals
NHS Foundation Trust and
University of Oxford
Oxford
UK

Dr Catherine Swales PhD FRCP
Consultant Rheumatologist and
Associate Director of Clinical Studies
Oxford University Hospitals
NHS Foundation Trust
Oxford
UK

Acknowledgements

The third edition of Medical Masterclass has been produced by a team. The names of those who have written and edited are clearly indicated, and along with all these contributors I gratefully acknowledge the contributions of those who wrote and edited the first and second editions. This third edition is based on their foundations, and some of their material has been retained. But my acknowledgements must not stop there, because the Medical Masterclass would not have been published without the efforts of many other people. Naming names is risky, but I must name Claire Daley, who has worked as editor of the third edition with a wonderful combination of quietness and efficiency, and with an attention to detail that has made me feel triumphant if I have ever spotted a misplaced comma in a proof.

Dr John Firth DM FRCP
Medical Masterclass Editor-in-Chief

© 2008, 2010, 2018 Royal College of Physicians of London

Cover image courtesy of: Dr P Marazzi / Science Photo Library

Published by:
Royal College of Physicians of London
11 St Andrews Place
Regent's Park
London NW1 4LE
United Kingdom

Typeset by Manila Typesetting Company, Makati City, Philippines

Printed by The Lavenham Press Limited, Suffolk

First edition published 2001
Reprinted 2004
Second edition published 2008
Updated and reprinted 2010
Third edition published 2018

ISBN: 978-1-86016-668-6 (this book)
eISBN: 978-1-86016-669-3 (this book)
ISBN: 978-1-86016-670-9 (set)
eISBN: 978-1-86016-671-6 (set)

Royal College of Physicians of London
11 St Andrews Place
Regent's Park
London NW1 4LE
United Kingdom
Tel: +44 (0)20 3075 1379
Email: medical.masterclass@rcplondon.ac.uk
Web: www.rcplondon.ac.uk/medicalmasterclass

Preface

This third edition of Medical Masterclass is produced and published by the Royal College of Physicians of London. It comprises 12 books and an online question bank. Its aim is to interest and help doctors in their first few years of training, to enable them to improve their medical knowledge and skills, and to pass postgraduate medical examinations, most particularly the MRCP(UK): Part 1, Part 2 and PACES (the practical assessment of clinical examination skills that is the final part of the exam).

The 12 textbooks are divided as follows: two cover the scientific background to medicine; one is devoted to general clinical skills, including medicine for older people, palliative care and specific guidance on exam technique for PACES; one deals with acute medicine; and the other eight cover the range of medical specialties.

The medical specialties are dealt with in eight sections:

> Case histories – you are presented with letters of referral that are commonly received in each specialty and led through the ways in which the patients' histories should be explored, and what investigations and/or treatments should follow, as in Station 2 of PACES.

> Physical examination scenarios – these emphasise solid and reliable clinical method, logical analysis of physical signs and sensible clinical reasoning ('having found this, what would you want to do next?'), as in Stations 1 and 3 of PACES.

> Communication and ethical scenarios – you are presented with difficult issues that can arise in each specialty. What should you actually say in response to the 'frequently asked (but nonetheless tricky) questions', as required in Station 4 of PACES?

> Brief clinical consultations – how should you take a focused history and perform a focused examination of a patient who has a medical problem when there isn't much time? This section explains how to do this while working as a medical registrar on take, or in Station 5 of PACES.

> Acute presentations – what are your priorities if you are the doctor seeing a patient in the emergency department or the medical admissions unit? The material in this section is relevant to all parts of the MRCP(UK) exam.

> Diseases and treatments – concise structured notes that are of particular relevance to the Part 1 and Part 2 exams.

> Investigations and practical procedures – short and concise notes.

> Self-assessment questions – in the form used in the Part 1 and Part 2 exams.

The online question bank, which is continually updated, enables you to take mock Part 1 and Part 2 exams, or to be selective in the questions that you tackle (if you want to do 10 questions on cardiology, or any other specialty, then you can do so). You can see how your scores compare with those of others who have attempted the same questions, which helps you to know where to focus your learning.

I hope that you enjoy using the Medical Masterclass to learn more about medicine. I know that medicine is tough at the moment, with hospital services under unprecedented pressure and the medical registrar bearing more than their fair share of the burden. But careers are a long game, and being a physician is a wonderful occupation. It is sometimes intellectually and/or emotionally very challenging, but with these challenges come great rewards, and few things give more substantial satisfaction than being a doctor who provides good care for a patient. The Medical Masterclass should help you do to that, as well as to pass the MRCP(UK) exam along the way.

Dr John Firth DM FRCP
Medical Masterclass Editor-in-Chief

Key features

We have created a range of icon boxes that sit among the text of the various Medical Masterclass books. They are there to help you identify key information and to make learning easier and more enjoyable. Here is a brief explanation:

This icon is used to highlight points of particular importance.

Key point

A patient with a normal physical examination, a normal ECG and a normal echocardiogram is at very low risk of significant arrhythmia.

This icon is used to indicate common or important drug interactions, pitfalls of practical procedures, or when to take symptoms or signs particularly seriously.

Hazard

Acute lymphoblastic leukaemia may present in an identical manner to infectious mononucleosis.

Case examples / case histories are used to demonstrate why and how an understanding of the scientific background to medicine helps in the practice of clinical medicine.

Case history

A man with a renal transplant is immunosuppressed with ciclosporin, azathioprine and prednisolone. He develops recurrent gout and is started on allopurinol.

Rheumatology

Authors

Dr A Aslam, Dr HJ Longhurst, Dr SA Misbah and Dr C Swales

Editor

Dr SA Misbah

Editor-in-Chief

Dr JD Firth

The rheumatology section of the second edition of Medical Masterclass was written by Dr WG Dixon, Dr B Griffiths, Dr HJ Longhurst, Dr N Snowden and Dr SA Misbah (editor). This third edition of Medical Masterclass contains entirely new material, but many sections from the second edition have been retained and updated, and we gratefully acknowledge the contribution of these authors.

Rheumatology and clinical immunology: Section 1

1 PACES stations and acute scenarios

1.1 History taking

1.1.1 Recurrent chest infections

Dear Doctor,

Re: Mr Ian Jones, aged 25 years

This young man, who works as a systems analyst, has been admitted to hospital with pneumonia three times in the past 2 years. He has also had several episodes of sinusitis. His only other symptom is diarrhoea, which might be related to antibiotics that he has had for his chest and sinuses. I wonder if he has some predisposition to infection and would be grateful for your advice.

Yours sincerely,

Introduction

Is this patient immunodeficient?
You must decide whether this man has an underlying immunological problem and, if so, determine what it is:

> If only one site (eg the respiratory tract) is affected, then local causes such as a tumour, foreign body or aspiration are most likely, but less common causes such as immune deficiency or ciliary dysfunction should be considered.

> Unusually severe or frequent infections, affecting different body sites, suggest the possibility of an immunodeficiency.

> Bacterial respiratory tract infections are most commonly associated with antibody deficiency, such as common variable immunodeficiency (CVID).

> Primary immunodeficiencies are uncommon but their diagnosis is often delayed for many years, leading to significant avoidable morbidity and mortality. The respiratory tract, gut and skin are the most common sites of infection in antibody deficiency.

History of the presenting problem

What pathogens has he been infected with to date?
Bacterial infections suggest an antibody deficiency. *Giardia* species are common bowel pathogens, as are persistent viral infections, particularly norovirus. Mild CD4 deficiency may occur in CVID and manifests as recurrent herpes simplex or zoster. Any suggestion of a more severe T-cell defect should prompt you to consider a combined T-cell and B-cell defect such as hyper-immunoglobulin M (IgM) syndrome or a 'leaky' severe combined immunodeficiency (SCID) (see Section 2.1.2). In routine clinical practice, although it will not available in PACES, check the patient's medical record for results of cultures: if pathogens have been isolated, this will help confirm the relative seriousness of the infections and will guide future antimicrobial therapy.

Severity

How long do infections last? How well do they respond to antibiotics? The need for surgery or excessive time off work is an indicator of severe disease. In antibody-deficient patients infections may be less acute, but are slow to clear.

Antibiotic response is often suboptimal unless high doses and longer duration of treatment (2 weeks is typical for an uncomplicated chest infection) are given.

Key point
The warning signs of immune deficiencies are:

> Frequent infections – what constitutes abnormally frequent infection will vary according to the patient, but in general, more than one hospital admission for infection in a year or more than six courses of antibiotics should trigger an investigation.

> Invasive infections – the definition of invasive depends on patient and organism factors: clearly a brain abscess in the absence of underlying risk factors would be of more concern than a cutaneous abscess.

> Unusual organisms – pneumococcal pneumonia can occur in healthy people, whereas *Pneumocystis* pneumonia suggests a severe immunodeficiency, usually HIV.

> Associated features – paradoxically, immunodeficient people are at greater risk of immunological complications such as granulomata, vasculitis or allergic reactions.

> Family history – many immune deficiencies are inherited, hence a known family history of immunodeficiency or unexplained infant deaths may be relevant.

When did the problem start?

CVID is acquired, often in early adulthood. If your patient has had a significant history of childhood problems, consider a late presentation of X-linked agammaglobulinaemia (XLA) (see Section 2.1.1) or a leaky SCID. Ask the patient specifically about common childhood illnesses.

Consequences of CVID

You need more details about this man's diarrhoea. It may simply be a result of chronic infection or bacterial overgrowth, but coeliac and inflammatory bowel disease-type enterocolitis may also occur. Ask about symptoms of bronchiectasis.

Other relevant history

What is his drug history?

Is the patient taking antiepileptics, eg phenytoin or carbamazepine? Is he on treatment for arthritis, eg gold, penicillamine, sulfasalazine or methotrexate? Has he required oral or high-dose inhaled corticosteroids? These are potentially reversible causes of hypogammaglobulinaemia. Antibody deficiency is a late complication of rituximab treatment.

Features associated with CVID

Does this man have a personal or family history of organ-specific autoimmunity? Ask about the following:

> Anaemia or thrombocytopenia – pernicious anaemia and autoimmune cytopenias are common in CVID.

> Arthralgia, which is often reactive but may be septic, is caused by *Mycoplasma* spp as well as by more conventional organisms.

> In CVID, granulomas may produce a sarcoid-like picture.

Key point

The mouth is a good place to look for signs of immunodeficiency:

> Tonsils (and other lymphoid tissue) are absent in antibody defects due to B-cell developmental abnormalities, such as XLA.

> Herpes, candidiasis or hairy oral leukoplakia are suggestive of a combined or T-cell defect.

> Periodontal disease occurs in chronic granulomatous disease and other neutrophil-killing or chemotaxis defects.

> Aphthous ulcers are a non-specific sign of immunodeficiency.

Key point

Primary or secondary antibody deficiency?

If this patient has antibody deficiency, is it primary or secondary? In a 25-year-old, once you have scrutinised his drug history, you are unlikely to find additional underlying pathology. You should, however, consider whether he may have intestinal lymphangiectasia, protein-losing enteropathy, severe nephrotic syndrome or a lymphoproliferative condition, all of which can cause secondary antibody deficiency.

Plan for investigation and management

After explaining to the patient that under normal circumstances you would carry out a thorough clinical examination, you would plan in the interim to undertake blood tests and scans to help with the following:

> define the immunological defect

> diagnose active infections

> assess structural damage

> initiate ongoing monitoring

> give appropriate treatment.

Define the immunological defect

Baseline investigations include full blood count (FBC), routine chemistry and immunoglobulins, including protein electrophoresis. Secondary causes of low immunoglobulins include lymphoproliferative disease (particularly myeloma), chronic lymphocytic leukaemia or lymphoma. Low albumin suggests the possibility of protein loss from the bowel or renal tract.

In future, genetic diagnosis is likely to be available in specialist centres. For further investigation see Section 3.3.

Diagnose active infections

This man has several potential sites of active infection:

> Respiratory system: request sputum microscopy and culture, and a chest radiograph if symptoms suggest active infection.

> Gastrointestinal (GI) tract: request repeated stool microscopy and culture, and polymerase chain reaction (PCR) for common stool viruses. Organise upper GI endoscopy including a duodenal biopsy and aspirate looking for *Giardia* spp, and also for bowel changes such as villous atrophy or, rarely, lymphoid interstitial hyperplasia / lymphangiectasia. Consider colonoscopy if inflammatory bowel disease is a possibility.

> Other sites: get samples for culture where possible. Remember that serology is likely to be unhelpful.

Assess structural damage and initiate ongoing monitoring

Get a baseline chest radiograph and computerised tomography (CT) scan of the chest (Fig 1) and sinuses. Take a radiograph of arthritic joints. Do baseline and annual lung-function tests. Take blood for baseline liver function and for hepatitis B and C markers if immunoglobulin replacement is contemplated.

Management

You should explain to the patient that the results of blood tests will be reviewed at the next outpatient visit.

Give appropriate treatment

> Acute infections require a prolonged course of antibiotics.

> If the patient is shown to have a severe antibody deficiency syndrome, long-term immunoglobulin replacement through the intravenous or subcutaneous route will be required (see Section 3.7). Immunoglobulin G (IgG) subclass or specific antibody deficiencies can often be managed with prophylactic antibiotics, such as azithromycin 500 mg once daily for 3 days every fortnight.

Further discussion

Key point

Consider other causes of a recurrent chest infection, many of which are associated with diarrhoea:

> common – foreign body, HIV, ciliary dysfunction caused by smoking and cystic fibrosis

> uncommon – immotile cilia syndrome and Young's syndrome (obstructive azoospermia and ciliary dysfunction).

Patients who have relatively rare conditions, such as CVID, are unlikely to meet others with the same condition. If the patient has this condition, then offer him the contact details of self-help organisations, such as UK Primary Immune-deficiency Patient Support (UKPIPS) (www.ukpips.org.uk) or Primary Immunodeficiency UK (PID UK) (www.piduk.org), that provide information and practical support.

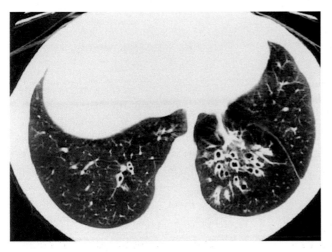

Fig 1 CT scan showing dilated and thickened airways that are characteristic of bronchiectasis.

1.1.2 Recurrent meningitis

Letter of referral to the immunology outpatient clinic

Dear Doctor,

Re: Mr Bill Taylor, aged 20 years

Thank you for seeing this student who has had two episodes of meningococcal meningitis. The first was at the age of 6 years and the second was 3 months ago. He has made a full recovery. I wonder if he has an underlying immunological defect and would be grateful for your opinion.

Yours sincerely,

Introduction

Meningococcal meningitis is a serious infection with significant morbidity and mortality rates. Your task is to determine whether there is an underlying reason for this man's infection and, if so, to advise on action to prevent a recurrence.

Underlying causes for recurrent meningitis:

> traumatic or congenital connection with the subarachnoid space causing a cerebrospinal fluid (CSF) leak

> deficiency of a component of a terminal pathway of complement (C5, C6, C7 or C8; C9 deficiency is usually asymptomatic), or properdin or factor D in the alternative pathway

> other immunodeficiencies: the patient's history will almost always reveal associated features

> recurrent aseptic meningitis (Mollaret's): some cases are associated with herpes simplex virus infection

> Behçet's disease (see Section 2.5.5)

> systemic lupus erythematosus (see Section 2.4.1).

History of the presenting problem

In routine clinical practice, ensure that you have enough information to confirm the diagnosis:

> Were meningococci cultured from blood or CSF?

> Were typical features of invasive meningococcal infection present?

Take this opportunity to ensure that appropriate antibiotic prophylaxis was given to your patient and his household contacts after treatment.

Are there any clues to suggest an external connection with the subarachnoid space?

This is the most common cause of recurrent meningitis, but it is uncommon for meningococci to cause infection in this setting and the causative organisms vary (*Streptococcus pneumoniae*, *Haemophilus influenzae*) (Fig 2).

Ask about the following:

> head injuries, especially fractures involving the base of the skull

> chronic sinusitis, mastoiditis or inner-ear disease

> previous brain or pituitary surgery.

Immunological cause

Deficiency of the terminal complement components, C5–C9, and deficiencies of the alternative pathway components, properdin and factor D, are strongly associated with an increased risk of neisserial infection and occasionally with *Escherichia coli* or other organisms. Infection may be recurrent and disseminated, but is often less intense in the presence of complement deficiency.

Other immunodeficiencies are sometimes associated with recurrent meningitis, hence ask the patient about features associated with antibody or cellular deficiencies (see Sections 2.1.1 and 2.1.2).

Other relevant history

Has the patient ever had gonorrhoea? If so, were there complications?

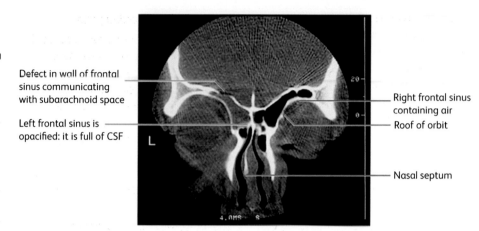

Fig 2 CT scan of a man who developed meningitis several years after a head injury. A defect in the frontal sinus communicates with the subarachnoid space. The left frontal sinus is opacified because it is full of CSF. (Reproduced with permission from Bannister BA, Begg NT, Gillespie SH. *Infectious Disease*, 2nd edn. Oxford: Blackwell Science, 2000.)

Labels in figure:
- Defect in wall of frontal sinus communicating with subarachnoid space
- Left frontal sinus is opacified: it is full of CSF
- Right frontal sinus containing air
- Roof of orbit
- Nasal septum
- L

Gonorrhoea is a neisserial infection and more likely to be disseminated to the joints or skin in the presence of a terminal complement deficiency.

Family history – if the history suggests an X-linked inheritance, properdin deficiency is most likely; autosomal recessive inheritance suggests one of the terminal pathway component deficiencies or, very rarely, factor D deficiency.

If the patient has terminal complement or properdin deficiency, he will be asymptomatic and have no physical signs between attacks.

Plan for investigation and management

After explaining to the patient that under normal circumstances you would carry out a thorough clinical examination, you would plan in the interim to investigate as follows.

CSF leak

The investigation of choice is magnetic resonance imaging (MRI). Increase the diagnostic sensitivity by making sure that the radiologist is fully informed about the clinical picture.

Complement deficiency

Fresh samples, sent on ice, are required.

> Haemolytic complement assays (CH50 or CH100) measure the ability of the classic complement pathway, C1–C9, to lyse red cells (Table 1).

> The AP50 (or AP100) measures lysis by the alternative pathway – factor B to complement C9.

The absence of red cell lysis implies the absence of one of the factors in the assayed pathway. If either of these

Table 1 Interpretation of haemolytic complement assays CH50 and AP50

	Classic pathway CH50	
	Normal	Abnormal
Alternative pathway AP50		
Normal	No abnormality of complement	C1–C4 abnormal
Abnormal	Factor B, D or properdin abnormal	C5–C9 abnormal

screening tests is abnormal, the test should be repeated to exclude a sample handling problem, and each relevant complement component should be measured individually. Occasionally, a non-functional complement component may be present. If no quantitative deficiency is found to account for absent lysis (and you are certain that the CH50 sample was handled correctly), then request functional studies.

Management

You should explain to the patient that the results of blood tests will be reviewed at the next outpatient visit.

Antibiotics

Prescribe long-term prophylactic phenoxymethylpenicillin 500 mg twice daily. Some organisms may, however, be resistant.

Immunisation

Conjugated vaccines against *Neisseria meningitidis* types A, C, Y and W-135 and type B should be given. Older unconjugated vaccines for types A, C, Y and W-135 give short-term protection and revaccination with conjugated vaccines should be arranged. Measurements of meningococcal antibody levels can help you decide when reimmunisation is necessary, although these may be unreliable. Bear in mind that higher antibody levels may be required for protection in complement-deficient individuals and that disease is often caused by uncommon serotypes not covered by immunisation.

> **! Hazard**
>
> Immunisation will reduce, but not eliminate, the risk of recurrent meningococcal meningitis for this man. For patients with early complement component or C3 deficiency, additional immunisation with pneumococcal conjugate and *Haemophilus* conjugate vaccines is indicated.

Replacement of missing factor

This is not usually practical, because the half-life of circulating complement is extremely short. Infusions of fresh frozen (or commercially available solvent-treated) plasma would be required, with significant expense, inconvenience and some risk to your patient.

CSF leak due to cranial anatomical defects

The demonstration of a cranial anatomical defect, either congenital or acquired (following trauma), will require neurosurgical intervention to plug the gap.

Further discussion

Genetic counselling

If a complement deficiency is identified, depending on the exact deficit, the CH50 or AP50 may be used for screening of relatives.

1.1.3 Recurrent facial swelling and abdominal pain

> **Letter of referral to the immunology outpatient clinic**
>
> **Dear Doctor,**
>
> **Re: Mrs Kathy Leighton, aged 30 years**
>
> This woman has had two episodes of angio-oedema. The most recent, which occurred following dental treatment, required overnight hospital admission. She also has recurrent abdominal pain, thought to be due to irritable bowel syndrome. I wonder if she has had an allergic reaction and would be grateful if you could help with establishing an underlying diagnosis.
>
> Yours sincerely,

Introduction

The combination of recurrent angio-oedema and abdominal pain should immediately raise the possibility of C1 inhibitor deficiency. You must, however, differentiate C1 inhibitor deficiency from drug-induced angio-oedema and anaphylaxis. Both C1 inhibitor deficiency and anaphylaxis present with facial and laryngeal oedema, but there are differences in these presentations. This is an important diagnosis to make – both disorders can present as medical emergencies with upper airway obstruction, but they require very different treatment and prophylaxis.

> **Key point**
>
> **C1 inhibitor**
>
> The C1 inhibitor limits activation of the early part of the classic complement cascade, as well as having a regulatory role in other inflammatory pathways, particularly the contact pathway. C1 inhibitor deficiency results in activation and consumption of the early components C4 and C2. Other regulatory mechanisms prevent C3 breakdown or further activation of the complement pathway. Increased local bradykinin levels result from reduced regulation of the contact pathway. Bradykinin is responsible for increased capillary permeability and the increased tendency to angio-oedema.

History of the presenting problem

The history is critical in distinguishing between C1 inhibitor deficiency and anaphylaxis.

Are there any features to suggest anaphylaxis?

How soon after the dental work did the reaction occur? How rapidly did the symptoms develop? Anaphylactic reactions usually occur immediately after the allergic stimulus, virtually always within 30 minutes, and the symptoms progress rapidly. The symptoms related to C1 inhibitor deficiency or other forms of angio-oedema usually build up over several hours and last for several days.

Urticaria, asthma and hypotension caused by generalised vasodilatation do not occur in angio-oedema due to C1 inhibitor deficiency, but they are common features of anaphylaxis (see Section 2.2.1).

Is C1 inhibitor deficiency the explanation?

This woman's abdominal pain may be the result of intestinal oedema. This strongly favours a diagnosis of C1 inhibitor deficiency and may be the presenting feature in children. Dermal swellings affecting limbs or genitals are common, but urticaria is not associated with this condition.

Key point

C1 inhibitor deficiency and bradykinin-mediated angio-oedemas do not improve with antihistamines, corticosteroids or epinephrine.

Precipitating factors
Symptoms following trauma

Even minor trauma such as dental work can precipitate symptoms in someone with C1 inhibitor deficiency. This may be mistaken for their being allergic to local anaesthetics. Ask about dermal swellings, which often follow minor knocks.

Are there any other triggers causing angio-oedema?

Ask about other precipitants of angio-oedema in those with C1 inhibitor deficiency: minor infections, emotional stress and endogenous oestrogens.

Is drug-induced angio-oedema the explanation?

Angiotensin-converting enzyme (ACE) inhibitors are a common cause of bradykinin-mediated angio-oedema. As symptoms do not follow immediately after taking the tablets, the patient may not link the symptoms with the medication. Most people with ACE inhibitor-induced angio-oedema do not have C1 inhibitor deficiency, although ACE inhibitors will precipitate attacks in affected people.

The following may be other drug-related causes of angio-oedema:

> anaphylactic (immunoglobulin E (IgE)-induced mast cell degranulation), eg penicillin allergy

> anaphylactoid (non-IgE-induced mast cell degranulation), eg radiographic contrast media

> immune complex mediated, eg blood products

> cytokine release, eg monoclonal antibodies.

Do not forget physical factors (cold, pressure and vibration). All of these may be associated with urticaria, which effectively excludes the diagnosis of C1 inhibitor deficiency. Idiopathic angio-oedema is common, is often associated with urticaria and does not normally require extensive investigation.

Other relevant history

Is there a family history of angio-oedema? C1 inhibitor deficiency may be congenital or acquired.

Congenital

Ask about the patient's family history. Congenital C1 inhibitor deficiency is inherited in an autosomal dominant manner. The onset of symptoms is usually in adolescence. If the diagnosis is confirmed, your patient will need genetic counselling and practical advice on the screening of any potentially affected relatives.

Hereditary angio-oedema with normal C1 inhibitor levels and function ('HAE, type 3')

Symptoms suggestive of hereditary angio-oedema, predominantly affecting women in an autosomal dominant pattern, are associated with gain-of-function factor XII mutations in some cases. Management, best undertaken in a specialist centre, is similar to that of C1 inhibitor deficiency.

Acquired C1 inhibitor deficiency

Autoantibodies to C1 inhibitor or paraproteins may result in the depletion or functional deficiency of C1 inhibitor. These occur as a result of autoimmune (systemic lupus erythematosus and rheumatoid) or lymphoproliferative disease.

Plan for investigations and management

After explaining to the patient that under normal circumstances you would carry out a thorough clinical examination, you would plan to proceed as follows.

Investigation
Diagnosis of C1 inhibitor deficiency

Screen for C1 inhibitor deficiency by checking serum C4 levels (Fig 3). If C4 is low, or if the history is suggestive of bradykinin-mediated angio-oedema, check C1 inhibitor level and function.

Key point

A low C4 level (with normal C3) is a hallmark of both hereditary and functional C1 inhibitor deficiency – even between attacks. Conversely, a repeatedly normal C4 makes the diagnosis unlikely.

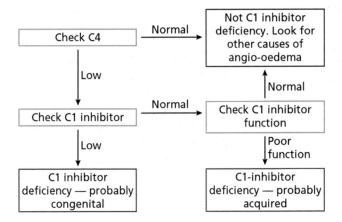

Fig 3 Algorithm for diagnosis of C1 inhibitor deficiency.

Associated disease

In acquired C1 inhibitor deficiency, check the following:

> FBC and film

> immunoglobulins

> serum and urine electrophoresis

> antinuclear antibody

> rheumatoid factor

> cryoglobulins.

Management

You should explain to the patient that the results of her blood tests will be reviewed at her next outpatient visit. If a diagnosis of C1 inhibitor deficiency is made, then the principles of management are as follows.

Treatment of acute attacks

For severe attacks, give C1 inhibitor concentrate or icatibant (a bradykinin B2 receptor antagonist) or, if this is not available, plasma. Epinephrine (adrenaline) is likely to be ineffective. Self-administration has been shown to improve outcomes and reduce hospital attendance, and training programmes are available in specialist centres.

Intercurrent prophylaxis

For hereditary C1 inhibitor deficiency:

> increase production by using modified androgens such as stanozolol or danazol, or

> decrease consumption by giving tranexamic acid, or

> increase C1 inhibitor levels by twice weekly C1 inhibitor infusion – this may be required in a minority of patients with very frequent attacks.

> **Hazard**

Long-term danazol therapy may be associated with hepatocellular adenomas, so monitor the patient's liver function at regular intervals and arrange ultrasonography of the liver every 2 years. Weight, blood pressure and cholesterol should also be monitored.

To reduce the incidence of androgenic side effects, a maximum dose of 100–200 mg daily is recommended for long-term use.

For acquired C1 inhibitor deficiency, treat the underlying cause. If prophylaxis is required, tranexamic acid is usually most effective.

Recommend that the patient wears a Medic-Alert bracelet, and alert her local accident and emergency department so that acute attacks can be appropriately treated.

ACE inhibitor-induced angio-oedema

Management involves permanent withdrawal of the drug. Angiotensin II antagonists are tolerated by most patients, but may themselves rarely cause angio-oedema.

Anaphylaxis

See Section 2.2.1.

Further discussion

Key point

Pregnancy and C1 inhibitor deficiency

A patient with this condition needs specific pregnancy advice:

> All androgens should be stopped before conception (to avoid the risk of virilisation).

> Tranexamic acid may be considered after 12 weeks' gestation.

> C1 inhibitor concentrate can be used for acute attacks, and may occasionally be required as twice weekly prophylaxis.

> Symptoms may improve or worsen during pregnancy.

> Prophylactic C1 inhibitor concentrate should be considered for patients giving birth by caesarean section.

Key point

Surgical or dental procedures and C1 inhibitor deficiency

> High risk: give C1 inhibitor concentrate preoperatively.

> Low risk: consider high-dose danazol (600 mg once daily) for 5 days before and 3 days after the procedure. Ensure that the C1 inhibitor concentrate or icatibant is available for emergencies; the patient will be at increased risk of attacks for 72 hours after the procedure.

1.1.4 Recurrent skin abscesses

Dear Doctor,

Re: Mr Danny Albright, aged 17 years

Thank you for seeing this 17-year-old boy who has had recurrent abscesses on a background of eczema. He has rarely been free of abscesses for the past 2 years, and on three occasions these have required incision and drainage. His father has also suffered from the occasional abscess.

I am concerned that he may have an underlying immunodeficiency and would be grateful for your help in investigating him and formulating an appropriate plan of management.

Yours sincerely,

Introduction

Is this patient likely to be immunodeficient?

Recurrent skin abscesses are common. They are distressing and expensive in time and resources, but are not usually associated with underlying immunodeficiency. However, they may occasionally be the presenting feature of a life-threatening condition, such as chronic granulomatous disease (CGD), hyper-IgE syndrome, Wiskott–Aldrich syndrome or common variable immunodeficiency {Section 2.1.1} (Table 2). You must be sure not to miss the occasional serious immunodeficiency, while providing practical advice for controlling the problem to those for whom that diagnosis is excluded. Although your list of differential diagnoses will include immunodeficiencies, the most likely explanation for this problem is staphylococcal colonisation.

Table 2 Differential diagnosis of recurrent skin abscesses

Common	Rare
Staphylococcal colonisation	CGD Neutrophil G6PD deficiency (common, but rarely presents with abscesses) Neutrophil MPD deficiency (common, but rarely presents with abscesses) Antibody deficiency Other immune deficiencies: hyper-IgE (Job's) syndrome, Wiskott–Aldrich syndrome, combined (antibody/cellular) immune deficiencies

CGD, chronic granulomatous disease; G6PD, glucose-6-phosphate dehydrogenase; IgE, immunoglobulin E; MPD, myeloperoxidase.

Key point

Chronic granulomatous disease (CGD)

Phagocytes of patients with CGD cannot efficiently kill organisms that they have engulfed, leading to granuloma or abscess formation and failure to clear the infection.

History of the presenting problem

What types of abscesses has he had?
Ask about the abscesses:

> Location – are they superficial and confined to the skin, or have they affected internal organs? If they have affected the skin only, then staphylococcal colonisation is by far the most likely diagnosis.

> How frequently do they occur?

> Are they large boils, needing surgical drainage, or smaller pustules?

> When did they start? A history of problems going back to childhood or infancy makes a congenital problem more likely.

> Does each abscess respond rapidly to conventional treatment? This makes immunodeficiency less likely.

Other relevant history

Is staphylococcal skin colonisation the explanation?
Ask about chronic skin conditions, particularly eczema (as in this case).

Does the patient have diabetes? Both of these common disorders increase the risk of abscesses, usually due to *Staphylococcus*.

Key point

Severe eczema causes damage to the protective barrier of the skin and is associated with staphylococcal colonisation. It is also a feature of two primary immunodeficiencies, although both are very rare, especially in adults.

Hyper-IgE (Job's) syndrome

Severe infections, especially skin and chest with pneumatoceles, failure to lose primary dentition, abnormal facies and grossly elevated serum IgE (this is not specific for the hyper-IgE syndrome because many patients with atopic eczema have comparable IgE levels).

Wiskott–Aldrich syndrome

X-linked combined (cellular and antibody) immunodeficiency, with severe infections. Thrombocytopenia with abnormally small platelets on the blood film.

Are there any other features to suggest immunodeficiency?
Ask about the following because the presence of any of these features would make an underlying immune deficiency more likely:

> Has there been associated invasive disease, abscesses of internal organs,

chronic periodontitis or persistent lymphadenopathy?

> Does he have inflammatory bowel disease or perineal abscesses?

> Did he have any problems with his Bacillus Calmette–Guérin (BCG) immunisation?

> Are there features of other immunodeficiencies (see Section 3.3).

> Has he been infected with unusual organisms? In routine clinical practice (but they will not be available in PACES), you should review notes and microbiology reports looking for evidence of *Aspergillus*, *Klebsiella*, *Serratia*, *Burkholderia* spp, as well as the more commonplace *Staphylococcus* spp, *E. coli* and *Salmonella* spp.

Key point

Recurrent infections with catalase-positive bacteria and *Aspergillus* spp are characteristic of serious neutrophil defects such as CGD (Fig 4).

Family history

Have there been any premature deaths in the family, or unusual infections? CGD is X-linked in 65% of cases, the rest being autosomal recessive. Abscesses resulting from staphylococcal colonisation often affect several members of the household.

Plan for investigation and management

After explaining to the patient that under normal circumstances you would carry out a thorough clinical examination, you would plan in the interim to investigate as follows.

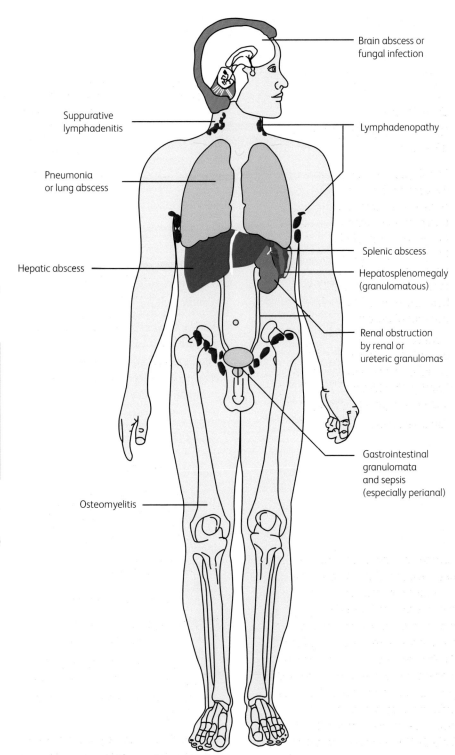

Fig 4 Common sites of pathology in chronic granulomatous disease (CGD).

Brain abscess or fungal infection

Lymphadenopathy

Suppurative lymphadenitis

Pneumonia or lung abscess

Splenic abscess

Hepatic abscess

Hepatosplenomegaly (granulomatous)

Renal obstruction by renal or ureteric granulomas

Gastrointestinal granulomata and sepsis (especially perianal)

Osteomyelitis

Investigation

Check his FBC, immunoglobulins and glucose. Take samples from his abscesses, looking for unusual organisms, and take swabs from his hairline, nose and perineum to look for *Staphylococcus aureus*.

If the history includes any features of immune deficiency then further investigation will be necessary to exclude CGD, using specialised tests that require discussion with the laboratory:

> Nitroblue tetrazolium (NBT) slide test – assesses the integrity of the neutrophil respiratory burst (nicotinamide adenine dinucleotide phosphate (NADPH) oxidase system). In neutrophil-killing defects (CGD, neutrophil glucose-6-phosphate dehydrogenase (G6PD) or myeloperoxidase (MPD) deficiency), neutrophils fail to reduce the NBT crystals that they have phagocytosed (Fig 5).

> Neutrophil respiratory burst by flow cytometry – the 'dihydrorhodamine fluorescence test' is replacing NBT testing in many laboratories.

If the NBT screening test suggests a defect:

> Check for the absence of individual NADPH subunits.

> If the NADPH system is intact, consider G6PD and MPD deficiency as alternative causes for the defective NBT test.

Management

You should explain to the patient that the results of his blood tests will be reviewed at his next outpatient visit.

If no immunological cause is found:

Treat eczema (in this case) and optimise control of diabetes (if relevant). Reduce staphylococcal skin colonisation with at least 2 weeks (often longer) of the following:

> Bath or shower daily using an antiseptic preparation such as chlorhexidine, with emollient if severe eczema is present, all over the body, including the hair.

> Each person in a household should use his or her own towel, which should be changed every day.

> In addition to the above, consider a short course (10 days) of a topical antibiotic, such as neomycin/chlorhexidine or (in resistant cases) mupirocin, to the nasal vestibule.

Key point

In cases of staphylococcal carriage, every member of the patient's household should be treated because recolonisation from untreated people will occur.

If CGD is the diagnosis, the principles of management are as follows:

> Prescribe prophylactic antibiotics (co-trimoxazole) and antifungal therapy (itraconazole), and give detailed instructions on the personal precautions to take to avoid infection (see Table 3).

> Acute infections – see Section 2.1.3.

> Refer to a specialist with an interest in CGD, who may consider interferon-γ prophylaxis or bone marrow transplantation in difficult cases.

Further discussion

Genetic counselling is important if a diagnosis of CGD is made. Carriers of the condition can be identified by the NBT test (see Fig 5), flow cytometric testing and by molecular analysis. Prenatal diagnosis is possible.

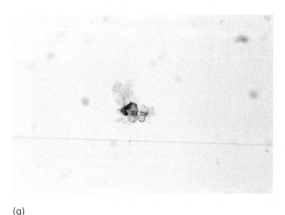

(a)

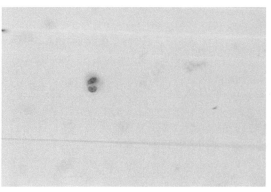

(b)

Fig 5 The nitroblue tetrazolium (NBT) test: activated neutrophils are tested for their ability to phagocytose and reduce NBT. **(a)** Reduced NBT is seen as dark-blue crystals. **(b)** Unstimulated neutrophils, or stimulated neutrophils from patients who have CGD, fail to reduce NBT. Blood from carriers of CGD contain a mixture of normal and abnormal neutrophils.

Table 3 Prevention of infection in CGD

Problem	Intervention
Avoid bacterial infection	Keep immunisations up to date Clean all cuts immediately and rinse with antiseptic or hydrogen peroxide (1.5% solution) Maintain meticulous dental hygiene and use hydrogen peroxide mouthwash after brushing teeth to reduce gingivitis Antibiotic prophylaxis is necessary for dental work
Avoid fungal spores	Avoid compost, hay, wood chips and grass clippings Do not enter barns or caves Do not repot houseplants For cut flowers, use a teaspoon of bleach in the water Avoid newly constructed or renovated buildings until they have been thoroughly cleaned
General	Do not smoke (tobacco or marijuana) Keep up to date with all killed vaccinations, including influenza vaccine

1.1.5 Flushing and skin rash

Dear Doctor,

Re: Mrs Celine Banks, aged 45 years

I would be grateful for your help in the investigation and management of this 45-year-old woman who presented with a 3-year history of episodic urticaria. The urticarial episodes occur weekly and are characterised by an intensely itchy rash affecting her trunk and limbs. Over the past year they have also been associated with intermittent facial flushing, which has been thought to be perimenopausal in origin.

Clinical examination during an acute episode revealed widespread urticaria.

Both the patient and myself are increasingly frustrated by her urticaria and would value your help in establishing a firm diagnosis.

Yours sincerely,

Introduction

Flushing in a 45-year-old woman could be due to a wide spectrum of disorders, ranging from an early menopause to disorders caused by release of endogenous vasoactive mediators (Table 4). In this case, where there is both flushing and urticaria, you need to consider whether the symptoms are triggered by an underlying allergy or if they reflect systemic mastocytosis (SM).

Key point

There are many causes of flushing, but the simultaneous occurrence of flushing and urticaria points to mast cell overactivity.

History of the presenting problem

Are there clues in the history to suggest an underlying allergic trigger for the urticaria?
The history is crucial in establishing an allergic trigger. A consistent link with foods, drugs or background atopy should suggest a possible allergy.

Could SM account for her symptoms?
Although flushing in this woman may well reflect the onset of menopause, it would be prudent in the face of intractable symptoms not to ignore the possibility of SM.

Ask about the following:

> Frequency of symptoms: completely asymptomatic phases between episodes may occur with either allergy or SM, although the most common rash of SM, urticaria pigmentosa, tends to be fixed.

> Itching: does scratching or mild trauma cause more urticarial lesions to appear (Darier's sign)? This is a characteristic feature of urticaria pigmentosa (Fig 6): a localised form of mastocytosis confined to the skin.

> Gastrointestinal symptoms: diarrhoea and abdominal pain. Symptomatic peptic ulcers occur in 50% of patients with SM.

> Palpitations: these are not uncommon with physiological flushing.

> Constitutional symptoms: include prolonged fatigue.

> Is the patient menopausal? Ask about the frequency and duration of her menstrual periods.

Other relevant history

Enquire about exaggerated reactions to drugs that release histamine. This is a frequent feature of mastocytosis and manifests as anaphylactoid reactions associated with the use of mast cell stimulators, such as opiates and certain neuromuscular blockers used in anaesthesia.

Table 4	Differential diagnosis of flushing	
Disorder	**Comments and key investigations**	**Frequency**
Physiological/idiopathic	Confined to exposed skin, eg face or neck Sometimes associated with palpitations and syncope No biochemical abnormality	Common
Menopause	Women aged >45 years with menstrual irregularities Males after orchidectomy Gonadotrophin levels are unreliable markers of the perimenopause	Common
Carcinoid	Often postprandial flushing associated with diarrhoea and/or wheeze Raised 24-h urinary 5-HIAA	Rare
Medullary carcinoma of the thyroid	Either sporadic or associated with multiple endocrine neoplasia syndromes Raised serum calcitonin	Rare
Mastocytosis	Flushing associated with urticaria, pruritus and/or diarrhoea Mast cell infiltration on skin / bone marrow biopsy Raised plasma tryptase Raised urinary methylhistamine	Rare
Drugs	Antidepressants, metronidazole (with alcohol) and nicotinic acid	Common

5-HIAA, 5-hydroxyindole acetic acid.

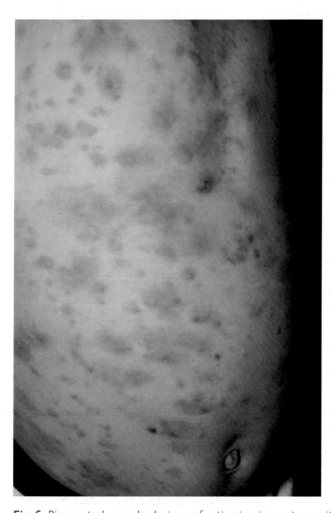

Fig 6 Pigmented macular lesions of urticaria pigmentosa with urtication. (Courtesy of Dr M Goodfield, Leeds General Infirmary.)

Hazard

Beware risk of severe adverse reactions with opioid analgesia and general anaesthesia.

Plan for investigation and management

After explaining to the patient that under normal circumstances you would carry out a thorough clinical examination, you would plan to investigate as follows.

Investigation

> Allergy: if the history suggests an allergic trigger, perform appropriate skin-prick tests and check allergen-specific immunoglobulin E (IgE). Although food allergy may occasionally cause widespread urticaria in isolation, it would be highly unusual for it to be associated with facial flushing. Nevertheless, should the history incriminate any foods as a consistent trigger, it would be worthwhile performing appropriate skin-prick tests for reactions to relevant foods and allergen-specific IgE.

> Mastocytosis: you need to demonstrate mast cell overactivity both histologically and biochemically. Check her plasma tryptase, an important mast cell mediator, and plan to proceed to bone marrow examination and/or skin biopsy if the tryptase is elevated.

Key point

Histological demonstration of mast cell hyperplasia in skin and/or bone marrow, combined with biochemical evidence of elevated mast cell mediators, is required to establish a diagnosis of SM. Measurements of mast cell mediators may be normal in mastocytosis confined to the skin.

Management

You should explain to the patient that the results of her blood tests will be reviewed at her next outpatient visit. If targeted skin testing suggests a possible allergenic trigger, give appropriate advice regarding allergen avoidance and ensure that she is on optimal antihistamine therapy to achieve symptomatic control of urticaria. Use a non-sedating antihistamine such as cetirizine or loratadine.

If mastocytosis is confirmed, the mainstay of management is histamine blockade using a combination of H_1- and H_2-receptor blockers to control cutaneous symptoms and gastric acid production, respectively. In addition to controlling gastric acid production, H_2-receptor blockers such as cimetidine or ranitidine have the added advantage of blocking histamine in the skin, because approximately 20% of cutaneous histamine receptors are of the H_2 class.

Further discussion

Mastocytosis is a myeloproliferative disorder: there are mutations in the c-kit receptor (a tyrosine kinase that functions as the receptor for stem cell factor, the most important growth factor for mast cells) in most patients with mastocytosis, and there is organ infiltration with mast cells (see Section 2.2.2).

1.1.6 Drug-induced anaphylaxis

Letter of referral to the immunology outpatient clinic

Dear Doctor,
Re: Mr Kevin Cook, aged 35 years

This man seems to have had a severe allergic reaction, and I'd be grateful for your help in unravelling the cause. He presented to the emergency department last week in anaphylactic shock, with hypotension, bronchospasm and widespread urticaria. Fortunately he responded rapidly to intramuscular adrenalin and intravenous hydrocortisone and chlorpheniramine.

Five days before he presented to the emergency department, he had developed pain, redness and swelling in the right foot. A diagnosis of cellulitis was suspected, and he was given a prescription for flucloxacillin, a drug he had taken in the past without problems. However, his foot symptoms failed to settle and, with a suspicion of gout, he was prescribed diclofenac. Within a few minutes of taking 50 mg of this drug, he developed the first signs of the allergic reaction described above.

He has previously been generally well, although in recent months he has had occasional self-limiting attacks of 'nettle rash' with no obvious cause.

Yours sincerely,

Introduction

In principle, nothing could be simpler than prevention of further attacks of drug-induced anaphylaxis: one merely has to identify the offending drug (Table 5) and avoid it. In practice, however, diagnosis and management are complicated by the following:

> Difficulty identifying the triggering drug, particularly where multiple drugs are used before the adverse reaction.

> The pathophysiology of the adverse reaction. These can be classic immunoglobulin E (IgF)-mediated type I hypersensitivity reactions, or non-IgE-mediated mast cell degranulation (as in the patient described here) where a non-steroidal anti-inflammatory drug (NSAID) has triggered severe mast cell degranulation in a patient with pre-existing mild chronic urticaria and angio-oedema.

> The pattern of cross-reactivity between different drugs, eg type I hypersensitivity to penicillins, will often be associated with the potential for similar reactions to cephalosporins.

History of the presenting problem

Key point

The history is the main diagnostic tool in the assessment of drug allergy. A painstaking history is therefore essential.

If a patient is acutely unwell, the priority is clearly the recognition and management of the anaphylactic reaction. Little or no history may be available at this stage. It is therefore vital to return to the patient when they have recovered, either on the ward or in the outpatients department (where this PACES scenario is set). Particular attention should be given to the following.

Table 5	Drugs most often associated with anaphylaxis	
IgE mediated		**Non-IgE mediated**
Cephalosporins		Radiographic contrast media
Penicillins		Aspirin and NSAIDs
Drugs used in general anaesthesia, especially		ACE inhibitors
neuromuscular blocking agents		
Proteins used as drugs, such as therapeutic antibodies		

ACE, angiotensin-converting enzyme; NSAID, non-steroidal anti-inflammatory drug.

> *Events immediately preceding and during the reaction.* The time course of these must be meticulously documented. In clinical practice an account may need to be obtained from witnesses if the patient's consciousness was impaired, but this will not be available in the PACES exam. However, does the history suggest anaphylaxis or some cause of collapse, such as a simple faint, cardiac syncope or epilepsy? Not all the components of a full-blown anaphylactic reaction need be present for a diagnosis to be made – it is just as important to identify isolated bronchospasm or severe angio-oedema. Dizziness/ pre-syncope (suggestive of hypotension) in the absence of bronchospasm/swelling/rashes can occur, but is more suggestive of a cardiac cause. Patients often report gastrointestinal symptoms (diarrhoea and abdominal pain) in addition to classical anaphylactic symptoms.

> *Previous use of any drugs.* Drugs taken without problems in the recent past are unlikely to be the cause, but have there been previous reactions to any drugs? Does the patient take any drugs that may trigger anaphylaxis, urticaria or angio-oedema by non-immunological means, such as NSAIDs or ACE inhibitors? And do they use any drugs that may worsen an anaphylactic reaction, especially beta-blockers?

> *Need this be drug induced?* Or could the reaction have been triggered by other environmental allergens, eg latex?

Other relevant history

> Is there (as in this case) a history suggestive of chronic idiopathic urticaria and angio-oedema: chaotic and unpredictable attacks of urticaria and angio-oedema (often facial/ perioral) occurring more often at night, with attacks occurring in clusters over time? Such patients are prone to NSAID-induced anaphylaxis and may also occasionally suffer spontaneous anaphylactic attacks (so-called idiopathic anaphylaxis).

> Does the patient have any other medical conditions that may increase the hazards of severe mast cell degranulation, such as unstable asthma or ischaemic heart disease?

Key point

The patient who gives a history of reactions to multiple drugs presents particular difficulties. Multiple drug allergies are extremely rare and most patients who report them have one of the following:

> Idiopathic urticaria and angio-oedema – reactions can be precipitated by some drugs (such as NSAIDs), but also occur spontaneously (when they are often wrongly attributed to outside events).

> A somatisation disorder – physiological changes caused by stress are perceived as being triggered by external events.

Plan for investigation and management

Explain to the patient that tests are of limited utility in determining the cause of this type of reaction.

Most attempts at investigation will take place in the convalescent stage, often in outpatients departments. Occasionally, in cases of acute illness, if there is uncertainty regarding the cause of an episode of collapse, then serial measurements of serum mast cell tryptase may be useful.

For some drugs, skin-prick and intra-dermal testing and measurement of specific IgE in serum may help to identify the triggering drug. These can be used only for IgE-dependent reactions, and even then, they are useful only in a small proportion of cases. Skin testing is difficult because the triggering allergen is often a subtle chemical modification of the administered drug, hence the use of simple solutions of the drug is likely to lead to false/negative results. It is of most use in the assessment of anaphylaxis associated with β-lactam antibiotics or general anaesthetic drugs, and in the latter case, these tests can be used to pinpoint the likely allergen out of a cocktail of administered drugs. The test involves scratching a tiny quantity of a drug into the upper layer of skin: when immediate hypersensitivity is present, an itchy wheal develops at the site of the scratch, which usually disappears within 30 minutes. Very occasional cases of generalised reactions to skin-prick testing have been reported, and treatments need to be on hand if this were to happen. Patients undergoing skin testing should not take antihistamines for 48 hours before, as these may cause false/ negative results.

In this patient, the close temporal relationship between the first dose of diclofenac and onset of anaphylaxis is highly suggestive of NSAID hypersensitivity. In the vast majority of patients, this is non-IgE mediated and a reflection of differential shunting of diclofenac, a cyclooxygenase-1 inhibitor

(COX-1), preferentially via the lipo-oxygenase pathway (Fig 7) leading to overproduction of leukotrienes, which are powerful mediators of bronchospasm. The diagnosis of NSAID hypersensitivity is made on clinical grounds and the mainstay of management is avoidance of COX-1 inhibitors and aspirin, which also exhibits strong COX-1 inhibitory activity. Most patients will be able to tolerate a selective COX-2 inhibitor (celecoxib, etoricoxib), but it would be prudent to ensure that the first dose is administered under medical supervision. IgE-mediated anaphylaxis to NSAID is exceptionally rare.

The cornerstone of management is avoidance of the suspected drug. Management of acute anaphylactic reactions is described in Section 2.2.1.

Key point

> The drug(s) to be avoided should be clearly recorded on the front of the patient's case notes.

> The patient should be encouraged to wear a Medic-Alert (or equivalent) necklace or bracelet giving details of the allergy.

1.1.7 Arthralgia, purpuric rash and renal impairment

Letter of referral to the immunology outpatient clinic

Dear Doctor,
Re: Mrs Matilda McGuire, aged 50 years

Thank you for seeing this 50-year-old woman who has a 2-year history of joint pains and an intermittent purpuric rash. On clinical examination the only abnormality is a purpuric rash involving her calves and thighs.

The results of initial investigations show a negative antinuclear antibody and a normal FBC, but impaired renal function with a plasma creatinine of 170 µmol/L (normal range 60–110).

I would value your help in establishing the underlying diagnosis and planning her further management.

Yours sincerely,

Introduction
The differential diagnoses for this constellation of clinical problems encompass lupus and the systemic vasculitides (Table 6). Lupus is effectively excluded by the negative antinuclear antibody. Of the vasculitides, type II mixed cryoglobulinaemia would fit her clinical problems well and should be considered the prime working diagnosis. Other small vessel vasculitides, such as Wegener's granulomatosis and microscopic polyangiitis (MPA), may also present in this manner.

History of the presenting problem
Skin rash
Since a purpuric rash on the legs on a background of renal impairment and joint pains suggests a multisystem disorder, such as cryoglobulinaemic vasculitis, you should characterise the rash bearing in mind the diagnoses listed in Table 6.

> Clarify distribution of the rash and any relationship to cold – a purpuric rash affecting the lower limbs is present in >90% of patients with mixed cryoglobulinaemia (Fig 8).

> Ask about leg ulcers, which are a feature of severe cutaneous vasculitis.

> Has there been poor circulation in the hands, feet and nose? Ask about Raynaud's phenomenon: although this is a common feature of cryoglobulinaemia reflecting peripheral vascular obstruction due to cryoglobulins, it also occurs frequently in lupus and scleroderma. In all of these conditions, patients may describe episodic symptoms on a background of permanently cold hands.

Joint pains
Ask about the following:

> Onset and course of pain: arthralgia associated with early morning stiffness may occur in most of the disorders listed in Table 6, but is particularly pronounced in patients with rheumatoid vasculitis.

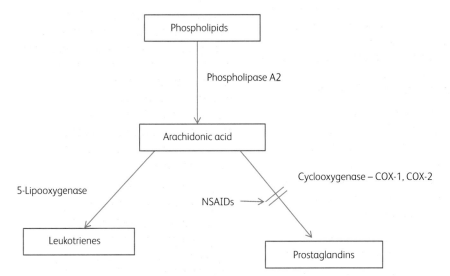

Fig 7 Schematic representation of arachidonic acid pathway. NSAIDs inhibit cyclooxygenase enzymes (also known as prostaglandin H synthases).

Table 6 Differential diagnosis of arthralgia, purpuric rash and renal impairment

Disorder	Key investigation
Lupus	Antinuclear antibody
Mixed cryoglobulinaemia	Cryoglobulins, C3, C4 and rheumatoid factor
Wegener's granulomatosis and MPA	ANCA and tissue biopsy
Rheumatoid vasculitis	Clinically apparent because it develops on a background of severe rheumatoid disease
Henoch–Schönlein purpura	Rare in this age group and with such a long history: tissue biopsy (skin, kidney) showing IgA deposition would make the diagnosis

ANCA, antineutrophil cytoplasmic antibody; C3, C4, complement factors 3 and 4; IgA, immunoglobulin A; MPA, microscopic polyangiitis.

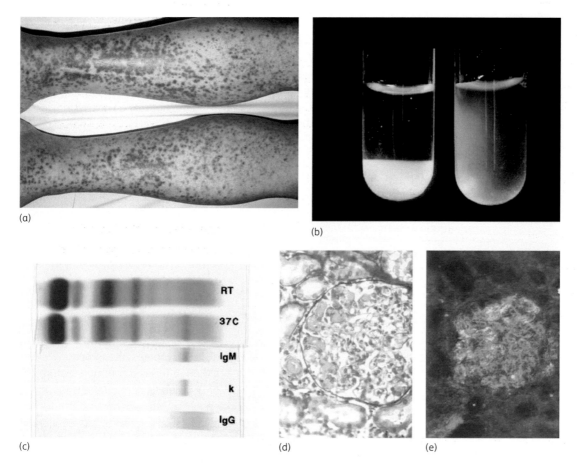

(a)

(b)

(c)

(d)

(e)

Fig 8 Clinical and laboratory manifestations of mixed cryoglobulinaemia in a patient with hepatitis C. **(a)** Palpable purpura caused by cutaneous vasculitis. **(b)** Stored serum showing cryoprecipitate after a 24-hour incubation at 4°C (left), and redissolving on heating to 37°C (right). **(c)** Zone electrophoresis of serum collected at 37°C shows the redissolved cryoprecipitate as a discrete band in the γ region, which on immunofixation is shown to be composed of monoclonal IgM κ and polyclonal IgG. Note the absence of γ band in the sample collected at room temperature (RT). **(d)** Renal biopsy showing eosinophilic glomerular deposits of cryoglobulin (pseudothrombi), corresponding to IgG deposits **(e)** on immunofluorescence. (Reproduced with permission from Graham A. *Arthritis Rheum* 1992;35:1106–7.)

> Distribution and symmetry: symmetrical arthralgia affecting the hands, knees, ankles and elbows is common in mixed cryoglobulinaemia, but rarely progresses to frank arthritis.

Renal impairment

The degree of renal impairment noted in this patient at presentation will not directly produce any symptoms, but is it a new finding related to her acute presentation or does she have unrelated chronic renal failure (chronic kidney disease stage 3)? Enquire about previous history of any renal problems including urinary tract infection, urinary stones, haematuria, tests of the urine for medicals or when pregnant, hypertension, family history of renal disorder and previous blood tests to measure renal function.

Rapidly progressive glomerulonephritis, which can cause advanced renal failure, may occur as part of the spectrum of antineutrophil cytoplasmic antibody (ANCA)-associated vasculitides, but in this case the length of the history suggests a more slowly evolving disorder such as mixed cryoglobulinaemia. Glomerulonephritis occurs in about 50% of cases of mixed cryoglobulinaemia (Fig 8) but remains asymptomatic in the early stages: oedema and hypertension

are common manifestations of advanced renal disease.

Are there features to suggest any of the alternative diagnoses listed in Table 6? Ask directly about:

> problems with the nose (bleeding and/or discharge) and ears (deafness and/or discharge), which would suggest Wegener's granulomatosis

> is there anything to support the diagnosis of lupus, (eg pleurisy, pericarditis or photosensitive rash)?

Other relevant history

Aside from a rapid screen of past medical history and a functional enquiry, ask about Sjögren's syndrome, lupus and rheumatoid arthritis because cryoglobulinaemic vasculitis can occur as a complication of any of these disorders.

Key point

Enquire about exposure to blood products, history of body piercing, tattooing or intravenous drug abuse because hepatitis C virus (HCV) infection now accounts for ~70% of cases of mixed cryoglobulinaemia.

Plan for investigation and management

After explaining to the patient that under normal circumstances you would carry out a thorough clinical examination to confirm the findings in the referral letter, you would plan to perform the following blood and urine tests to arrive at a diagnosis.

Immunological tests
Cryoglobulins

The key to detecting cryoglobulins is meticulous attention to detail. Collect a clotted sample of blood at 37°C and transport immediately and at the same temperature to the immunology laboratory. Once a cryoglobulin has been detected (see Fig 8), it is essential to characterise the type in view of the different disease associations (Table 7).

Serum complement C3 and C4

Like any immune complex, mixed cryoglobulins activate the classic complement pathway, hence C4, but not C3, is reduced in their presence.

Table 7	Classification of cryoglobulins	
Type	**Composition**	**Disease associations**
I	Composed entirely of monoclonal immunoglobulin, usually IgM or IgG	Waldenström's macroglobulinaemia Myeloma Lymphoproliferative disease
II	Monoclonal IgM rheumatoid factor plus polyclonal IgG	Infections, particularly HCV Autoimmune Lupus Sjögren's syndrome Rheumatoid arthritis A minority of cases are labelled 'idiopathic' (mixed essential cryoglobulinaemia)
III	Polyclonal IgM rheumatoid factor plus polyclonal IgG	

Types II and III cryoglobulins have overlapping disease associations.
HCV, hepatitis C virus; IgG, immunoglobulin G; IgM, immunoglobulin M.

Key point

A markedly low C4 occurs in ~ 90% of patients with mixed cryoglobulinaemia as a result of classic pathway activation.

Rheumatoid factor

Check the rheumatoid factor because it forms an integral part of mixed cryoglobulins.

Key point

> The IgM component of mixed cryoglobulins exhibits strong rheumatoid factor activity, which taken together with the low C4 is an important clue pointing towards mixed cryoglobulinaemia.

But by contrast:

> Wegener's granulomatosis and MPA are characterised by normal or elevated complement levels as part of the acute phase response.

ANCAs

Check ANCAs in view of the possibility of Wegener's granulomatosis / MPA.

Other tests

> urine: dipstick for proteinuria and haematuria; use microscopy of sediment for red cell casts as evidence of active glomerulonephritis

> renal function: determine whether or not this has changed since referral

> liver function: performed in view of the strong association between HCV and mixed cryoglobulinaemia

> viral serology, especially hepatitis C. If negative, proceed to polymerase chain reaction analysis of cryoprecipitate for HCV RNA

> chest radiograph: this may show changes compatible with Wegener's granulomatosis; lung involvement is unusual in mixed cryoglobulinaemia.

Explain to the patient that the results of any investigations will be reviewed at the next outpatient visit. It would also be appropriate to briefly discuss the need for a renal biopsy to confirm the diagnosis of cryoglobulinaemic vasculitis and rule out other causes of renal dysfunction, eg drug-related interstitial nephritis. The glomerulonephritis in mixed cryoglobulinaemia has distinctive features, being characterised by the marked deposition of immunoglobulin and complement (see Fig 8). By contrast, a pauci-immune glomerulonephritis (little or no complement or immunoglobulin deposited in the glomeruli) would favour ANCA-positive systemic vasculitis.

Further discussion

Symptoms in mixed cryoglobulinaemia are the result of a combination of immune complex-induced vasculitis and vascular obstruction by cryoglobulin. Most cases (60–80%) of cryoglobulinaemic vasculitis associated with a mixed cryoglobulin are now known to be driven by HCV infection. Prior to the 1990s these cases were categorised under the term mixed essential cryoglobulinaemia. Although the role of hepatitis C in causing liver infection is plausible, its role in driving a monoclonal population of plasma cells is less clear. Recent evidence suggests that the HCV may do this by using CD81 (a cell-surface glycoprotein found on both lymphocytes and hepatocytes) as a receptor to gain entry into these cells. See Section 2.5.4 for discussion of management.

1.1.8 Arthralgia and photosensitive rash

Dear Doctor,
Re: Miss Hannah Cole, aged 22 years

I would value your opinion on this 22-year-old nurse who presented with a 6-month history of joint pains and a facial rash. The rash has been intermittent and appears to be predominantly associated with outdoor activities. Clinical examination was essentially normal, but she is particularly concerned about the possibility of systemic lupus erythematosus (SLE) because her mother had cutaneous lupus diagnosed 5 years ago. Is SLE the diagnosis in this case?
Yours sincerely,

Introduction

The combination of joint pains and a facial rash (Fig 9) in a young woman certainly raises the possibility of SLE, more so in the presence of a family history of lupus, as in this case. However, although SLE should be the main diagnosis under consideration, you should be aware of other disorders that present with joint pains and a rash:

> Viral infection*, eg parvovirus infection, may mimic SLE.

> Dermatomyositis may present with arthralgia and a photosensitive rash in the 'V' of the neck and upper trunk.

> Lyme disease* and rheumatic fever* are both characterised by distinctive skin rashes that appear in association with arthralgia and systemic disease; they should not cause difficulties in differential diagnosis.

> Psoriatic arthritis*.

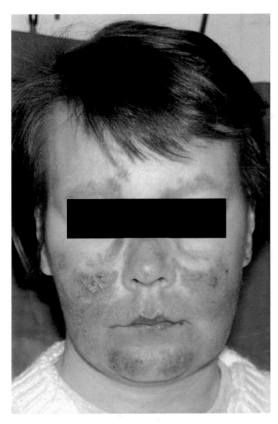

Fig 9 Patchy facial erythema with scarring and marked eyebrow involvement in a patient with SLE. (Courtesy of Dr M Goodfield, Leeds General Infirmary.)

*Photosensitivity is not a feature of these disorders; each has characteristic features that enable them to be distinguished from SLE on clinical grounds. Proceed to serology in cases of diagnostic doubt.

History of the presenting problem

Is SLE the explanation? The aim must be to clarify the presenting symptoms, and also to ask relevant questions regarding the involvement of other organ systems.

Joint pains

Ask about:

> Onset and course of the pain: non-specific joint pains associated with early morning stiffness may occur with any inflammatory disorder and will not help in differentiating between lupus, parvoviral infection and psoriatic arthritis.

> Distribution and symmetry: is it proximal or distal? An asymmetrical distal arthropathy may occur with both lupus and psoriatic arthritis, but is distinguished in psoriasis by characteristic distal interphalangeal

joint involvement accompanied by skin changes. Large joint involvement tends to occur more frequently in psoriatic arthropathy.

> Morning stiffness? This is a non-specific feature of any inflammatory joint disorder.

Key point

Joint involvement occurs in 90% of patients with lupus and is characterised by a symmetrical, distal and non-erosive arthritis. Frank deforming arthritis is rare and occurs in a small minority of patients.

Rash

Ask about the distribution of the rash. Does it predominantly affect sun-exposed areas of the body? Does sunlight precipitate or aggravate the rash? Skin manifestations of lupus may occur either on their own (discoid lupus erythematosus (Fig 10) and subacute cutaneous lupus erythematosus) or in association with systemic disease. In subacute cutaneous lupus erythematosus a photosensitive malar rash (Fig 11) affecting the bridge of the nose and the cheeks is characteristic. Photosensitivity is a characteristic

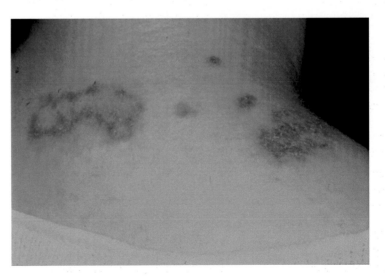

Fig 10 Rash of discoid lupus in a patient with isolated cutaneous lupus.

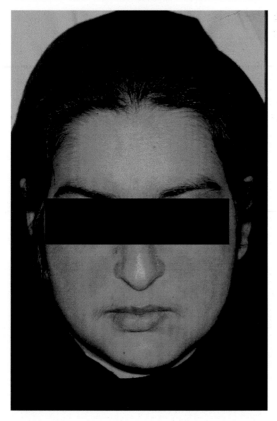

Fig 11 Photosensitive malar rash in a patient with systemic lupus.

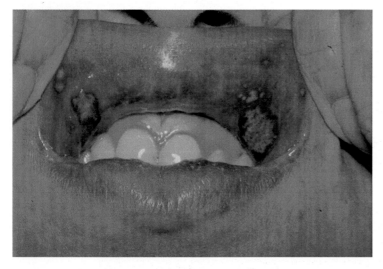

Fig 12 Mouth ulcers in a patient with active lupus.

feature of the skin rash of lupus, which is probably due to the induction of keratinocyte apoptosis by ultraviolet light and the consequent exposure of lupus autoantigens to the immune system.

Other relevant history

Since SLE is a multisystem disease, ask about the following pointers towards the diagnosis and activity of lupus:

> hair loss

> livedo reticularis

> Raynaud's phenomenon

> mouth ulcers (Fig 12)

> chest or abdominal pain (serositis), and dyspnoea

> headaches

> seizures

> drug history – to exclude the possibility of drug-induced lupus. More than 80 drugs have been reported to trigger lupus, with common culprits being sulfasalazine, hydralazine and minocycline.

Plan for investigation and management

After explaining to the patient that under normal circumstances you would carry out a thorough clinical examination to confirm the findings in the referral letter, you would plan to perform the following tests.

Investigations: immunological
Antibodies to nuclear antigens

As SLE is the main diagnosis under consideration, the patient's antinuclear antibody (ANA) status is crucial.

Key point

Using human epithelial cells as a substrate:

> ANA positivity (titre >1:80) occurs in >99% of patients with untreated SLE.

> A negative ANA effectively excludes systemic lupus.

As a positive ANA can occur in a variety of other disorders, it is important to characterise its specificity, ie is it directed against double-stranded DNA and/or other extractable nuclear antigens (ENA) (individual specificities known as Ro, La, Sm and ribonucleoprotein)?

Key point

Antibodies to DNA and ENA are specific for lupus or lupus overlap disorders and occur in 30–90% of patients.

Serum complement levels

Check C3 and C4 levels. Patients with lupus may be hypocomplementaemic as a result of active disease and/or possession of one or more C4 null alleles.

Antiphospholipid antibodies

Check for anticardiolipin antibodies and lupus anticoagulant. These antibodies occur in 30% of lupus patients and act as markers for thrombosis (Fig 13).

Other tests

Check the following:

> urine: dipstick to check for proteinuria and haematuria. If there is proteinuria, quantitate by estimation of urinary albumin to creatinine ratio; if there is haematuria, use microscopy of sediment for red cell casts as evidence of active glomerulonephritis

> renal function

> liver function

> FBC: looking for cytopenia

> C-reactive protein: marker of inflammation/infection. This is often normal in active uncomplicated lupus despite an elevated erythrocyte sedimentation rate or plasma viscosity.

It would be worthwhile pointing out that further investigations may be required should the diagnosis of lupus be confirmed. If renal function is significantly impaired and/or there is an active urinary sediment, then it is likely that a renal biopsy will be required to determine prognosis and guide treatment decisions. Skin biopsies are seldom performed in the assessment of SLE, although the demonstration of a 'lupus band' is useful in the diagnosis of cutaneous lupus erythematosus (Fig 14).

Further discussion

Given the multisystem nature of the disease, the American College of Rheumatology have drawn up a list of criteria to help in the diagnosis of SLE. Although these are helpful for research and disease classification, it is important to recognise that rigid adherence to them in clinical practice may, on occasions, lead to the delayed diagnosis of lupus.

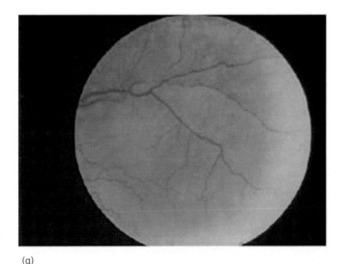

(a)

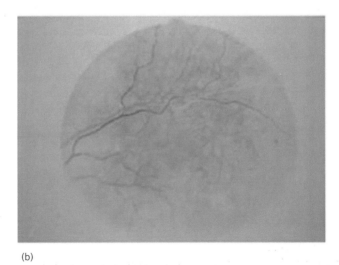

(b)

Fig 13 (a) Branch retinal artery occlusion in a patient with SLE and the antiphospholipid syndrome; the defect is more pronounced in the subtraction angiogram **(b)**.

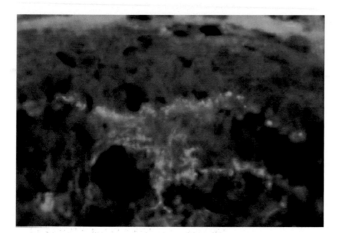

Fig 14 Granular immunoglobulin G deposits at the dermoepidermal junction (lupus band). (Courtesy of Dr W Merchant, Leeds General Infirmary.)

Key point

American College of Rheumatology criteria for the diagnosis of SLE:

> malar rash

> discoid rash

> photosensitivity

> oral ulcers

> non-erosive arthritis

> serositis (pleuritis/pericarditis)

> renal disease (persistent proteinuria / casts)

> neurological disorder (seizures/psychosis)

> haemolytic anaemia / leukopenia / thrombocytopenia

> antinuclear antibody

> antibodies to double-stranded DNA / anti-ENA / antiphospholipid antibodies.

To establish a diagnosis of SLE, four or more criteria are required serially or simultaneously during any period of observation.

If this patient is shown to have lupus, it would be worthwhile excluding primary complement deficiency in view of the positive family history. Homozygous deficiency of early complement components (C1q, C1r and C1s, C4 and C2) is strongly associated with the development of SLE. See Section 2.4.1 for discussion on management.

1.1.9 Cold fingers and difficulty swallowing

Letter of referral to the rheumatology outpatient clinic

Dear Doctor,

Re: Mrs Hannah Adams, aged 50 years

Thank you for seeing this woman who presented with a 9-month history of cold, painful fingers. She has had some mild swallowing difficulties that have started recently, but is otherwise well. She has no past medical history of note. Please would you advise as to whether she requires any further investigation or ongoing follow-up?

Yours sincerely,

Introduction

It is important to clarify both of these symptoms, because cold fingers mean different things to different people and the meaning of difficulty in swallowing can range from occasional benign choking to true dysphagia. The following are key questions to consider:

> Are her cold fingers a result of Raynaud's phenomenon, and if so, is it primary or secondary (see Table 8)?

> If the diagnosis is scleroderma, the commonest of the connective tissue diseases (CTDs) associated with Raynaud's, is it limited cutaneous systemic sclerosis (LCSSc) or diffuse cutaneous systemic sclerosis (DCSSc)?

> Is there evidence of internal organ involvement?

Key point

Causes of secondary Raynaud's phenomenon

> Connective tissue diseases (CTDs): scleroderma, systemic lupus erythematosus (SLE), rheumatoid arthritis (RA) and inflammatory myositis

> occlusive arterial disease: thoracic outlet syndrome, atherosclerosis/embolism and thromboangiitis obliterans

> occupational: vibrating tools

> drugs/toxins: ergotamine, beta-blockers and polyvinyl chloride (PVC)

> intravascular coagulation or aggregation: cryoglobulinaemia, cold agglutinin disease and polycythaemia rubra vera.

History of the presenting problem

Are the cold fingers caused by Raynaud's phenomenon? Consider the following, which also help to distinguish primary from secondary causes:

> Is there a colour change? Well-demarcated pallor, then cyanosis and then rubor (white → blue → red)

Table 8 Comparison of primary and secondary Raynaud's phenomenon

Characteristics	Primary Raynaud's phenomenon	Secondary Raynaud's phenomenon
Age (average) (years)	Teenage	>50
Sex	Female	Female
Tissue damage	Absent	Digital ulcers and gangrene
Symmetry	Symmetrical attacks	Can have asymmetrical attacks
Nailfold microscopy	Negative	Positive
Antinuclear antibody	Negative	Positive
Associated disease	No associated disease	Scleroderma, SLE and lupus overlap

SLE, systemic lupus erythematosus.

are the typical triphasic colour changes of Raynaud's phenomenon, although many patients will describe only biphasic changes.

> What are the precipitating factors? Raynaud's phenomenon is usually provoked by exposure to cold and emotional stress, and is terminated by rewarming – although it may abate spontaneously.

> Where? Usually in the fingers (Fig 15), but other areas affected are toes and ears.

> How bad and for how long?

> Is the problem associated with trophic changes/ulcers in the fingers?

Key point

Obstruction of major arteries

Consider obstruction of major upper arm arteries (atherosclerosis, thrombosis and embolism), which may mimic Raynaud's phenomenon.

> Colour changes may be similar to those in Raynaud's.

> Symptoms are more likely to be unilateral.

> Arm claudication is characteristic.

> There will be low blood pressure (BP) and reduced peripheral pulses in the affected arm.

> Arteriography demonstrates the arterial lesion.

Explore the history of dysphagia.

Other relevant history

Does the patient have one of the causes of secondary Raynaud's phenomenon? Consider the following.

Systemic sclerosis

This is clearly the most likely diagnosis in this case, so pursue symptoms commonly seen in this condition:

> skin – sclerodactyly, digital ulceration, calcinosis and telangiectasia

> gastrointestinal (GI) – dysphagia, indigestion/heartburn, weight loss and faecal incontinence

> respiratory – shortness of breath, which may reflect lung fibrosis or pulmonary hypertension.

Also note that cranial neuropathies, in particular facial pain secondary to trigeminal neuralgia, are rarely seen.

If the patient has systemic sclerosis (SS), ask about the timing of Raynaud's in relation to sclerodactyly: Raynaud's can precede skin changes by many years in LCSSc.

Other connective tissue disorders
Ask about arthralgia/arthritis, photosensitivity, rashes, oral ulcers, alopecia and proximal muscle weakness; also enquire regarding any family history of connective tissue disease (CTD).

Other issues
Drug history: beta-blockers, anti-migraine compounds and cytotoxics can exacerbate Raynaud's.

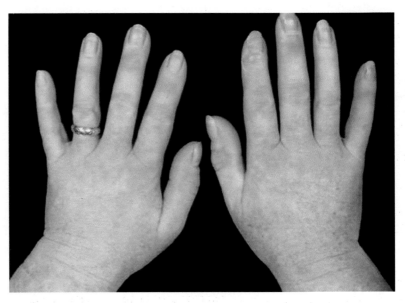

Fig 15 Finger pallor during an attack of Raynaud's phenomenon.

Occupation, eg use of vibrating tools and exposure to PVC / organic solvents.

Smoking is an obvious risk factor for obstructive arterial disease.

Plan for investigation and management

After explaining to the patient that under normal circumstances you would carry out a thorough clinical examination to confirm the findings in the referral letter, you would plan to perform the following tests.

Investigation

Diagnosis/prognosis

> Antinuclear antibodies: these are typically negative in primary Raynaud's phenomenon. Anti-centromere is associated with LCSSc and anti-topoisomerase / anti-Scl70 are present in DCSSc.

> Inflammatory markers: the erythrocyte sedimentation rate (ESR) and C-reactive protein (CRP) are usually normal in primary Raynaud's phenomenon, but may be elevated in secondary Raynaud's phenomenon if there is tissue inflammation/damage. In SLE, the ESR is characteristically elevated in the presence of a normal CRP (unless there is serositis or superadded infection).

> Radiology: request a chest radiograph to look for basal fibrosis, followed by a high-resolution CT of the chest if this fibrosis is present. Use cervical rib views if hand/arm symptoms are unilateral.

> Nailfold capillary microscopy: this is useful in differentiating primary from secondary Raynaud's phenomenon. Abnormal nailfold capillary morphology depicting dilatation and drop out (Fig 16) indicates secondary disease and predicts the presence or future development of autoimmune rheumatic disease (see Section 2.4).

> Cold challenge test: abnormal rewarming is seen in SS but is unusual in primary Raynaud's.

Assessment of organ damage

> FBC: patients with secondary Raynaud's phenomenon may be anaemic as a result of the chronic disease itself, GI blood loss and/or malabsorption. A rare cause of GI blood loss in DCSSc is gastric antral vascular ectasia (GAVE), a form of arteriovenous malformation that gives rise to the characteristic 'watermelon stomach' sign on endoscopy.

> Urine dipstick for protein and blood (with estimation of urinary albumin to creatinine ratio and urine microscopy for casts if positive) and estimation of

renal function: abnormalities would not be expected in primary Raynaud's phenomenon and would suggest renal problems related to a secondary disorder.

Key point

Even though 5% of the general population have Raynaud's phenomenon, only a minority eventually develop an associated CTD. The following are the frequencies of Raynaud's phenomenon in those with autoimmune rheumatic disease:

> scleroderma: 95%

> SLE: 20%

> Sjögren's syndrome: 20%

> myositis: 20%

> RA: 5%.

Other tests that might be considered, depending upon clinical findings and the outcome of initial tests, include an echocardiogram to assess right-sided heart pressures as pulmonary hypertension can occur in both forms of SS: pulmonary hypertension due to LCSSc is driven by a pulmonary vasculopathy; in DCSSc it is due to interstitial lung disease.

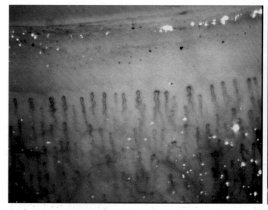

Normal capillaroscopy image (size 3x2 mm)

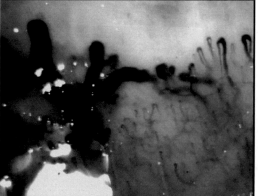

Dilated capillary structure to the grade of mega-capillary

Fig 16 Abnormal nailfold capillary morphology, characterised by dilatation and loss of capillaries, depicted on microscopy with normal appearances for comparison. (Courtesy of Dr John Allen, Freeman Hospital.)

Management

For any patient with troublesome Raynaud's phenomenon, it will be appropriate to consider the following:

> general measures: patient education and keep their hands warm

> smoking cessation: this should be strongly advised

> vasodilators, eg nifedipine; alternatives for severe disease include sildenafil and iloprost

> careful control of BP

> where possible avoid (or at least minimise) corticosteroid use, as it may precipitate sclerodermic renal crisis, particularly in Scl-70-positive individuals.

No other treatment is required for most patients with primary Raynaud's and regular follow-up in hospital is generally not needed. Some causes of secondary Raynaud's may be amenable to specific treatment, but unfortunately options for patients with SS (the likely condition in this case) are limited (see Section 2.4.3).

Further discussion

Absence of signs or symptoms of CTD in a patient with late onset Raynaud's does not mean the Raynaud's is primary. The presence of abnormal nailfold microscopy or positive autoantibodies is strongly predictive of an associated CTD. Raynaud's may precede other symptoms by many years in cases of LCSSc.

LCSSc and DCSSc are differentiated clinically according to the extent of skin involvement (cut-off at elbows and knees). A common misconception is that in LCSSc there is no internal organ involvement, which is not true: although less common than in DCSSc, there can be very serious internal complications such as pulmonary artery hypertension.

1.1.10 Dry eyes and fatigue

Dear Doctor,

Re: Mrs Beth Stokes, aged 53 years

Thank you for seeing this woman who has had dry eyes for over 6 months. These are uncomfortable and appear to be interfering with her work. She has also been troubled by facial swelling, increasing fatigue, breathlessness and pain in her hands.

On examination it seems as though her parotid glands are enlarged, but I cannot convince myself of any other physical signs.

Please can you see her and advise regarding appropriate investigation and management.

Yours sincerely,

Introduction

Dry eyes are caused by insufficient tear production. Possible causes are:

> ageing, especially in post-menopausal women

> medication: diuretics, anticholinergics, antihistamines, beta-blockers and the oral contraceptive pill

> Sjögren's syndrome: primary or secondary

> damage to the eyes/eyelids

> blepharitis

> idiopathic.

In this case, the associated fatigue and facial swelling caused by enlarged parotid glands point towards Sjögren's syndrome, with arthralgia suggesting a secondary cause of this.

History of the presenting problem

Assess the severity of the patient's sicca symptoms by asking the following questions:

> Do you feel a gritty sensation in your eyes?

> Do you have sore eyes or difficulty in wearing contact lenses?

> Do you have difficulty in trying to eat dry foods (cracker sign)?

> Do you need to take liquids to aid swallowing?

> Do you wake up at night with a dry mouth and have to take sips of water?

Consider other causes of parotid swelling (Table 9), although it would be uncommon for the other disorders listed in the table to cause sicca symptoms.

Once the diagnosis of Sjögren's seems likely, establish whether this is primary or secondary (ie associated with an established connective tissue disease). The presence of hand pain in this case should lead you to ask questions directed towards an overlap with rheumatoid arthritis (RA; see Section 1.1.14), which commonly coexists with Sjögren's syndrome. Enquire about disease manifestations beyond the dry eyes and mouth, which can be divided into exocrine and non-exocrine (Table 10).

Other relevant history

Dental caries is increased in Sjögren's, so ask the patient questions regarding dental health and frequency of dental appointments.

The impact of ocular and oral dryness upon quality of life is substantial. It has an effect upon social interactions, particularly as meal times are a focal point for socialising. Likewise, the impact of dyspareunia on relationships and psychosexual health should not be underestimated.

Table 9 Causes of bilateral parotid enlargement

Disorder	Comments
Viral infection (mumps, EBV, coxsackie virus A, CMV, HIV)	Usually acute in onset on a background of systemic ill-health
Sarcoidosis	Occurs on a background of systemic disease
Sjögren's syndrome	Positive ANA, rheumatoid factor and antibodies to Ro and La
Miscellaneous group: diabetes, hyperlipidaemia, alcohol abuse, acromegaly and chronic renal failure	Other clues to primary diagnosis usually present

ANA, antinuclear antibodies; CMV, cytomegalovirus; EBV, Epstein–Barr virus.

Table 10 Manifestations of Sjögren's syndrome

Exocrine	
Eyes	Dry
Mouth / upper respiratory tract	Dry, hoarseness and oral candidiasis
Gastrointestinal	Dysphagia (can also be secondary to dysmotility)
Pancreas	Rarely clinically apparent
Vagina	Dyspareunia / vaginal dryness
Non-exocrine	
Musculoskeletal	Arthralgia, arthritis and myalgia (60–70% of cases)
Skin	Raynaud's (in ~20–40% of cases of primary Sjögren's) Purpura (mixed cryoglobulinaemia) Vasculitis (5–10% of cases)
Lungs	Interstitial pneumonitis (10–20% of cases) NB Suspect lymphoma if chest radiograph shows hilar/mediastinal lymphadenopathy
Renal	Interstitial nephritis May rarely present as distal renal tubular acidosis with renal colic and hypokalaemic muscle weakness
Neurological	Peripheral neuropathy (secondary to vasculitis)

Plan for investigation and management

To confirm Sjögren's syndrome

> Use Schirmer's test to measure objectively how dry the eyes are: insert a small strip of filter paper under the patient's lower eyelid: wetting of less than 5 mm in 5 minutes is considered pathological.

> Check antinuclear antibodies (ANA) and antibodies to Ro and La antigens: these are present in 40–90% of patients with Sjögren's syndrome.

Biopsy of minor salivary glands can reveal histological evidence of focal lymphocytic infiltrates, but is rarely required because of the ease of detecting antibodies to Ro and La.

Other investigations

Keratoconjunctivitis sicca, a consequence of reduced tear production, is diagnosed using rose bengal staining of the cornea. Severity of xerostomia can be assessed using salivary gland scintigraphy and sialometry, but these investigations are rarely performed in routine practice.

Other autoimmune and inflammatory markers: rheumatoid factor is positive in 90% of cases of Sjögren's; C3 and C4 levels are usually normal; and erythrocyte sedimentation rate is usually elevated (a direct consequence of polyclonal hypergammaglobulinaemia) but C-reactive protein is often normal.

Check thyroid function in view of the strong association between Sjögren's and hypothyroidism.

Other tests as clinically indicated, eg in light of the breathlessness in this case, pulmonary function tests and/or high-resolution CT may be warranted depending on the findings on clinical examination; also consider investigations specific to RA if it is suspected following history and examination (see Section 1.1.14).

Management
Therapy for Sjögren's syndrome is limited to symptomatic relief and limitation of the damaging local effects of the sicca complex using the following:

> artificial tears, eye drops and ointments and moisture chamber spectacles to reduce tear evaporation; if severe, referral to ophthalmology for punctal plug insertion is an option

> saliva production can be encouraged with sugar-free candies and chewing gum. Some patients find pilocarpine beneficial

> vaginal lubricants, oestrogen creams or hormone replacement therapy

> meticulous dental hygiene

> avoidance of diuretics and anticholinergic agents that worsen sicca symptoms.

Immunosuppressive therapy is of little value in uncomplicated Sjögren's syndrome, but patients with arthralgia (even in the absence of coexistent RA) may benefit from conventional disease-modifying agents such as hydroxychloroquine or methotrexate.

There is a modest increased risk of Hodgkin's lymphoma with Sjögren's syndrome, so surveillance may be prudent; any patient with new or changing lymphadenopathy should be investigated swiftly.

1.1.11 Breathlessness and weakness

Letter of referral to the rheumatology outpatient clinic

Dear Doctor,

Re: Mrs Brenda Wilde, aged 35 years

This woman presented with a 6-week history of breathlessness, aching thighs and shoulders, and insidiously progressive weakness. She now finds it difficult to climb stairs or rise from a low chair. Her previous medical history is unremarkable. I would be grateful for your help with diagnosis and management.

Yours sincerely,

Introduction
The history raises an immediate suspicion of a proximal myopathy. This should trigger a hierarchy of diagnostic questions. Is the weakness real, or could the primary problem be pain rather than weakness? Weakness is usually more prominent than pain in primary muscle disease. Is this true proximal weakness, or could there be another cause of symmetrical leg weakness (eg spinal cord pathology).

If a myopathic pattern of weakness is present, consider the diagnoses listed in Table 11. If dermatomyositis (DM) or polymyositis (PM) is likely, consider a search for associated malignancy. Also, remember to be alert for non-muscular manifestations of connective tissue disease (CTD).

Key point

In suspected myositis think about:

> alternative causes of weakness

> malignancy

> changes in other systems, especially the lungs.

History of the presenting problem
Muscular/neurological
Gain a picture of the pattern of symptoms and their rate of progression. Ask the patient about the following.

> When did the weakness start? A very long history might suggest an inherited muscle dystrophy presenting in an adult. Although the history is said to be of 6 weeks' duration, could it be longer than this? A year ago, could she walk as far and as fast as other people? Has she ever been able to do this?

> What are the functional consequences of the weakness? Can the woman get up stairs at all and, if so, how does she do it? Can she brush her hair? Is there anything to suggest defective control of swallowing or the upper airway? Has she choked when drinking?

> Is pain a prominent feature? If it is, this might indicate osteomalacia or fibromyalgia.

> Does the history suggest a rapid onset of fatigue with repeated movement, possibly as a result of myasthenia?

> Has the patient had headaches? This woman is too young but, in an older patient, have there been headaches that might indicate temporal arteritis / polymyalgia rheumatica (PMR)?

Table 11 Causes of proximal muscle weakness developing over a few weeks

Disorder type	Disorder	Comments
Inflammatory (idiopathic)	PM/DM	DM associated with heliotrope rash affecting eyelids and Gottron's papules (see Fig 17) Other features of autoimmune rheumatic disorder 25% of cases associated with malignancy
	PMR	>55 years only Weakness secondary to pain General malaise Anaemia of chronic disorder Raised inflammatory markers No other organ involvement Negative serological tests
Endocrine/metabolic	Cushing's syndrome	Look for associated features of steroid excess Exogenous steroids are a very common cause of proximal myopathy
	Thyrotoxicosis	Look for associated features of steroid excess Exogenous steroids are a very common cause of proximal myopathy
	Osteomalacia	Rare in this age group, when the problem is likely to be the result of malabsorption
	Diabetes mellitus	Diabetic amyotrophy affects the quadriceps, causing pain and weakness Usually asymmetrical Does not affect shoulder girdle
Other	Myasthenia gravis	Critical clinical feature is fatiguability
	Carcinomatous neuromyopathy	Usually found in patients with known malignancy, but can be a presenting feature
	Trichinella spiralis	Acquired from eating improperly cooked pork Weakness caused by muscular pain, a feature of the larval migration stage

DM, dermatomyositis; PM, polymyositis; PMR, polymyalgia rheumatica.

> Are there any other neurological symptoms, particularly sensory changes that would suggest a non-myopathic cause?

Other systems

> Ask specifically about the breathlessness. Is exercise limited by weakness of the legs or by the breathing? Breathing difficulty could be caused by myopathy of the respiratory muscles or be associated with lung disease (alveolitis).

> If information does not emerge spontaneously, pursue the following, which may give important clues about a systemic disorder. Think about the conditions listed in Table 11 as you do so.

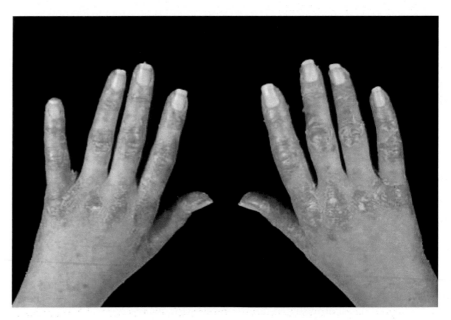

Fig 17 Scaly patches (known as Gottron's papules) on the dorsal surface of the hands in dermatomyositis.

> General: weight loss or weight gain, and preference for hot or cold weather – these could be clues to malignancy, Cushing's syndrome or thyrotoxicosis.

> Skin: has there been a rash, especially a photosensitive rash, which might be found in both systemic lupus erythematosus and DM?

> Joints: has there been any pain or swelling?

> Hands: does the woman have Raynaud's phenomenon?

> Eyes and mouth: has she had any problems with gritty eyes or a dry mouth? These might indicate Sjögren's syndrome (see Section 2.4.2).

> Respiratory: has there been pleuritic pain or haemoptysis?

> Gastrointestinal: have there been any new symptoms?

> Pregnancy history: multiple fetal losses might indicate the presence of an antiphospholipid antibody.

> Previous vascular or thromboembolic disease: this also might indicate the presence of an antiphospholipid antibody.

Plan for investigation and management

After explaining to the patient that under normal circumstances you would carry out a thorough clinical examination to look for evidence of disorders that may be responsible for her symptoms, you would plan to carry out the following blood and muscle tests to arrive at a diagnosis. It would be prudent to warn the patient at this stage that you may wish to proceed to muscle biopsy.

Investigations

The diagnosis may be clear from the history and examination, in which case investigations should be appropriately tailored; otherwise, the following issues need to be addressed.

Muscle disease

> Creatine kinase (CK) estimation is the most useful marker of muscle damage, but remember that myopathies may occur with a normal CK, and that CK may be raised in the absence of muscle disease (eg after heavy exercise).

> Other enzymes (such as aspartate transaminase and alanine transaminase) may be raised, leading to the potential for confusion with liver disease if myopathy is not initially suspected.

> Electromyography provides useful evidence to confirm myopathy and to exclude denervation as a cause of weakness.

> Muscle biopsy remains the only tool for definitive differential diagnosis of myopathy.

> MRI is useful in patchy myositis to identify a site for biopsy.

Identifying the underlying cause

The extent of investigation for malignancy is determined by clinical suspicion and the patient's age. A minimal screen would be a chest radiograph and abdominal and pelvic ultrasonography. Endocrinological investigation (for steroid excess and vitamin D studies) should be considered, depending on the clinical picture.

Are immunological markers of inflammatory myositis present? Consider appropriate tests in suspected lupus and other CTDs (see Sections 1.1.8 and 3.2). Antibodies to Jo-1 (histidyl-tRNA synthetase) occur in 30–50% of

patients with DM and PM, and act as a marker for interstitial lung disease.

Key point

Antibodies to Jo-1
Antibodies to Jo-1 identify a distinct group of patients with inflammatory myositis, designated the anti-synthetase syndrome (myositis, fever, interstitial lung disease, Raynaud's phenomenon and symmetrical non-erosive arthritis).

Management

You should explain to the patient that the results of blood and muscle tests will be reviewed at an urgent follow-up visit. It would be sensible to warn her that she may require hospital admission for the initiation of immunosuppressive treatment if the diagnosis turns out to be inflammatory myositis.

Beware of respiratory failure in patients severely affected by PM/DM. Swallowing and the airway may be compromised with the risk of aspiration. Any patient with severe muscular weakness will require physiotherapy to minimise wasting and prevent contractures. Management otherwise depends on the cause. Treatment of inflammatory muscle disease is with corticosteroids and immunosuppressants, eg methotrexate or azathioprine.

Further discussion

Be alert to the possibility that DM may present as a paraneoplastic manifestation of underlying malignancy, such as carcinoma of the ovaries, gastrointestinal tract, lung or breast and non-Hodgkin's lymphoma. The quest for detection of underlying malignancy has been helped by the detection of antibodies to a transcription factor (anti-TIF-1-Υ) as a marker of cancer-associated DM (see Section 2.3.5).

1.1.12 Low back pain

Dear Doctor
Re: Mr Manny Vass, aged 35 years

Thank you for seeing this man who has recently had to stop work as a plasterer because of low back pain. His symptoms began in his early twenties and have progressed to a near-constant pain. He has recently developed a sharp shooting pain down his right leg. His sleep is now disturbed and he is increasingly depressed and frustrated. I suspect his back pain is mechanical in origin but would value your opinion.

Yours sincerely,

Introduction

Most low back pain is mechanical in nature, requiring little or no investigation. However, a few patients have serious, progressive pathology that needs rapid access to appropriate investigations and management. When considering back pain, try to categorise the differential diagnosis into the following major groups: mechanical, metabolic, inflammatory, referred and infiltrative (Table 12). Note that patients may have more than one disease process going on simultaneously.

The categories may be differentiated by some of the features listed in Table 13.

History of the presenting problem

What was the progression of his symptoms?

The natural history of mechanical back pain – the commonest cause of low back pain – is initially short, infrequent episodes of disabling pain, usually of

Table 12	Differential diagnosis of low back pain
Category	Disease process
Mechanical (common)	Facet joint arthropathy Degenerative disc disease Vertebral fractures
Inflammatory	Ankylosing spondylitis Sacroiliitis
Infiltrative	Malignancy Infection (osteomyelitis, discitis or abscess)
Radicular	Foraminal stenosis Herniated intervertebral disc
Metabolic	Paget's disease Osteomalacia
Referred	Intra-abdominal pathology, eg aneurysm, ovarian cysts and endometriosis

Table 13	Features of mechanical, inflammatory and infiltrative causes of low back pain		
	Mechanical	**Inflammatory**	**Infiltrative**
Onset	Episodic Acute becoming chronic	Subacute	Insidious May be a sudden onset if there is a pathological fracture
Site	Diffuse	Diffuse May be localised to sacroiliac joints or referred to buttocks or back of thighs	Focal, though muscle spasm may lead to diffuse pain
Exacerbating factors	Variable. Often related to increasing forces, eg lifting or bending	Worse with inactivity and at night	Worse at night – can prevent sleep
Alleviating factors	Rest	Exercise	None
Morning stiffness	Mild	Severe (>1 hour)	None
Systemic features	None	Peripheral arthritis, iritis, colitis and psoriasis	Fever, weight loss and change in bowel habit

sudden onset, interspersed with episodes of good health. The episodes become more frequent over time and ultimately the patient may develop constant chronic low back pain, often with superimposed exacerbations.

When did it start?
Mechanical low back pain usually starts between the ages of 20 and 40. New onset back pain over the age of 55 is a 'red flag' (see below).

What is the character of the leg pain?
Sharp, lancinating pain suggests direct nerve root involvement, eg a herniated intervertebral disc, whereas pain referred from other lumbar-innervated structures tends to be more dull and aching.

What is the distribution of the leg pain?
Is there any associated altered sensation / loss of sensation / weakness? Are there exacerbating/ alleviating factors?

Nerve roots are commonly compressed in spinal pathology. Unilateral nerve root compression is indicated by referred pain with a radicular distribution, lower limb dermatomal sensory disturbance or lower limb motor disturbance. Peripheral nerve compression, such as entrapment of the sciatic nerve in the piriformis fossa, can give similar symptoms. Features of nerve root lesions are shown in Fig 18 and Table 14.

Neuropathic pain that is made worse with exertion is typical of spinal claudication. This may be differentiated from true intermittent claudication by the association of back pain, or by the pattern of resolution with spinal claudication. In some cases, resting alone can be insufficient to alleviate the pain, but it may be eased by sitting or

lying with the hips and knees flexed. Pain that is exacerbated by raising a straight leg suggests sciatic nerve root irritation (L4–S1), and pain exacerbated by hip extension suggests femoral nerve root involvement (L2–4).

Other relevant history
It is important to explore the suggestion of psychosocial distress in the referral letter. Psychosocial 'yellow flags' indicate barriers to recovery and a poor prognosis.

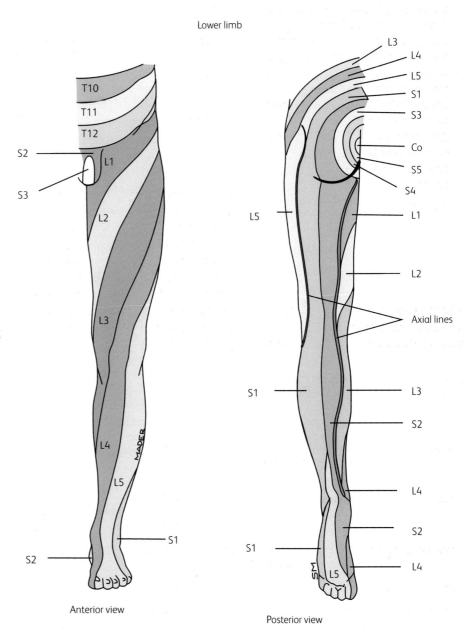

Fig 18 Lower limb dermatomes and peripheral nerves.

Table 14	Features of nerve root lesions	
Nerve root	Weakness	Reflex
L2	Hip flexion and abduction	
L3	Knee extension	Knee
L4	Knee extension and ankle dorsiflexion	Knee
L5	Knee flexion, great toe dorsiflexion and foot inversion	
S1	Knee flexion, ankle plantarflexion and foot eversion	Ankle

Hazard

Psychosocial 'yellow flags':

> past or present depression

> tendency to somatise

> belief that serious disease is present and the prognosis is poor

> secondary gain from the 'sick role', including ongoing litigation

> tendency to view problems in a catastrophic fashion.

Plan for investigation and management

Investigation
Investigation is unlikely to be helpful in this patient. Plain radiographs may even cause iatrogenic harm by revealing incidental radiological features of doubtful clinical significance, which often reinforce the patient's belief that they have a serious and irreversible problem with their back. However, on occasions, patients may find negative investigations reassuring.

Therapeutic options and pain management
In chronic low back pain, exercise and a multidisciplinary pain management approach are beneficial in improving pain and function. Analgesics, NSAIDs, back schools, behavioural therapy, massage and trigger-point injections may all provide some benefit. Other treatments are of unproven benefit. Drugs such as amitriptyline or gabapentin may be of benefit for neuropathic pain.

1.1.13 Chronic back pain

Letter of referral to the rheumatology outpatient clinic

**Dear Doctor,
Re: Mrs Tina Forbes, aged 68 years**

This woman has had chronic low back pain for over 25 years, but recently the pain has affected the thoracic spine and become more severe, leading to poor sleep. She is very worried and is losing weight.

She is a heavy smoker and has a history of long-standing chronic obstructive airways disease and glaucoma.

Is anything serious going on, or does she simply require better analgesia?

Yours sincerely,

Introduction
The general practitioner's (GP's) referral letter describes four definite 'red flags', suggesting a probable sinister cause of her back pain and meaning that she requires rapid investigation and/or treatment of a potentially serious underlying condition.

Hazard

'Red flags':

> age under 20 or over 55

> non-mechanical pain (capsular pattern)

> history of malignancy, steroids, HIV or other significant past history

> systemic symptoms such as weight loss or night sweats

> progressive neurological deficit, eg saddle anaesthesia, sphincteric disturbance and other motor or sensory deficits

> structural deformity

> persistent night pain

> thoracic pain.

The differential diagnoses to explore in this case are:

> infiltrative cause, eg malignancy or infection

> osteoporosis and vertebral fracture – steroid use is likely given the history of long-standing chronic obstructive airways disease

> worsening of chronic low back pain.

History of the presenting problem
What is the nature of the pain? How did it start and how has it progressed? Pain from infiltrative lesions is severe, often prevents sleep and is not eased by

movement. Pain from vertebral fractures may also be severe. The two may be differentiated by the onset: osteoporotic vertebral fractures begin acutely, sometimes precipitated by lifting something heavy; infiltrative lesions start more insidiously. The pain from osteoporotic fractures improves slowly over months, whereas infiltrative lesions tend to progress into a more serious problem.

Is there any neurological involvement? If so, is it progressive and how fast is the progression?

Progressive neurological symptoms are suggestive of a worsening or expanding lesion and require urgent investigation. Ask specifically about both power and sensation in the legs, and also about the function of the bladder and bowels.

Key point

Cauda equina syndrome (altered perineal sensation +/- bowel or bladder paralysis) is a neurosurgical emergency.

Other relevant history

Are there associated symptoms suggestive of the underlying cause?

> Malignancy – quantify the weight loss and ask about night sweats. Are there symptoms of a primary on systems review? In this case, be particularly aware of lung cancer (as the patient has a strong smoking history). Is there bony pain at any other sites? Are there any symptoms of hypercalcaemia?

> Infection – is it a fever / systemic illness? Note any past history of serious infections, particularly tuberculosis.

> Osteoporosis – has the woman used steroids for her chronic obstructive

pulmonary disease, and does she have any other of the following osteoporotic risk factors:

> female gender

> increasing age

> ethnicity – Caucasian or Asian

> positive family history

> sex hormone deficiency – including early menopause, late puberty and nulliparity

> past history of low-trauma fracture

> slender build

> drugs, eg steroids

> endocrine disorders, eg hyperthyroidism and hyperparathyroidism

> neoplasia, eg multiple myeloma

> gastrointestinal disorders, eg coeliac disease

> rheumatic diseases, eg rheumatoid arthritis and ankylosing spondylitis

> smoking

> excessive alcohol consumption

> low calcium intake

> poor weight-bearing exercise.

The referral letter states that the patient is worried: try to find out why. Is it the severity of the pain, is she concerned about what might be causing it or does she have other worries? A detailed discussion of such matters would be the preserve of Station 4 in PACES, but some acknowledgement of these concerns would be appropriate and necessary in Station 2 as it would clearly be required when taking a history in routine clinical practice.

Plan for investigation and management

Explain to the patient that although she has had back pain for a long time, it is a concern to you that the nature of the

back pain has changed and that the severity is such that she is not able to get a good night's sleep. Because of this, you need to perform some investigations.

If you suspect cord compression or a cauda equina syndrome then arrange admission for an urgent MRI and neurosurgical opinion. If there are no symptoms or signs to suggest these conditions, then tests to be organised from outpatients are:

> plain radiology – lumbar spine and chest radiographs

> blood tests – FBC, renal function, liver and bone profiles, inflammatory markers, blood cultures, myeloma screen

> further imaging – discuss these with radiological colleagues:

> > MRI – good for imaging discs, bone marrow, neural tissue, the spinal canal, ligaments and paraspinal tissues

> > CT – good for spinal stenosis, bone tumours and fractures, and osteophytes.

If after the investigations listed above it seems likely that there has been an osteoporotic fracture, then arrange a dual-energy X-ray absorptiometry bone density scan.

Further discussion

The challenge in assessing patients with back pain is to sort the wood from the trees using clinical acumen. Very few patients – as is likely in this case – have a serious, progressive pathology and need rapid access to the appropriate investigations and management. Most patients have mechanical back pain and require little or no investigation: they are best served by a rehabilitative approach with minimal medical intervention.

1.1.14 Recurrent joint pain and stiffness

Dear Doctor,
Re: Mr Bobby Williams, aged 42 years

Thank you for seeing this self-employed labourer who has recently stopped work because of pains in his hands and shoulders. He also has pains in his feet. He feels constantly tired and stiff, particularly in the mornings.

His father had recent hip surgery for osteoarthritis (OA) and he is worried he may also have the same condition, although I am concerned he may have rheumatoid arthritis (RA).

Please will you see him and advise regarding probable diagnosis and appropriate management.

Yours sincerely,

Introduction

When considering polyarthralgia (pain in more than five joints), first consider inflammatory versus non-inflammatory arthropathies:

> Inflammatory joint disease is associated with pain, swelling, tenderness and stiffness. Early morning stiffness of more than 60 minutes is usual in severe active RA. Tiredness, lethargy and feeling generally unwell are features of active disease.

> Non-inflammatory arthritis can also be seen after inactivity, but it lasts for only a few minutes.

It is not associated with significant morning stiffness. The pain of non-inflammatory arthritis tends to get worse with increased use of the affected joint and is worse in the evenings rather than the mornings.

The differential diagnosis can then be narrowed down according to the distribution of involved sites and associated disease characteristics.

Key point

Inflammatory joint disease:

> RA

> seronegative spondyloarthropathies, eg psoriatic arthritis, reactive arthritis and enteropathic arthritis

> polymyalgia rheumatica (PMR; in older patients)

> crystal arthritis, eg gout

> connective tissue diseases (CTDs), eg systemic lupus erythematosus (SLE)

> post-viral arthritis (especially parvovirus).

Non-inflammatory/mechanical arthritis:

> osteoarthritis (OA)

> fibromyalgia / chronic widespread pain

> soft tissue rheumatism.

History of the presenting problem

You will clearly want to explore the duration, site and character of the pain, but note the following particularly:

> Do the symptoms change with movement? Non-inflammatory conditions will tend to get worse, whereas patients with inflammatory conditions may say that things improve as they get 'warmed up'.

> Are they stiff in the mornings, and how long does it last for? As stated above, prolonged early morning stiffness is typical in RA, but not in OA.

> What is the pattern of joint involvement? Is it monoarticular, oligoarticular or polyarticular? Additive or migratory? RA often presents in an additive polyarticular and symmetrical distribution. The commonest sites of initial joint involvement are the metacarpophalangeal joints, wrists, proximal interphalangeal joints and metatarsophalangeal joints. The distal interphalangeal joints are characteristically spared in RA, but commonly involved in psoriatic arthritis. See Section 1.3.1 for further discussion.

> How fast did it come on? Most cases of RA develop insidiously over weeks or months.

> Are there any extra-articular manifestations of RA, such as subcutaneous rheumatoid nodules and secondary Sjögren's? Has the patient had any respiratory or neurological problems that might be caused by RA or another CTD? Any rashes to suggest psoriatic disease or SLE?

> Has the patient had any preceding infections?

> Seek out the specific risk factors for RA – a family history of RA and smoking.

Key point

Different patterns of onset of RA:

> acute polyarthritis

> subacute, insidious polyarthritis

> polymyalgic presentation, particularly in older people; it is important to differentiate this from PMR (see Section 2.5.1)

> acute monoarthritis (rare, see Section 1.4.4).

Explore the differential diagnoses for an inflammatory arthritis. Bear in mind the conditions listed in the 'key point' box as you enquire about specific areas including:

> eyes – inflammatory eye disease and dry eyes

> skin – psoriasis, other rashes, Raynaud's phenomenon and sclerodactyly

> nails – characteristically involved in psoriatic arthritis (pitting, ridging, onycholysis)

> gastrointestinal (GI) – inflammatory bowel disease

> infection – recent diarrhoea or urethritis, viral illness

> risk factors for gout – alcohol and diet, medication history, renal disease

> drug history – what analgesia has been tried so far? Has the patient taken any drugs that might have precipitated the problem, eg diuretics causing gout or drug-induced SLE (minocycline)?

Other relevant history

It is important to explore the functional limitations caused by the arthritis, and the impact of these limitations on the particular patient. Ask 'Can you wash and dress yourself without any difficulty?' and 'Can you walk up and down stairs without any difficulty?'. Also enquire about examples of daily tasks that the patient struggles with or needs help with (and what help is available to them). Ask the patient what effect the arthritis is having on his job (a severe arthritic condition is likely to have a devastating impact on a self-employed labourer) and on his finances, home life and relationships.

As always, it is sensible to ask (both in PACES and in routine clinical practice) whether the patient has any specific issues that you have not already addressed.

Plan for investigation and management

Explain to the patient that his story is in keeping with an inflammatory arthritis, such as RA. You plan to examine him and then request some tests to support your diagnosis. Explain that if the investigations support your clinical suspicions, then it is likely that he will need to start long-term medication (see Section 1.2.5).

Key point

The diagnosis of RA is based on a collection of features rather than a specific pathognomonic abnormality.

Investigations

Diagnosis

> Rheumatoid factor (RhF): this is positive in 70% of cases of RA and usually negative in OA, but remember that around 5% of a healthy general population are RhF-positive. Seronegative arthropathies are RhF-negative by definition.

> Anticitrullinated peptide antibodies (ACPA or anti-CCP (cyclic citrullinated peptide)) have much higher specificity for RA than RhF, in the region of 90%. Patients with both RhF and CCP antibodies generally have the worst prognosis.

> Inflammatory markers: erythrocyte sedimentation rate and C-reactive

protein are expected to be high in inflammatory arthritis and normal in OA; they also contribute to calculation of the disease activity score (DAS) (see below).

> Radiology: on X-ray, changes in RA (marginal erosions) are most commonly seen in the hands, wrists and feet. However, radiographs may be normal in the early stages of the disease. Ultrasound is increasingly used to quantify synovitis and to detect small erosions that are not evident with plain radiography.

> Arthrocentesis: examination of the patient's synovial fluid may be useful in selected cases to differentiate RA from non-inflammatory arthritis and crystal arthritis (see Section 3.5).

Damage / disease activity / prognosis

> Significant erosive disease within the first year of symptoms is a predictor of a poor prognosis. Serial radiographs of the affected joints provide a useful clue to disease progression and response to treatment (see Section 2.3.3).

> Renal and liver function tests: likely to be normal, but important to establish a pretreatment baseline.

> Each patient has a DAS calculated. This is based on the number of swollen and tender joints from a total of 28 (shoulders, elbows, wrists, metacarpophalangeal joints (MCPs), proximal interphalangeal joints (PIPs) and knees), the acute phase response, and the patient's own assessment of their disease activity. Treatment regimens, especially the use of biologic treatments such as tumour necrosis factor (TNF) blockade, are predicated on this score.

Complications

A FBC may show anaemia of chronic disease or highlight occult GI blood due to NSAID use. A thrombocytosis is common in active disease.

Management

Management is multidisciplinary and includes the following:

> Medical – a target for treatment should be agreed with the patient. This is usually remission, based on the DAS, but it may be functional, depending on the patient's needs and preferences. Treatment involves early use of combination disease-modifying antirheumatic drugs (DMARDs) and judicious use of steroids (usually intramuscular). Review is regular and frequent until such time as the agreed treatment target is met.

> Preservation of function and maintenance of the patient's normal lifestyle if at all possible (using physiotherapy, occupational therapy, podiatry and social support).

> Patient education regarding their chronic disease.

> Surgical correction of severe structural damage.

Further discussion

Current management strategies for RA involve early aggressive treatment with one or more DMARDs and a treat-to-target approach. Failure of conventional synthetic DMARDs may lead on to the use of biologic agents targeting key pathogenic cells or cytokines (such as TNF blockade – see Section 2.3.3).

RA is a chronic disease and, despite considerable advances in therapy, a significant proportion of patients fail to respond to available treatment and may suffer progressive disability. RA is associated with a two-fold increase in standardised mortality rate, with increased mortality from cardiovascular, malignant and infectious causes.

1.1.15 Fever, myalgia, arthralgia and elevated acute phase indices

Letter of referral to the rheumatology outpatient clinic

**Dear Doctor,
Mr Frank Marsden, aged 50 years**

This man presented with a 4-month history of fever and weight loss. He has also been suffering from testicular and abdominal pain, and on examination he has a palpable purpuric rash (Fig 19).

His inflammatory markers are elevated: erythrocyte sedimentation rate (ESR) 110 mm/h (normal threshold <20 mm/1st hr) and C-reactive protein (CRP) 80 mg/L (normal threshold <10). His immunology is negative: antinuclear antibody (ANA) negative, antineutrophilic cytoplasmic antibody (ANCA) negative and rheumatoid factor negative.

I am unsure of the diagnosis and would appreciate your opinion.

Yours sincerely,

Introduction

Persistent episodic fever, systemic symptoms and a marked acute phase response in a middle-aged patient may be caused by a wide range of disorders (Table 15). Of the vasculitides, Wegener's granulomatosis and microscopic polyangiitis (MPA) are rendered unlikely (but not excluded) by the negative ANCA, and the negative ANA effectively excludes lupus. Polyarteritis nodosa (PAN) remains a diagnostic possibility (see Table 20 in Section 1.3.10) and is compatible with the clinical presentation and the results of initial investigations.

**Key point
Polyarteritis nodosa**

The American College of Rheumatology criteria for the classification of polyarteritis nodosa (PAN) are listed below. The diagnosis should be *considered* as a diagnosis if a patient has at least three of these criteria:

> weight loss

> livedo reticularis

> testicular pain or tenderness

> myalgia

> mononeuropathy or polyneuropathy

> diastolic blood pressure >90 mmHg

> renal impairment

> hepatitis B antigenaemia (particularly in Asian patients, who have a high background prevalence of hepatitis B)

> arteriographic abnormality (aneurysms and arterial occlusion)

> biopsy of small- or medium-sized artery-containing polymorphs.

History of the presenting problem

Is PAN the likely diagnosis?
Clarify the nature of the following:

> pyrexia and systemic symptoms

> abdominal pain: recurrent postprandial central abdominal pain may indicate critical bowel ischaemia ('mesenteric claudication').

Also ask about the following:

> Skin rash – is this compatible with cutaneous vasculitis? Is there a history to suggest critical digital ischaemia, such as digital gangrene (Fig 20)?

> Has he had numbness, paraesthesiae or muscle weakness that might indicate mononeuritis multiplex?

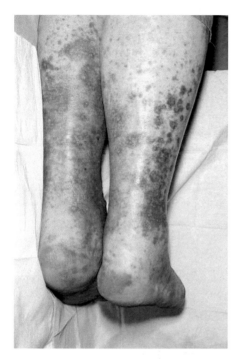

Fig 19 Necrotic purpuric rash in PAN.

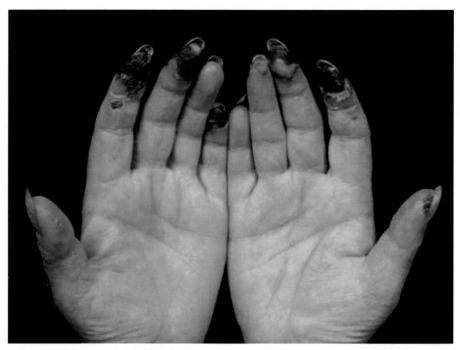

Fig 20 Digital gangrene in PAN.

Table 15	Differential diagnosis of persistent fever (>2 weeks), systemic symptoms and a marked acute phase response in an adult who is not immunosuppressed	
Type of disorder	**Comment**
Infection	Bacterial: > Subacute bacterial endocarditis and TB are the most likely > Consider liver abscess Viral: > Infection with EBV and CMV can be persistent Other: > Consider malaria in anyone who might have been exposed to it > Consider wider differential in anyone who has been to the tropics or who is immunosuppressed for any reason
Inflammatory disorders	Autoimmune rheumatic disorders: > Adult onset Still's disease > Lupus and lupus overlap disorders > Rheumatoid arthritis Other: > Sarcoidosis > Vasculitis – giant cell arteritis, MPA, Wegener's granulomatosis and PAN > Drug fever
Malignancies	Haematological – lymphoma Renal
Other	A very few cases will be factitious

CMV, cytomegalovirus; EBV, Epstein–Barr virus; MPA, microscopic polyangiitis; PAN, polyarteritis nodosa; TB, tuberculosis.

Is there a history of exposure to recreational drugs?

> Exposure to recreational drugs, particularly in a younger patient (eg cocaine-induced vasculitis) may mimic PAN.

Other diagnoses

Consider the diagnostic possibilities listed in Table 15 when taking the history: are there any leads to one or other of these conditions? Dental extraction 4 months previously might have led to endocarditis, masked by two courses of antibiotics given for fever, etc. Haematuria might indicate hypernephroma.

Other relevant history

Is there a history of tuberculosis exposure, cardiac abnormality, risk factor for endocarditis, travel abroad, blood transfusion or a known malignancy? Ask about hepatitis B infection because hepatitis B surface antigenaemia is a feature of 10–20% of cases of PAN and may affect management.

Plan for investigation and management

After explaining to the patient that under normal circumstances you would carry out a thorough clinical examination to verify the physical signs noted in the referral letter and to look for new signs, you would plan to carry out the following blood tests, special scans and a possibly tissue biopsy to arrive at a diagnosis. It would be sensible to warn the patient regarding the likely need to perform visceral angiography and sural nerve biopsy in order to make a definitive diagnosis.

Investigation

PAN seems the most likely diagnosis on clinical grounds. The following investigations are useful in establishing

this and/or excluding other conditions listed in Table 15:

> FBC – neutrophilia is expected, and eosinophilia occasionally occurs

> check acute phase markers – both erythrocyte sedimentation rate (ESR) and C-reactive protein (CRP) will be elevated and reflect disease activity

> electrolytes, renal, liver and bone function tests

> autoimmune / vasculitic serology – already performed in this case

> hepatitis B status

> blood cultures – several

> urine dipstick – looking for proteinuria and/or haematuria. If positive, proceed to microscopy for casts and estimation of albumin to creatinine ratio (urinary)

> echocardiogram – if normal and there is a high suspicion of endocarditis, consider a transoesophageal study

> CT scan of the chest, abdomen and pelvis – looking in particular for lymphadenopathy and at the kidneys

> visceral angiography for evidence of aneurysms and arterial occlusion

> tissue biopsy – consider sural nerve biopsy in patients with neuropathy and skin biopsy in patients with cutaneous features

> 18F-fluorodeoxyglucose (FDG) positron emission tomography (PET) can also be helpful in the diagnosis of large vessel vasculitis

> other investigations may be indicated depending on clinical suspicion, eg thick film for malaria.

Management

If the diagnosis of PAN is confirmed, immunosuppressive therapy with steroids and cyclophosphamide will be required for treatment of severe cases. Patients with disease confined to the skin may respond to steroids alone.

Where PAN is associated with hepatitis B infection, antiviral treatment using a combination of vidarabine/lamivudine with interferon-α is often helpful.

Further discussion

The rarity of PAN has contributed to difficulties in differentiating it from MPA, an ANCA-associated predominant small-vessel vasculitis.

Key point

PAN versus MPA

In a patient with systemic vasculitis the following features favour MPA rather than PAN:

> glomerulonephritis

> ANCA positivity

> normal visceral angiography.

1.1.16 Non-rheumatoid pain and stiffness

Letter of referral to the rheumatology outpatient clinic

Dear Doctor,

Re: Mr Alexander Jacobs, aged 55 years

This mechanic has been complaining of increasing widespread pain over the past year, particularly affecting his hands, knees and lower back. He is having some functional difficulty at work because of his hand problems and has noticed bony lumps developing over his finger joints.

I suspect that he is developing early osteoarthritis (OA), but would be grateful for your views. Am I missing something else?

Yours sincerely,

Introduction

The first thing to establish in cases of polyarthralgia is whether the symptoms sound inflammatory or non-inflammatory: see Section 1.1.14 for relevant discussion.

History of the presenting complaint

What is the location of the pain?

Primary OA, like rheumatoid arthritis, has a tendency to affect certain joints more than others (Table 16). Involvement of the thumb carpometacarpal joints (CMCs), with pain on opening jars or wringing out cloths, is highly suggestive.

What is the pattern of the pain?

The pain of OA tends to get worse with movement and better with rest. Is there any joint stiffness? There may be morning stiffness, although it is less severe and prolonged than in inflammatory arthritides, and inactivity stiffness (or gelling) is common, particularly in the knees.

Have your joints changed shape?

Bony swellings over the distal interphalangeal joints (DIPs) and proximal interphalangeal joints (PIPs) are typical in nodal OA, sometimes with palmar and/or lateral deviation of the distal phalanx. Severe knee OA may be associated with valgus or varus deformities.

Have you noticed your joints creaking, crunching or grinding?

Crepitus is a common feature of OA, most commonly experienced in the knees.

Other relevant history

If there is OA in an atypical joint distribution, consider secondary causes (see Sections 1.3.2 and 2.3.2).

Ask about family history (this is often strongly related in cases of generalised nodal OA) and previous trauma. The patient's occupation may be relevant, and also note obesity – a risk factor for OA of the knee.

What are the functional limitations secondary to the arthritis? How well is the patient able to continue his job? Are there options for alternative employment? Are there financial implications? Explore psychological factors associated with function and chronic pain.

Plan for investigation and management

Explain that his story and pattern of joint involvement is suggestive of OA, and that you plan some tests to confirm this diagnosis.

Investigation

Plain radiographs

In OA (Fig 21) these reveal the following:

> loss of joint space

> sclerotic bone on either side of the joint

> bony spurs (osteophytes) at the joint margin.

Less frequently they may show:

> cystic changes in subchondral bone

> chondrocalcinosis – suggesting calcium pyrophosphate disease.

Table 16 Likelihood of involvement of particular joints in primary OA

Joints typically involved	Joints typically *not* involved
DIPs	MCPs
PIPs	Wrists
First CMCs	Elbows
Acromioclavicular joints	Shoulders
Hips	Ankles
Knees	
First MTPs	Second to fifth MTPs
Facet joints	

CMCs, carpometacarpal joints; DIPs, distal interphalangeal joints; MCPs, metacarpophalangeal joints; MTPs, metatarsophalangeal joints; PIPs, proximal interphalangeal joints.

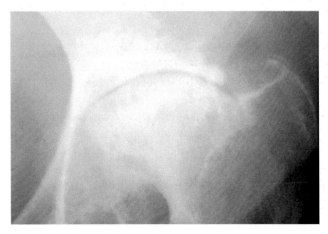

Fig 21 Radiograph showing severe OA of the hip with loss of joint space, subchondral sclerosis and osteophyte formation. (Courtesy of Dr M Pattrick.)

Synovial fluid analysis

If a joint is swollen, then joint aspiration may reveal characteristic features of OA: fluid from a non-inflammatory arthropathy is typically clear, straw-coloured and viscous, and aspiration also helps to exclude sepsis and crystal arthritides.

Blood tests

These are not often necessary, but a normal C-reactive protein and/or erythrocyte sedimentation rate help exclude an inflammatory arthritis. Ferritin, serum iron and total iron binding capacity should be checked if haemochromatosis is suspected (see Section 2.3.2).

Management

The management of OA should be based around:

> education – the patient should understand that the goal of treatment is pain relief and the maintenance of function, but not an alteration to the natural history

> reducing pain and stiffness – analgesia (oral and topical), intra-articular therapy (steroids and viscosupplementation), paraffin/wax baths for hands, superficial heat packs, insoles to improve foot posture and hydrotherapy

> maintaining muscle strength, fitness and joint mobility

> supporting unstable joints, eg wearing a knee brace

> minimising disability – using walking aids, splints and tools; also managing psychological distress

> surgery – arthroplasty and osteotomy.

1.1.17 Widespread pain

Letter of referral to the rheumatology outpatient clinic

Dear Doctor,

Re Mrs Wendy Hawkins, aged 38 years

This woman has a 4-year history of widespread musculoskeletal pain, fatigue and tiredness. She is now unable to work and is becoming increasingly dependent upon her family. She spends much of her day in bed and is now asking for the provision of a wheelchair.

She has seen several physicians and orthopaedic surgeons over the past few years, but extensive investigation has shown no evidence of any serious neurological or musculoskeletal disease. She appears low in mood and angry to me, but denies that she is depressed and has declined a trial of antidepressant treatment.

Am I missing any serious organic condition here? How can we best help her?

Yours sincerely,

Introduction

Widespread pain and fatigue have many causes. The case description given here points strongly towards the syndrome known as fibromyalgia, but diagnostic thoughts should be cast wider than this, particularly if 'red flag' features are present. Fibromyalgia is discussed in more detail in Section 1.2.4.

Hazard

'Red flag' features in widespread pain

> onset age >50 years

> recent onset and progressive history

> weight loss or night sweats

> previous history of malignancy or immunosuppression

> focal versus diffuse pain

> fever

> any abnormal physical signs other than tenderness

> abnormal blood tests.

History of the presenting problem

Although it seems very likely that this woman has fibromyalgia, it would be wrong to assume this immediately without the benefit of a full systems enquiry. Are any 'red flag' features present? Also remember that fibromyalgia is not an exclusive diagnosis: fibromyalgic pain may (and often does) coexist with other rheumatological causes of pain such as rheumatoid arthritis, osteoarthritis and mechanical spinal pain.

Pain

Document the pattern of pain and its progression over time. Pain in fibromyalgia is very widespread but usually predominantly axial rather than peripheral, and typically inexorable but rarely progressive (Fig 22). By presentation, most patients have had widespread pain for many months, if not many years. The patient will usually feel that 'everything hurts', but will usually identify the muscles rather than the joints as the main sites of pain. Descriptions of the pain will often lead

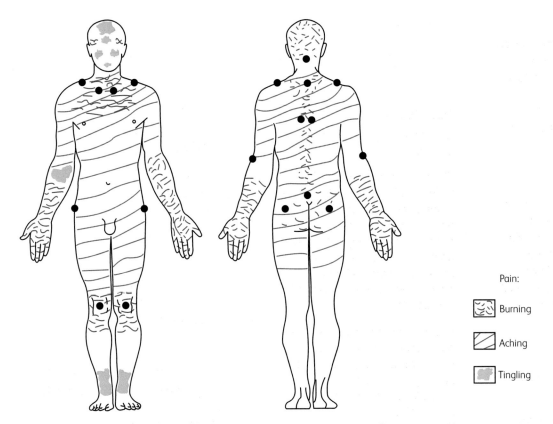

Pain:

☒ Burning

☒ Aching

☒ Tingling

Fig 22 Pain diagram showing classic tender points (filled circles) in fibromyalgia plus a patient's own illustration of the site and nature of pain.

rapidly onto other non-pain symptoms, especially fatigue and low mood. Numbness and other sensory disturbances are often described, but these are usually flitting in site, transient in duration and have no obvious neuroanatomical correlates.

Fatigue
Ask what the patient means by fatigue. Is this localised muscle weakness (raising suspicions of neurological disease) or, typical of fibromyalgia, a more generalised feeling of tiredness or lack of energy ('tired all the time')? In fibromyalgia, this is often associated with other cognitive symptoms such as difficulty concentrating and a feeling of 'muzzy-headedness'. Other neurological symptoms may be present – particularly flitting paraesthesia.

Disability
Gain a picture of the patient's degree of disability and the impact on her life. High degrees of disability are usually reported, but this often relates to fatigue and poor stamina, rather than difficulty performing any specific activities. What is the patient's current exercise capacity?

Depression and related conditions
Ask about sleep patterns and sleep disturbance: is sleep refreshing (poor quality, unrefreshing sleep is virtually universal)? Is there evidence of depression currently? Note that other cognitive symptoms may occur and are often associated with depression. Is there a history of other functional syndromes (see 'key point' box)? Has the patient had any previous psychiatric illness?

Key point
A review of the past medical history (and in routine clinical practice of the case notes, along with discussion with the GP) may be particularly helpful. Look for the following:

> irritable bowel syndrome

> chronic fatigue syndrome / myalgic encephalopathy

> unexplained breathlessness or chest pain

> unexplained gynaecological symptoms

> unexplained headache or dizziness

> multiple 'allergies' in the absence of objective evidence.

Key point

Most patients with fibromyalgia will give an immediate impression of distress and depression – this in itself is striking and significant. The psychological state of patients with most illnesses depends heavily on their personality and coping strategies: a patient with rheumatoid disease can be cheerful, stoical, anxious or depressed, but a patient with fibromyalgia will invariably be weary and sad. Despite this unhappiness, the patient usually appears physically well.

Plan for investigation and management

After explaining to the patient that under normal circumstances you would carry out a thorough clinical examination, you will need to carry out a few investigations to exclude diseases that can present in this way.

Investigation

This requires a balance between the need to exclude serious pathology and the harm that can be done by over-investigation. Patients with fibromyalgia (and other functional syndromes) will often have undergone repeated episodes of negative investigation. This process strongly reinforces a belief that their symptoms have a serious physical cause, which would be identified if only the right tests were done. However, as further negative investigations are performed, patients come to feel that the doctor does not believe that their symptoms are real ('you think it's all in my mind'). This results in the deterioration of the doctor–patient relationship, and the patient may move on to repeat the process elsewhere. It is therefore more helpful to try and make a positive diagnosis of fibromyalgia at an early stage based on the clinical picture, rather than a negative diagnosis of exclusion after negative investigation.

The need for investigation should be determined by the degree of clinical suspicion that the diagnosis is not fibromyalgia. Pay attention to the 'red flag' features listed in the 'hazard' box earlier in this section. Unfortunately, however, investigation is often driven by insecurity, lack of experience and a fear of 'missing something'.

It is very important that the rationale for investigation be explained to the patient. If you feel that the results are likely to be negative, say so and explain why. A minimalist approach to investigation might include the following:

> FBC

> renal, bone and liver biochemistry, calcium and blood glucose

> creatinine kinase

> thyroid function

> acute phase markers – C-reactive protein and erythrocyte sedimentation rate

> myeloma screen in patients >50 years

> vitamin D

> chest radiograph, especially in smokers.

Management

Further explanation of the diagnosis and management plan is discussed in Section 1.2.4.

1.2 Communication skills and ethics

1.2.1 Collapse during a restaurant meal

Scenario

Role: you are a junior doctor working on a general medical ward.

Scenario: you have admitted a 19-year-old female student following a severe anaphylactic reaction to peanuts. Following emergency treatment she is well. She has no significant past medical history and lives in a university flat with two fellow students, one female and one male.

Your task: to explain to the patient the diagnosis of nut allergy as the cause of her anaphylaxis; and avoidance measures and the use of self-injectable epinephrine (ie EpiPen). There is no specialist allergy service in your hospital, but one of the pharmacists would be able to show the patient how to use the EpiPen and you would be able to make an outpatient referral to the regional allergy service.

Key issues to explore

It will obviously be appropriate to ask the patient if she has any particular concerns and to address these, but the most important issue that must be tackled is to find out what she understands about her anaphylactic reaction. Understanding is important if she is to feel confident about minimising future risk. Lifestyle issues will be important:

> She will need to know how to minimise the risk of ingesting 'hidden' sources of peanut if eating out.

> She will need to read food labels if buying pre-prepared food.

> Does she have a partner, flatmates or family? They could be important allies in avoiding peanuts and may be able to assist in an emergency if given the appropriate information.

Key points to establish

After an appropriate introduction, let the patient know that the purpose of your interview is to discuss what happened so that the chance of it happening in future is minimised. Say that you will also discuss a simple but effective treatment that she can give herself in case of emergency. You must try to give her confidence in her ability to manage the situation.

Explain how to avoid future reactions
Emphasise that she should continue to live a normal life, but that she must take appropriate precautions. Discuss potentially difficult or risky situations: parties, restaurants and choosing peanut-free food when shopping. Allow her time to express her concerns.

Discuss self-management of anaphylaxis
Discuss the need to carry two epinephrine devices at all times, the recognition of anaphylaxis and measures which should be taken if it happens again. Be aware that she may be afraid of using injectable epinephrine and encourage her to discuss this. Encourage her to discuss her peanut allergy with her friends – who may be trained in the use of the epinephrine, if appropriate – but you should ensure that she gains the confidence to

self-inject in an emergency: her friends will not always be with her.

Appropriate responses to likely questions

Patient: why did this happen? I've eaten peanuts lots of times before.

Doctor: that's a good question, and I'm afraid that I don't have a good answer. All I can say is that this often happens: for some reason we don't know, people can become allergic to peanuts – and to other things – and their body starts to react in this dangerous way if they are exposed to them.

Patient: is it just peanuts I'm allergic to?

Doctor: that's another good question and at the moment I can't be sure. Sometimes people who react to peanuts also react to other nuts, so my advice for now is that it's very important that you avoid all nuts. But I will, with your agreement, refer you to the regional allergy service as an outpatient. They will do various tests to find out whether it's just peanuts that you're allergic to, or other nuts as well.

Patient: I couldn't possibly inject myself. How can I? I'm scared of needles.

Doctor: it's natural to feel that way at first, but you can overcome your fear. You will feel safer knowing that you know what to do in an emergency. One of the pharmacists in the hospital can show you how to use a device that does all the work for you: you don't actually see the needle and you can practice using a 'trainer' pen, which doesn't actually inject you. We could also show your flatmates how to use it too, if you wanted that and they were willing to learn.

Patient: how will I know when to use the epinephrine?

Doctor: the epinephrine is only for severe reactions like the one you had today. If you think you may be having an allergic reaction, you should take epinephrine if you feel any throat tightness, wheezing or faintness.

Patient: I'll be too frightened to eat out in a restaurant: what if the same thing happened again?

Doctor: I can understand why you are worried about that, but you can minimise the chances by taking simple measures. Most restaurants are aware of the difficulties faced by people with allergies – some have allergy information on the menus. However, you should always ask the waiter to check specifically with the cook in the kitchen whether what you're thinking of ordering contains any nuts at all.

Patient: what about travelling abroad? Should I cancel my holiday?

Doctor: there is no need to cancel your holiday, but be cautious about unfamiliar foods that may contain nuts and always check in restaurants, as I've said before. Make sure that you carry your epinephrine with you and, to avoid difficulties on the plane and at customs, it would be wise to carry a doctor's letter explaining what it is and why you need it. I can write one of these for you.

Patient: what if the epinephrine doesn't work?

Doctor: in any situation that you need to use the epinephrine, an ambulance should also be called. The aim of the epinephrine is to give time for the ambulance to get to you. The epinephrine will work, but if the effect is insufficient, or if your symptoms start to come back, you should use your second epinephrine syringe. By that time medical help is likely to be there.

1.2.2 Cold fingers and difficulty swallowing

Scenario

Role: you are a junior doctor in a rheumatology outpatient clinic.

Scenario: Mrs Hope Adams, aged 50 years, has recently been referred to the outpatient clinic with cold fingers. The clinical suspicion from the initial consultation that she has secondary Raynaud's phenomenon in association with systemic sclerosis (SS) has been supported by the detection of anti-centromere antibodies in her blood.

She tells you that despite her doctor's concern, the Raynaud's does not trouble her too much and she can control her symptoms by avoiding cold weather and wearing gloves.

Your task: to explain to Mrs Adams the diagnosis of SS, including the uncertain prognosis and lack of curative treatment.

Key issues to explore

How does she currently view her problems? Does she appreciate that she may have a serious, chronic condition, and that the disease may progress beyond the symptoms of her Raynaud's? Approach this by asking what she was told at the last clinic appointment: was it mentioned that her cold fingers could be a feature of a more widespread disease? This is a 'warning shot' before explaining the diagnosis.

Key points to establish

> Tests have suggested that she may develop more than cold fingers in the future: they are associated with a disease called SS, or scleroderma, which means 'hard skin'. In this condition the skin, usually of the hands and feet, swells and thickens and becomes stiff, tight and shiny.

> This 'hardening' or fibrosis can also affect internal organs, which can cause a variety of symptoms depending upon which organ is involved.

> As and when other symptoms develop, they can be addressed and treated. However, there is no effective treatment for the underlying condition.

> Regular reviews are required to direct symptomatic treatments, anticipate problems with screening tests and provide support.

> If the patient does develop other problems, referral to a regional centre with a relative special interest may be appropriate.

Appropriate responses to likely questions

Patient: I feel completely well other than the cold fingers. Why do you think I have anything more serious than cold fingers?

Doctor: that's a good question: it's because of the blood tests. They show that you have an antibody that is linked with a condition called scleroderma, and it is common for people with this condition to have cold hands – Raynaud's – for many years before they develop skin thickening or any other problems.

Patient: so what will scleroderma do to me?

Doctor: I'm afraid that I cannot say for certain – not because I'm hiding anything, but because I don't know. Sometimes it just causes very slow thickening of the skin, especially of the hands and feet. But sometimes it causes thickening of the tissues of internal organs, and that can lead to a variety of problems.

Patient: what sort of internal problems can scleroderma cause?

Doctor: I don't want to cause you unnecessary concern because all these things certainly don't happen to every patient, but it can cause problems with the gut – in particular difficulty with swallowing; a variety of problems with the lungs; and problems with the kidneys, including very high blood pressure.

Patient: I have never heard of this disease. How can I find out more?

Doctor: I can give you a leaflet on scleroderma today, and also the contact details for the Raynaud's and Scleroderma Association.

Patient: what can you do if the scleroderma starts causing serious problems?

Doctor: I'm afraid that we don't have any good treatment that will cure the scleroderma: we don't have anything that will make it go away, but what we can do is to help the problems that it causes. For instance, if it causes problems with indigestion or swallowing then there are tablets that we can recommend – strong anti-indigestion tablets – that can help. If it causes problems with your blood pressure, then it's important to try and control this very carefully to prevent serious complications.

Patient: if you can't treat this disease, then why are you telling me about it?

Doctor: as I said, we don't have any treatment that will cure scleroderma, but we can do things that will help. By monitoring you in clinic we can try to pick up any problems early on, rather than waiting until things have got really bad. For instance, we would keep a careful check on your blood pressure and your lungs, and we would recommend treatment if problems were developing. Good treatment of blood pressure would be very important in cutting down the chances of your developing kidney failure, or other problems.

1.2.3 Back pain

Scenario

Role: you are a junior doctor working on a general medical ward.

Scenario: you have admitted a 58-year-old woman for urgent investigation. She has a 2-week history of low back pain which is now keeping her awake at night. Over the past 2 days she has noticed progressive numbness and weakness of both legs, and also sphincteric weakness.

She had breast cancer with axillary node involvement 4 years ago, but was told at her last outpatient appointment in the oncology clinic 6 months ago that 'she was fine'.

On examination she has bilateral lower limb sensory impairment and lower motor neurone weakness.

A plain radiograph of the spine shows at least one suspicious lesion.

Your task: to explain to her that:

> She has cord compression – cause uncertain, but with a strong suspicion of malignancy.

> The plan will be for her to have imaging (MRI spine) and that surgery will probably be recommended, but that this will not be curative.

Key issues to explore

Your discussion with the patient should cover the following areas:

> her understanding of the problem

> your explanation of her symptoms

> the probable underlying cause

> the treatments available

> the likely prognosis.

Key points to establish

> That there is a problem with the patient's spine: it is pressing on her spinal cord and causing a blockage of the nerve signals to the lower half of her body.

> That this is a serious problem, probably related to her breast cancer, which needs urgent investigation and may require surgical intervention.

> That, even in the worst case, there will always be support and a plan of management.

In routine clinical practice (and in PACES, although the offer will inevitably be declined) encourage the presence of a close friend or relative if the patient wishes it. As well as providing support, this will spare the patient the necessity of repeating the explanation and may improve their overall understanding of their problem.

Appropriate responses to likely questions

Patient: it's not the breast cancer come back, is it?

Doctor: I don't know, but I'm afraid that there is a good chance that it could be the cancer. We won't know for certain until we have done some tests. We'll start off with a scan – an MRI – of the spine and then probably perform an operation to relieve any pressure on the spine and take samples for analysis. If it is the cancer, we will arrange for you to see the cancer specialist to talk about further treatment.

Patient: but at the clinic a few months ago, the oncologist told me that everything was fine.

Doctor: I know, because at that time you hadn't got any back pain or any problems with your legs. If this is the cancer coming back, then it seems as though that's happened just in the past few months.

Patient: if the oncologist had done a scan of my back when I saw them in the clinic a few months ago, would they have found anything?

Doctor: that's a good question, but I'm afraid that I don't know the answer. Scans of the spine aren't organised as a routine, only if there seems to be a problem. However, this is something that you could discuss with the oncologist if and when you see them.

Patient: I'm afraid to have surgery in case it makes things worse – are there any alternatives?

Doctor: you're right in saying that all surgery has risks, but this is not something we're going to race into. The surgeons will look at your scans very carefully and will discuss things with you before you make the final decision. They will only recommend going ahead if they agree that there is a good chance of success. If you didn't have surgery, your legs might get worse and it would be difficult to know what was causing the problem or how to treat it. Is there anything in particular about the surgery that is worrying you?

Patient: if it's the cancer, will they be able to remove it during the operation?

Doctor: if it is possible to remove it, then the surgeons will do so. However, trying to remove the whole tumour may well damage your spinal cord so it's likely that the surgeons will just take enough to relieve any pressure. If further treatment is necessary, then radiotherapy treatment or medication will probably be recommended – but this is something on which the oncologists would advise.

Patient: does this mean that I can't be cured, that I have terminal cancer?

Doctor: if it is cancer, then you are right in thinking that we probably won't be able to get rid of it completely. But having said that, there are treatments that can work pretty well and it is possible for some people to live a relatively healthy and normal life for some time, even though the cancer is not completely removed.

Further comments

It is important that you are realistic in your explanations. This patient will undoubtedly need to have trust and confidence in her medical team in the future. Although it is important to be as positive as you reasonably can be in your attitude, a falsely over-optimistic assessment at this stage is likely to result in increased distress and loss of trust in the medical team in the future.

1.2.4 Widespread pain

Scenario

Role: you are a junior doctor in a rheumatology outpatient clinic.

Scenario: you are seeing a 38-year-old woman who is attending the clinic for her first follow-up appointment. She was first seen in the clinic 6 weeks ago (by the consultant), when she gave a 3-year history of widespread pain, profound fatigue and poor-quality sleep. These symptoms were associated with significant disability, and she reported spending much of her day in bed and being heavily dependent upon her family.

The notes record that she was 'sad, withdrawn and angry'. Examination revealed very widespread tenderness with numerous tender 'trigger points', but movement of her joints was unrestricted and no neurological abnormality could be detected.

The consultant felt that a diagnosis of fibromyalgia was likely, with some evidence of associated depression. Various investigations including an FBC, erythrocyte sedimentation rate, C-reactive protein, bone/liver/kidney/muscle biochemistry, thyroid function tests, a screen for autoimmune/vasculitic disease and a chest radiograph were performed, and all were normal.

Your task: to explain the diagnosis of fibromyalgia to the patient and suggest a graded exercise programme, and also the possible benefits of treatment for depression.

Key issues to explore

This consultation is likely to be difficult, even for an experienced clinician. It is important to:

> find out what the patient thinks is causing her problems, and what their expectations are – discussions are likely to be easier if you are aware of the patient's perspective

> pursue the role that depression and other psychological factors might be playing in the illness.

Key points to establish

It is essential to establish an atmosphere of trust, taking the patient's physical symptoms seriously and acknowledging their reality.

> Explain fibromyalgia as a pattern of muscular pain, which can be severe and distressing, but which is not associated with any tissue damage.

> Explain that factors such as sleep disturbance, loss of physical fitness (conditioning) and low mood can perpetuate the pain and make it worse. Some patients find it difficult to accept that depression can cause pain, but most will see how pain and sleep disturbance can cause depression. It is rarely productive to get drawn into a 'chicken or egg' argument about pain and depression, and it is usually easier and more helpful to explain how vicious circles between these factors can worsen the pain (see Fig 22), viewing low mood as a practical problem to be solved in helping to overcome the pain.

> Explain that treatment is not easy and that a complete, rapid cure is unlikely, but also that addressing the

perpetuating factors can improve function and quality of life for most patients.

Appropriate responses to likely questions

Patient: *you are saying all the tests are normal and that there is nothing wrong with my muscles. Are you saying it is all in my mind?*

Doctor: no, your pain is real and is clearly causing you distress and affecting your life. Many kinds of rheumatic pain do not lead to changes in the blood or abnormalities on X-rays. Nevertheless, it is good that fibromyalgia is not associated with any long-term damage to the tissues.

Patient: *I don't see how I can do more exercise when exercise just makes the pain worse.*

Doctor: this is a very common concern for people with fibromyalgia, because exercise can certainly make the pain and tiredness worse. Nevertheless, we know that graded exercise programmes are one of the most helpful treatments for patients with fibromyalgia. The key thing is to approach exercise in the right way, and this usually needs help from a physiotherapist. You need to start with an amount of exercise that you can cope with easily, repeat this regularly, and just gradually increase the amount you are doing. You will only improve if you are able to exercise three times a week or more. At first the exercise will cause some discomfort, but if you are able to come back and do the same again within a day or two, then this is fine. However, if you get so much pain after exercise that you cannot do anything for a week, then you have started at too high a level.

Patient: *I know that amitriptyline is an antidepressant – are you suggesting that I take it because you think my main problem is depression?*

Doctor: you are right that amitriptyline is an antidepressant, but low doses of amitriptyline and similar drugs are often used in the treatment of long-standing pain – particularly when the pain disturbs sleep. The doses used to manage pain are much lower than those used in cases of depression. I'm suggesting that you take it simply because I think it might help.

Patient: *do you think my main problem is depression?*

Doctor: I honestly find it very difficult to know. For obvious reasons, people with painful conditions often become depressed and depression makes any sort of pain worse. Treating depression can sometimes be easier than treating pain and it can certainly do a lot to improve your quality of life.

Patient: *if I take amitriptyline, I'll become addicted to it and I'll get side effects, won't I?*

Doctor: no, it isn't addictive. It's generally safe and well tolerated, although it can cause morning drowsiness in some people, especially at the beginning of treatment.

Patient: *what about my other problems with irritable bowels? How will they be affected by your treatments? Lots of tablets upset my stomach.*

Doctor: people with fibromyalgia often have a lot of pain in other parts of their bodies, and irritable bowel syndrome is very common. In most cases, treatments for fibromyalgia, such as amitriptyline, tend to improve irritable bowel syndrome.

Patient: *it isn't just the pain – the fatigue is just as bad. Why am I so tired?*

Doctor: tiredness is one of the most distressing symptoms in fibromyalgia, and is also a big problem in many other painful conditions. One of the most important causes of the tiredness is sleep disturbances due to

pain, and these often improve with drugs such as amitriptyline.

1.2.5 Explain a recommendation to start a disease-modifying antirheumatic drug

Scenario

Role: you are a junior doctor in a rheumatology outpatient clinic.

Scenario: Mrs Susan Terrell, a 40-year-old secretary, has recently been diagnosed with erosive rheumatoid arthritis after she presented with a 3-month history of disabling joint pains affecting her wrists and fingers. She has a strongly positive rheumatoid factor and anti-CCP (cyclic citrullinated peptide) antibodies and has had a persistently elevated serum C-reactive protein (CRP) of 40–75 mg/L (normal threshold <10) since presentation, all of which are adverse prognostic factors. Although it has been explained to her that treatment with a disease-modifying antirheumatic drug (DMARD) – methotrexate – is her best hope of preserving joint function in the long term, she is unconvinced of the need to start treatment with this drug at this juncture on account of its possible adverse effects.

Your task: to explain to Mrs Terrell why it is in her best interests to take methotrexate.

Key issues to explore

The decision whether or not to take any drug should depend on the balance of benefits and risks. Anxiety about drug-induced adverse effects is entirely understandable, and methotrexate can certainly be toxic; but the key issues to explore here are the patient's perceptions of the benefits and risks to her.

Key points to establish

> Do not be dismissive of the patient's concerns – recognise her anxiety regarding the impact of the diagnosis and what the future might hold.

> Explain the reasoning behind the recommendation to commence methotrexate rather than to use symptomatic treatments alone, ie she has active disease with adverse prognostic indices comprising radiological evidence of joint erosions coupled with a persistently elevated CRP and positive autoantibodies (rheumatoid factor, anti-CCP).

> Emphasise that the risk–benefit ratio of treatment in this situation is heavily tilted towards treatment.

> Explain the potential long-term consequences of not undertaking treatment with a DMARD.

> Offer to introduce her to a clinical nurse specialist in rheumatology for more detailed discussion.

Appropriate responses to likely questions

Patient: *how confident are you that methotrexate will not cause me any problems?*

Doctor: as you know, it's impossible to guarantee that any drug will not cause problems. Deciding whether or not to recommend any drug is always a matter of balancing benefits and risks, but most people who take methotrexate do not get any problems with it and it's a very effective drug for treating rheumatoid arthritis in many cases.

Patient: *but how many people get problems with it?*

Doctor: adverse effects such as nausea, loss of appetite and diarrhoea occur in up to one in 10 patients, but most of these individuals usually get better on their own without the need to stop treatment. Low blood counts may occur in up to one in 20 patients, but these should be detected by routine monitoring – which is necessary for anyone taking the drug – before they cause a problem.

Patient: which adverse effects would you be most concerned about?

Doctor: like any medication which dampens the activity of the immune system, methotrexate may suppress production of white blood cells in the bone marrow and increase your susceptibility to infections. It also has the potential in a few patients, less than 5% of cases, to cause liver problems or lung inflammation.

Patient: if I get these problems, do they always get better if the drug is stopped?

Doctor: yes, in most patients both bone marrow suppression and liver or lung problems are reversible. Regular follow-up and blood-test monitoring means that we would pick up evidence of any problems at an early stage. It would be equally important that you told us if you felt unwell or developed a cough or shortness of breath while you were on the drug, so that we could check things over promptly.

Patient: are there any other drugs that attack the disease that I could take instead?

Doctor: yes, there are other drugs which modify disease activity, but all of them have side effects, many similar to those of methotrexate. Methotrexate is the one that's been around the longest and none of the other drugs are clearly better, so that's why we recommend methotrexate in the first instance.

Patient: if you were afflicted with rheumatoid arthritis, would you take methotrexate?

Doctor: yes, I would take methotrexate or one the other disease-modifying antirheumatic drugs if I had evidence of an active, erosive disease, because of the strength of evidence showing that early treatment prevents further joint damage.

Patient: why can't I wait and see how things go?

Doctor: you can wait if you want to, but that's not what we recommend. Damage is occurring in your joints – we can see it on the X-rays – and if that damage gets worse, then there isn't any treatment that will turn the clock back.

1.2.6 Explain a diagnosis of rheumatoid arthritis

Scenario

Role: you are a junior doctor in a rheumatology clinic.

Scenario: Mrs McClinton, a 52-year-old teacher, was referred with inflammatory joint symptoms in her hands and feet. She has been diagnosed with seropositive rheumatoid arthritis. She is rheumatoid factor (RhF)- and cyclic citrullinated peptide (CCP)-positive, but X-rays have revealed no erosions. She is a smoker, but there are no other risk factors for inflammatory arthritis.

Your task: to explain the new diagnosis of rheumatoid arthritis (RA).

Key issues to explore

> Check what the patient understands by inflammatory arthritis, and contrast it with degenerative disease (or other causes of musculoskeletal pain) that would need different treatment. Tell them that RA is the most common of the inflammatory forms of arthritis.

> Find out what they know about RA. Many patients will have looked on the internet and will be frightened by the images of end-stage destructive disease. Some will have relatives with RA – ask about them and their experiences, as that will affect your patient's feelings about the diagnosis and their future.

Key issues to establish

> Reassure them that the prognosis for patients with RA is much better than previously, and that many people are able to live a normal life in remission, albeit on medication.

> Point out that there is much more psychosocial support, both in the hospital (eg clinical nurse specialists, doctors) and in the community (local National RA Society (NRAS) groups). Emphasise that they are not alone.

> There are a lot of very effective treatments for RA, but these will need to be taken long term, so it's very important to establish your patient's beliefs around medication (the side effects of steroids and immunosuppression can make patients particularly anxious).

> Agree with the patient the clinical target you are both aiming for (for most people this will be remission), and stress to them that you will regularly assess them and modify their treatment until they reach that target.

Appropriate responses to likely questions

Patient: why did I get this?

Doctor: we don't know exactly why some people get rheumatoid arthritis (RA) and others don't. Family history plays a role, because we know there are some at-risk genes that can be inherited. Smoking also increases your chances of developing RA, but there are still a lot of things we don't fully understand about how the disease starts.

Patient: will it ever go away?

Doctor: I'd like to say something different, but it's very unlikely to disappear altogether, and it will need treatment to keep the symptoms at bay and prevent any damage to the joints. But some people have milder disease than others, and everyone will experience flares of disease every now and again. Our aim is to use medications that not only suit you, but also keep you active and pain-free long term.

Patient: *am I one of the patients in a bad disease group?*

Doctor: I'm afraid that we still can't predict precisely what will happen to an individual patient with RA. However, the fact that you have both antibodies that go with classic RA suggests that your disease might be a bit harder to control than those who have one or other or neither; but we have lots of ways of doing that, and we will find the right combination for you. The good news is that your joints have not been damaged by the disease, so we've caught it early.

Patient: *how soon will I feel better?*

Doctor: very soon. The standard way to approach things now would be to give you a steroid injection into a muscle: this will have the effect of damping down all the inflammation in the body immediately. That will make you feel much better in the next few days, and for the next few weeks – and will give you support while the longer-acting treatments kick in over the next couple of months.

Patient: *how often do I need to come to the hospital?*

Doctor: in the first instance, quite frequently, maybe every 4–6 weeks or so – but not always to see the doctor. The clinical nurse specialists will be an important point of contact for you and will help you to understand the disease, how to manage it, the new treatments and the monitoring they need; if they think it's necessary, they can suggest changing the dose of your medicine. Once your disease is under control, with medication that suits you and all the monitoring is fine, then we'll end up only seeing you every few months or even yearly.

Patient: *can I still exercise, or should I rest?*

Doctor: it's very important that you maintain your fitness. Obviously you'll need to strike a balance between pacing yourself a bit and keeping active, but you'll come to know where that tipping-point is for you – and we can help you with that too. The most important thing to remember is that you will not damage your joints with sensible exercise; there's been a lot of research done in this area, and all the studies indicate that exercise is very beneficial and not harmful in patients with RA.

1.3 Brief clinical consultations

1.3.1 Hands (general examination)

Introduction

All hand examinations should follow a routine structure: each disease involving the hands will have specific findings for each subheading of the structure.

Although occasionally limited to the hands, musculoskeletal diseases are often more widespread, affecting other joints or organs. The patient's attitude or posture, and the environment around them (walking aids, orthotics and medication), will give you clues as to what you might expect to find when examining their hands, as will their gait as they walk into the consulting room in routine clinical practice.

Hand examination

Key point
A quick look at the hands and the pattern of joint involvement will often give a 'spot diagnosis', targeting what else to look for on closer examination.

Figs 23–27 show the five main hand diagnoses likely to be seen (including systemic sclerosis).

Look systematically for the features shown in Table 17.

If asked to do so by the examiner, be prepared to examine other sites or systems relevant to the case.

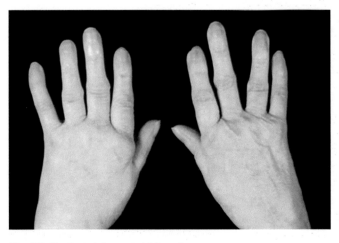

Fig 23 Typical rheumatoid hands.

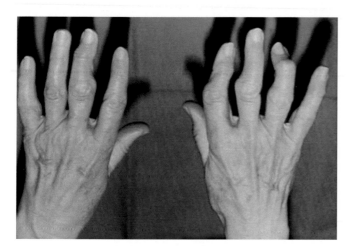

Fig 24 Classic nodal osteoarthritis.

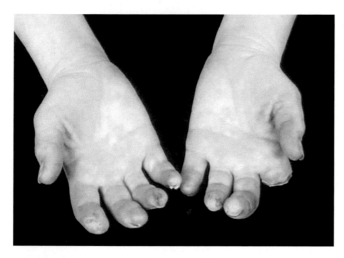

Fig 25 Severe digital ischaemia leading to multiple autoamputations in a patient with diffuse cutaneous systemic sclerosis.

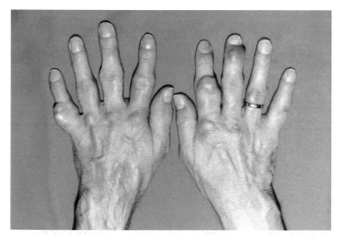

Fig 26 Tophaceous gout in the hands of an older woman on diuretics.

1.3.2 Hand osteoarthritis

Scenario

Mrs Lancaster, a 54-year-old woman, presented to a rheumatology outpatient clinic with a history of worsening pain and swelling of numerous joints in both hands (see Fig 24) What is the likely diagnosis?

Introduction

Swelling and pain of the small joints of the hand are a common presentation. There is a wide differential diagnosis for these symptoms that spans both inflammatory and non-inflammatory causes. Swelling can be a consequence of synovitis of the joint capsule or can be bony in nature due to osteophytes that typify nodal osteoarthritis. Swelling and pain may also arise from outside the synovial-lined joint capsule due to inflammation of the tendon and tendon sheaths.

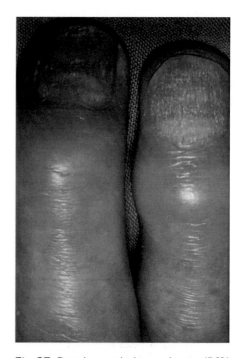

Fig 27 Distal interphalangeal joint (DIP) and nail involvement in psoriatic arthropathy. (Courtesy of Dr M Pattrick.)

Table 17	Features to look for systematically in a routine hand examination	

Tissue	Note	Comment
Skin and subcutaneous tissues	Texture	Eg waxy and thin/bruised
	Rashes	
	Digital ulcers and fissuring	
	Scars	
	Subcutaneous lumps: nodules/tophi/calcinosis	
Nails	Nail disease	Eg pitting and onycholysis
	Nailfold infarcts	
	Capillary loops	
Muscles and tendons	Wasting	
	Rupture	
Joints (look, feel and move only *after* ensuring there is no pain)	Pattern of joints involved (Table 18)	MCP/PIP/DIP/first CMC 'Row' or 'ray' distribution?
Deformity	Symmetry	
	Subluxation	
	Angulation	
Swelling	Inflammatory/non-inflammatory	Firm or soft? Tenderness
	Site, origin and extent of swelling	
	Function	Ability to make a fist Power grip Pinch grip
Sensation	Evidence of carpal tunnel syndrome / ulnar neuropathy / peripheral neuropathy / cervical spine disease	

CMC, carpometacarpal joint; DIP, distal interphalangeal joint; MCP, metacarpophalangeal joint; PIP, proximal interphalangeal joint.

Key point

The most common disorders that cause symmetrical, painful and swollen joints are osteoarthritis and rheumatoid arthritis.

Beginning the encounter

Doctor: hello, my name is Dr A, I understand that you have been suffering from painful and swollen hands?

Patient: yes, I've been having pain and swelling for the past few months.

Doctor: before we get into the details of that, can you tell me if you have any major medical problems? Any problems with psoriasis or inflammatory bowel disease?

Patient: [gives list (with the doctor politely but firmly discouraging lengthy detail).]

Doctor: and are you on any tablets or medications?

Patient: [gives details (and will probably have been asked to produce a written list).]

These introductory questions will provide useful clinical context and may immediately give a clue to the likely diagnosis, eg any drugs that could cause hyperuricemia, or a history of diseases that are associated with inflammatory arthritides.

Focused history

Doctor: can you tell me more about your hand pain and swelling?

Table 18	Pattern of joint involvement in various conditions affecting the hands		
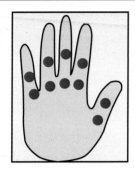	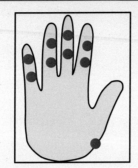	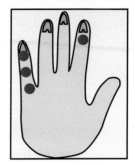	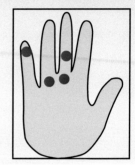
Rheumatoid arthritis	**Osteoarthritis**	**Psoriatic arthritis**	**Gout**
Row distribution MCPs and PIPs	Row distribution PIPs and DIPs First CMC	Ray distribution DIPs next to dystrophic nails	Asymmetrical

Patient: *it's worse soon after getting up in the morning, and I'm having great difficulty with opening lids and unscrewing bottle tops.*

It is important to determine if the joint pain is inflammatory or non-inflammatory. Inflammatory joint symptoms are worse in the morning and are associated with stiffness for at least 30 minutes. The pain and stiffness eases with use and worsens with rest. Non-inflammatory joint symptoms, typically, are worse with use and if early morning stiffness is present, it does not last long. Inflammatory joint pain has a more rapid onset, overnight for gout, weeks to months for rheumatoid arthritis, whereas the onset for non-inflammatory pain is over months to years.

Doctor: how are these symptoms affecting your daily life?

Patient: *they're causing me great difficulty in carrying out day-to-day tasks ranging from preparing and eating meals to carrying shopping bags.*

It is important to determine the extent of disability as this will influence treatment decisions.

Specific questions about symptoms that would be helpful in this case are:

> Are your hands stiff when you wake and, if so, how long before the stiffness eases?

> Are your hands worse in the morning or the evening?

> Are your hands worse with use or rest?

> Have you ever suffered from gout?

> Have you or any member of your immediate family suffered from psoriasis, inflammatory bowel disease or inflammatory arthritis?

Focused examination

General – look for the following:

> walking aids or splints (particularly carpometacarpal) – are any visible?

> signs of other joint involvement – eg varus/valgus knee deformities, knee brace, knee effusion, quadriceps wasting or any scars of joint replacement surgery.

> gait – if you have the opportunity to see the patient walk, then does she have a Trendelenburg (waddling) gait?

Hands – look systematically for the following features:

> Skin and subcutaneous tissues

> > depigmentation from intra-articular steroid injections to first carpometacarpal joints (CMCs)

> Joints

> > pattern of joints involved: distal interphalangeal (DIP)/proximal interphalangeal (PIP)/first CMC

> deformity: palmar and/or lateral deviation of distal phalanx; squaring of the thumb

> Swelling – look for the following:

> > firm bony swelling, limited to joints

> > Heberden's nodes in DIPs

> > Bouchard's nodes in PIPs. Early nodes may be tender, but usually pain-free once established.

> Function: the patient's ability to make a fist may be impaired. Their power grip may also be reduced.

Questions from the patient

[On the assumption that the likely diagnosis is primary generalised osteoarthritis:]

Patient: *my hands are very painful. Is there anything that would help?*

Doctor: for osteoarthritic pain, treatment is symptomatic. First, we would suggest trying simple painkillers like paracetamol. If this isn't enough, then the next step would be to consider anti-inflammatory drugs, which can be applied as a gel or cream directly on your hands, or taken by mouth instead. For bothersome joints, we can try localised injections of steroid which can provide relief for months and can be repeated. If your pain is limiting your ability to do specific functions, an assessment by an occupational therapist may help.

Questions from the examiner

Examiner: how do you differentiate between inflammatory and non-inflammatory joint pain?

Doctor: inflammatory arthritis is typically associated with stiffness more than pain. The presence and duration of early morning stiffness will help to distinguish between inflammatory and non-inflammatory joint pain: early morning stiffness for more than 30 minutes is typical of inflammatory arthritis. Synovitis is the hallmark of inflammatory arthritis and swollen, boggy joints will be found on examination, whereas swelling in non-inflammatory arthritis is bony and due to osteophytes.

Examiner: which joints are most affected in primary generalised osteoarthritis?

Doctor: the typical distribution involves the PIP, DIP and first CMC joints.

Examiner: if there was MCP (metacarpophalangeal joint) involvement, what might you think of?

Doctor: this is common in rheumatoid arthritis, but it can also occur in haemochromatosis.

Examiner: supposing the diagnosis was haemochromatosis and you did an X-ray of the hand, what might you see?

Doctor: chondrocalcinosis – this can be seen in the triangular fibrocartilage complex of the wrist on plain X-rays.

Further discussion

Bony erosions are the X-ray changes that typify the inflammatory arthritides, but these will not be present if the history of arthritis is short. In such cases, if there is difficulty in determining the presence or absence of inflammatory arthritis clinically, ultrasonography can be helpful as it can identify synovial inflammation and can also detect bony

erosions and the presence of crystals, as well as inflammatory involvement of tendons.

Consider examining for secondary causes of non-inflammatory degenerative arthropathies (see Section 2.3.2), especially if there is evidence of osteoarthritis in atypical joints.

1.3.3 Rheumatoid arthritis

Scenario

Mrs Taylor, a 27-year-old business manager, presented to the rheumatology clinic with painful and stiff hands and swollen fingers, which had developed over a number of weeks and started to affect her activities of daily living. What is the most likely diagnosis?

Introduction

Joint pain and stiffness in a young person is suggestive of inflammatory arthritis, with rheumatoid arthritis (RA) being the commonest cause of persistent arthritis (affecting 1% of the population worldwide).

The differential diagnosis of polyarthritis includes:

> RA

> psoriatic arthritis

> post-infectious arthritis (eg post-viral or post-streptococcal)

> systemic lupus erythematosus (SLE)

> (rarely) vasculitis.

The history must efficiently do three things:

> confirm an inflammatory rather than a biomechanical aetiology

> determine the functional impact on the patient, and

> identify the risk factors for, or symptoms suggestive of, a particular arthritis to generate the most likely diagnosis.

Beginning the encounter

Doctor: hello, my name is Dr A. I understand your hands have become uncomfortable, is that right?

Doctor: before we get into the details of that, can you tell me if you have any major medical problems? Any problems with psoriasis or inflammatory bowel disease?

Patient: [gives list (with the doctor politely but firmly discouraging lengthy detail).]

Doctor: and are you on any tablets or medications?

Patient: [gives details (and will probably have been asked to produce a written list).]

Now moving onto the problem with the hands ...

Patient: [gives details, offering an inflammatory story of early morning pain, soft tissue swelling and stiffness.]

Doctor: how long does it take for your hands to improve in the morning?

Patient: I tend to feel better after 1 hour [>1 hour symptoms is part of the classification criteria for the diagnosis of RA].

Doctor: what sort of things can't you do?

Patient: [lists impact on activities of daily living (ADLs). (It is crucial to pursue the emotional impact and effect on work and/or caring responsibilities.)]

Doctor: are your feet or any other joints affected too?

Patient: [lists involved areas.]

These first few questions will indicate whether the pain is inflammatory, and whether it is a polyarthritis, oligoarthritis or monoarthritis, which will help you rank the most likely diagnoses. It will also help gauge the severity of disease.

Focused history

Doctor: have you been well in the run up to this? Or has anyone in the family suffered with something similar? Have you taken any tablets for it?

These questions may give a clue to the diagnosis (eg clear history of streptococcal throat beforehand, or a strong family history of RA). In theory, NSAIDS should be more effective in inflammatory joint pain than standard analgesia such as paracetamol.

Doctor: is it both hands? Which bits exactly?

RA is characteristically symmetrical and affects wrists and metacarpophalangeal joints (MCPs) most commonly. Other patterns of joint disease are listed below.

Specific features suggesting RA:

> symmetrical, with predilection for wrists and MCPs; proximal interphalangeal joints (PIPs) also involved, but distal interphalangeal joints (DIPs) characteristically spared

> family history of RA

> smoker.

Psoriatic arthritis is associated with:

> personal or family history of psoriasis

> nail abnormalities (pits, ridges, onycholysis)

> dactylitis (involvement of whole digit – 'sausage' finger or toe)

> history of tendinopathy or plantar fasciitis.

Do a quick screen for SLE:

> history of oral ulcers?

> unusual skin reactions to sunlight or other rashes?

> episodes of pleuropericarditis?

> alopecia and Raynaud's phenomenon are not very specific, but lend weight to the diagnosis if seen in this context.

Focused examination

General – note the following, but bear in mind that many of these features will not be present at first presentation:

> Is the patient wearing any aids: soft collar, wrist splints or orthotic shoes?

> Is there scleritis, episcleritis or nodular eye disease?

> Is there generalised or focal muscle wasting?

> Is there evidence of chronic steroid use: thin skin, bruising and kyphosis?

> What other joints appear affected from the end of the bed: is there fixed flexion of the elbows, knee swelling or foot deformities?

Look around the patient's chair or bed for walking aids, soft collar and orthotic shoes (and if the shoes are off, look for insoles).

Hand – look systematically for the following features:

> Skin and subcutaneous tissues:

> > rheumatoid nodules

> > thin fragile skin, reflecting long-term steroid use

> > surgical scars:

> > > MCP joint replacement

> > > removal of ulnar styloid and/or extensor tendon repair

> > > wrist fusion

> > > carpal tunnel release

> Nails:

> > nailfold vasculitis

> Muscles/tendons:

> > thenar eminence wasting – carpal tunnel syndrome

> > tenosynovitis

> > tendon rupture (inability to extend fingers)

> Joints:

> > pattern of joints involved – MCPs, PIPs and wrists

> > deformity – usually symmetrical (Fig 23):

> > > MCP subluxation

> > > ulnar deviation

> > > swan-neck, Boutonniere and Z-deformity of the thumb

> Swelling – is the disease active or not? The presence of tenderness and swelling would indicate that it is active, but be careful to ensure that the patient is not in pain when palpating joints – look at their face at all times, not just at their hands. And remember where the MCP joint line is – distal to the metacarpal heads (Fig 28).

> Function – the pinch grip is often modified, using the lateral border rather than the tip of thumb/index finger.

> Sensation – carpal tunnel syndrome.

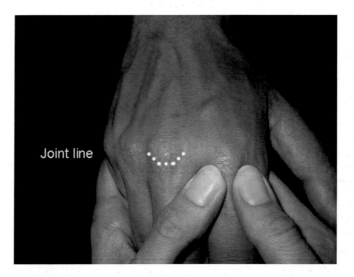

Fig 28 Surface markings and examination of the MCP joint.

System	Clinical feature
Eye	Episcleritis, scleritis, keratoconjunctivitis sicca and scleromalacia perforans (see Fig 29)
Skin	Rheumatoid nodules, vasculitis, palmar erythema and pyoderma gangrenosum
Haematological	Anaemia, splenomegaly, Felty's syndrome, lymphadenopathy and cryoglobulinaemia
Respiratory	Pleurisy with effusion, pulmonary fibrosis and Caplan's syndrome
Cardiovascular	Raynaud's phenomenon, pericarditis, myocarditis, cardiac nodules and mitral valve disease
Neurological	Carpal tunnel syndrome, peripheral neuropathy, mononeuritis multiplex and cervical myelopathy

Table 19 Non-articular manifestations of RA

Other relevant examination – if given the opportunity to extend your examination beyond the hand, then look for:

> other affected joints
> extra-articular manifestations of RA (see Table 19 and Section 2.3.3):
>> nodules
>> vasculitis
>> inflammatory/nodular eye disease
>> lung disease (interstitial lung disease, pleural effusions and bronchiectasis)
>> ischaemic heart disease (coronary artery bypass grafting and peripheral vein harvesting)
>> anaemia
> side effects of treatment:
>> steroids – osteoporosis, thin skin/bruising and Cushingoid appearance
>> anaemia.

Questions from the patient

[On the assumption that the likely diagnosis is rheumatoid arthritis:]

Patient: what's wrong with me?

Doctor: from what you're telling me, and from what I can see in your hands, there's no doubt that you have active inflammation in the joints in your hands, so I'm not surprised that they're sore and stiff. We'll need to do some blood tests and X-rays to confirm exactly what type of inflammation it is, but I suspect that this is rheumatoid arthritis.

Patient: what's the treatment?

Doctor: if, as I suspect, this is rheumatoid arthritis, then you will be on medication long term to make you feel better and try to avoid any damage to your joints.

Questions from the examiner

Examiner: what are the key features of inflammatory joint pain?

Doctor: early morning exacerbations of pain, stiffness and swelling; the swelling is soft tissue, ie synovitis, rather than the bony swelling of osteoarthritis (OA); inflammatory disease is often accompanied by constitutional upset of malaise or fatigue.

Examiner: what investigations would you request?

Doctor: I would order investigations that to confirm the diagnosis and assess disease severity. For diagnosis I would like an autoantibody screen in the form of RhF, CCP and ANA; I would also request X-rays of the hands and feet looking for erosions, and a chest X-ray to rule out lung involvement. In terms of disease activity assessment, I would like to know the CRP/ESR [as these contribute to the disease activity score (DAS) – see Section 2.3.3 on rheumatoid arthritis]. I would also request an FBC to look for anaemia of chronic disease and thrombocytosis, plus kidney and liver biochemistry prior to starting disease-modifying antirheumatic drugs (DMARDs).

Examiner: assuming she's a new seropositive RA patient, what would you do?

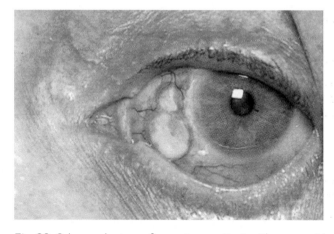

Fig 29 Scleromalacia perforans in a patient with seropositive RA. (Reproduced with permission from Dieppe PA, Kirwan J, Cooper C. *Arthritis and rheumatism in practice.* London: Gower Medical Publishing, 1991.)

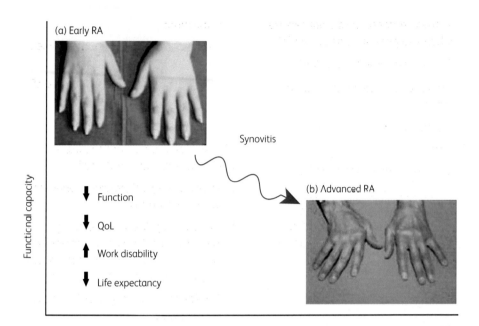

(a) Early RA

Functional capacity

Synovitis

↓ Function

↓ QoL

↑ Work disability

↓ Life expectancy

(b) Advanced RA

Time

Fig 30 **(a)** Early RA with synovitis but no deformities. **(b)** Established RA with characteristic deformities. QoL, quality of life.

Doctor: the approach to RA management is multidisciplinary. I would refer them to a clinical nurse specialist, occupational therapist and physiotherapist for patient education and support. In terms of medical management, I would give them a depot steroid injection 120 mg intramuscular (IM) to kick-start their treatment and start them on combination DMARD therapy in the form of methotrexate and hydroxychloroquine. The exception to this would be if the patient were planning a family.

Examiner: *which DMARDs are contraindicated in pregnancy?*

Doctor: methotrexate and leflunomide.

Further discussion

Patients with early disease, or well-controlled disease, may have none of the classic deformities of RA and may simply have wrist and MCP synovitis, leading to spindle-shaped fingers. This contrasts with established disease, in which bony deformities may be pronounced (see Fig 30a and b).

There is compelling evidence demonstrating that patients with RA have a better outcome with early diagnosis and swift treatment with combination DMARD therapy. They need close support at the point of diagnosis, and frequent assessment of disease activity, altering treatment to meet the agreed target (usually remission). Close liaison is needed between primary and secondary care, and many of the DMARDs need regular blood tests to monitor for bone marrow suppression and transaminitis. The psychosocial impact of RA is often underestimated and some patients go on to develop coexistent depression and/or fibromyalgia.

Key point

RA is the commonest form of small joint polyarthropathy. The most salient risk factors are smoking and a family history. Always explore the impact on work and relationships, and be sure to check on plans for starting a family which may have implications for drug treatment.

1.3.4 Psoriatic arthritis

Scenario

Mr Johnson, a 52-year-old pilot with a history of psoriasis, presented to the rheumatology department with a painful swollen knee and ankle. The pain has only partially responded to anti-inflammatories. What is the likely diagnosis, and how should he be managed?

Introduction

Of patients with a diagnosis of psoriasis, 10–15% develop inflammatory joint symptoms, which can occur independently of both the timing and the severity of the skin disease. In some individuals there may be no rash apparent, but on close questioning there is a family history of psoriasis.

Key point

Psoriatic arthritis can cause almost any pattern of disease:

> rheumatoid arthritis (RA)-like pattern in the hands (ie wrists and metacarpophalangeal joints (MCP) / proximal interphalangeal joints (PIP) predominant disease)

> osteoarthritis (OA)-like pattern in the hands (ie predominantly PIP/distal interphalangeal joints (DIP) disease)

> monoarthritis or oligoarthritis

> spondyloarthritis

> arthritis mutilans.

Beginning the encounter

Doctor: hello, my name is Dr A, I understand you have psoriasis but recently your knee and ankle have become sore. Is that right?

Doctor: before we get into the details of that, can you tell me if you have any major medical problems?

Patient: [gives list (with doctor politely but firmly discouraging lengthy detail).]

Doctor: and are you on any tablets or medications?

Patient: [gives details (and will probably have been asked to produce a written list).]

Now moving onto the problem with the joints …

Patient: [gives details of classic rash or treatment for psoriasis, and new history of inflammatory oligoarthritis.]

Doctor: when is it worst and what does it stop you doing?

Patient: [gives details.]

Focused history

Doctor: are your nails ok? Have you ever had swelling of a whole finger or toe? Is there any pain in the sole of your foot or your heels when you walk, especially first thing in the morning? Do you have back or buttock pain?

The main priority is to differentiate psoriatic arthritis from another form of inflammatory arthritis in a patient with coexistent psoriasis. Key features to elicit that would point to a diagnosis of psoriatic arthritis would include:

> presence of nail disease (pitting, ridging, onycholysis)

> history of dactylitis

> features of tendinopathy, plantar fasciitis, enthesitis.

Focused examination

General features – note the following:

> Is there any psoriasis visible on the scalp/elsewhere?

> Is the patient tanned from psoralen ultraviolet A treatment?

> Are any topical treatments obvious on the skin?

> Is there suggestion of axial disease when the patient turns or bends?

> Is there ocular inflammation?

> Are functional aids / orthotics in evidence?

Hand examination – look for the following:

> Skin and subcutaneous tissues:

> > psoriatic plaques – check elbows, scalp/hairline (and if further examination is permitted later on in the station, the umbilicus or natal cleft)

> Nails – pitting, onycholysis, hypergryposis and dystrophy

> Joints:

> > pattern of joints involved:

> > > psoriatic arthritis more commonly affects 'rays', ie DIP, PIP and MCP of one digit, rather than 'rows', ie all MCPs (use Table 18)

> > > is there one of these five classical patterns (Moll and Wright classification)?

> > > > DIP involvement

> > > > rheumatoid-like pattern

> > > > asymmetrical oligoarthritis

> > > > axial disease

> > > > arthritis mutilans

> > deformity:

> > > rheumatoid-like pattern clinically indistinguishable from RA

> > > digital telescoping, subluxation and 'flail' joints in arthritis mutilans

> > swelling:

> > > differentiate soft tissue swelling from firm bony swelling of Heberden's nodes in OA

> > > DIP swelling of psoriatic arthritis is often associated with nail changes at that adjacent nail

> > > tenosynovitis along a digit may present as dactylitis (more common in the feet)

> function:

> > pinch/grip is often weak if index DIP is involved.

> > function is very poor in cases of arthritis mutilans.

Questions from the patient

[On the assumption that the likely diagnosis is psoriatic arthritis:]

Patient: is the joint problem connected with my psoriasis?

Doctor: yes, I think it is. We always need to consider whether or not two medical problems are connected, but in your case I think that they are.

Patient: will my joints get better if my skin improves?

Doctor: not necessarily, we have patients with arthritis who have very mild skin involvement. But the good news is that many of our treatments work well for both the joints and the skin at the same time.

Patient: can I have some steroid tablets? Steroids work very well on my skin.

Doctor: we do need to consider using steroids, either as tablets or as an intramuscular injection, but it's always a matter of balancing benefits and risks, so this is something I'd like to talk about with a rheumatology specialist (psoriasis can flare badly as the effects of intramuscular steroid wear off).

Questions from the examiner

Examiner: would you expect this patient to be seropositive or negative?

Doctor: classically they should be seronegative for RhF (rheumatoid factor); a small proportion might be positive for CCP (cyclic citrullinated peptide).

Examiner: which disease-modifying antirheumatic drug (DMARD) would you suggest?

Doctor: methotrexate, sulfasalazine and leflunomide are all used in psoriatic arthritis.

Examiner: *is there any pattern of disease that doesn't respond so well to standard DMARD?*

Doctor: yes, spondyloarthritis tends not to respond as well as peripheral arthritis to standard DMARDs – the best therapeutic option in that case is anti-tumour necrosis factor alpha (TNF-α).

Examiner: *what other inflammatory arthritis can be provoked by severe psoriasis?*

Doctor: gout (due to purine load from high skin turnover rate).

Further discussion

The classic X-ray features of psoriatic arthritis are subtly different to RA. True psoriatic arthritis may demonstrate:

> relative paucity of periarticular osteopaenia

> ankylosis

> whittling of the terminal phalanges

> pencil-in-cup deformities.

It is also worth remembering that the acute phase response is less pronounced in psoriatic arthritis compared with RA. Psoriatic arthritis occurs in a few patients with Crohn's disease. The latter association is interesting in view of the overlap in genetic control of inflammation in both disorders and the therapeutic benefit of anti-TNF-α treatment in both psoriatic arthritis and Crohn's disease.

Key point

The most important outcome from the history and examination is to establish whether the patient has psoriatic arthritis or another inflammatory arthritis on the background of psoriasis. Key features pointing towards psoriatic arthritis would include dactylitis, prominent inflammatory DIP disease and nail involvement.

1.3.5 Systemic sclerosis

Scenario

Miss Rose, a 33-year-old woman, presented to the rheumatology clinic with deterioration in her long-standing Raynaud's phenomenon and skin changes. What is the likely diagnosis?

Introduction

Idiopathic Raynaud's phenomenon is common, primarily affecting young women from puberty. In 10–15% of cases it is associated with a connective tissue disease, most commonly systemic lupus erythematosus (SLE) or systemic sclerosis (scleroderma). Features in the history that might point to an underlying condition would include a late onset or recent deterioration/worsening of pre-existent Raynaud's.

Systemic sclerosis is characterised by tightening and thickening of the skin, and can be divided clinically according to the extent of the skin changes (and thereafter serologically with differing autoantibody profiles). Internal organ involvement is variable, with pulmonary hypertension and renal crisis being the most feared complications.

Beginning the encounter

Doctor: hello, I'm Dr A. I understand you've had Raynaud's phenomenon for some time but things have changed of late, is that right?

Doctor: before we get into the details of that, can you tell me if you have any major medical problems?

Patient: [gives list (with doctor politely but firmly discouraging lengthy detail).]

Doctor: and are you on any tablets or medications?

Patient: [gives details (and will probably have been asked to produce a written list).]

Now moving onto the problem with the hands …

Patient: [gives details about change in the severity or frequency of attacks (if not volunteered, doctor should ask about skin integrity or development of ulcers).]

Doctor: and you feel that your skin has changed too, can you tell me about that? Where have you noticed it's a problem?

Patient: [gives details, which may point to a subtype of systemic sclerosis (diffuse versus limited).]

Focused history

Doctor: have you noticed any other changes at all? Do you have any trouble swallowing for example? Or shortness of breath?

Once the possibility of scleroderma is raised, the purpose of the remainder of the history should be centred on establishing the extent of disease (ie diffuse versus limited), and the severity of any internal organ involvement, although some complications of systemic sclerosis may be clinically occult and require investigations to identify/quantify.

Key point

In limited cutaneous systemic sclerosis (LCSSc) the skin changes of scleroderma and sclerodactyly typically end at the elbow; in diffuse cutaneous systemic sclerosis (DCSSc) the skin manifestations are more severe and extensive, progressing above the elbow and across the face.

Questions to screen for internal organ involvement would include looking for gastrointestinal and pulmonary involvement:

> Have you had any problems with swallowing?

> Have you had any diarrhoea or faecal incontinence?

> Have you become short of breath or lost exercise tolerance?

Focused examination

General features – aim to differentiate between primary and secondary Raynaud's by looking for evidence of diseases associated with the latter, in particular systemic sclerosis. Check:

> the patient's face – for telangiectasia, microstomia and 'beaked' nose

> the patient's respiratory system – is the patient short of breath or cyanosed?

> the patient's gastrointestinal system – is there evidence of long-term intravenous access for parenteral feeding?

> for collateral clues – look around for gloves (if so, are they heated?); parenteral nutrition bags; and medication (particularly ambulatory iloprost for pulmonary hypertension).

Hand examination – check the following:

> Skin and subcutaneous tissues:

> sclerodactyly – take note of:

> tight, shiny and waxy skin

> assess the extent of its involvement by working from distal phalanges, proximally. If sclerodactyly is limited to distal limbs (ie below elbows and knees), then this is suggestive of LCSSc; if the spread is more proximal, then it is suggestive of DCSSc

> digital ischaemia (worse in LCSSc), is indicated by:

> digital ulceration or digital pitting (healed ulcers) at finger pulps. Also look for distal interphalangeal and proximal interphalangeal joint involvement, and examine for signs of infection

> digital pulp atrophy

> gangrene

> autoamputations

> Raynaud's

> calcinosis – more prominent in LCSSc

> telangiectasia

> Fingernails:

> increased curvature of nails can be seen, secondary to the resorption of distal phalanges

> dilated tortuous nailfold capillaries are suggestive of connective tissue disease as a cause of secondary Raynaud's. These are best appreciated by examination with ×20 magnification using an ophthalmoscope (see Fig 16) – but use of this would not be expected in PACES (and indeed most examiners would regard it as eccentric, which would be a bad thing).

> Muscles/tendons. The involvement of these is more common in DCSSc; check for:

> friction rubs in active disease

> contractures.

> Joints – the problems this patient has with her hands may be associated with inflammatory arthritis.

> Function – find out of the patient has an:

> impaired ability to make a fist – assess fingertip to palmar crease distance

> impaired pinch grip secondary to sclerodactyly and pain of digital ulceration.

Cardiovascular and respiratory – check blood pressure and look for signs of pulmonary hypertension (elevated jugular venous pressure (JVP), loud second heart sound, parasternal heave, evidence of peripheral oedema); in DCSSc pulmonary fibrosis may be audible; LCSSc is driven by vasculopathy, so auscultation may be normal.

Questions from patient

[On the assumption that the likely diagnosis is DCSSc:]

Patient: isn't this just a problem with my Raynaud's?

Doctor: I understand why you say that, but from what you've told me and what I find when I examine you, I think that something else is going on. We need to do some more tests to find out for sure.

Patient: what do you think it might be?

Doctor: I think it's most likely to be due to a condition called scleroderma, and we need to do some tests to find out, and – if it is scleroderma – work out which sort of scleroderma it is.

Patient: can you treat it?

Doctor: there are lots of options for treating Raynaud's phenomenon, but if, as I suspect, this is being driven by another condition called systemic sclerosis, there's no single treatment that will deal with that – so we need to see what problems the systemic sclerosis is causing, and deal with each of them when or if they arise.

Questions from examiner

Examiner: how would you investigate?

Doctor: the purpose of further investigations is to confirm the diagnosis and subtype of scleroderma and to identify/quantify the extent of internal organ involvement. I would begin investigation by requesting an antinuclear antibody (ANA) (plus anti-centromere and anti-SCL70 antibodies), performing an echocardiogram and spirometry to look for the development of pulmonary hypertension and restrictive lung disease, and assessing renal function.

Examiner: what other conditions are associated with Raynaud's phenomenon?

Doctor: Systemic lupus erythematosus (SLE) would also feature in the differential diagnosis, but this would be characterised by non-erosive arthralgia, photosensitive rashes, oral ulcers and a history of serositis. These patients would also have a positive ANA result, but a different pattern of extractable nuclear antigens (such as double-stranded DNA and Sm).

Further discussion

In secondary Raynaud's disease vasospasm can be severe, leading to ulceration and even autoamputation (see Section 1.1.9 for a discussion of the investigation and management of patients presenting with Raynaud's phenomenon).

Key point

In a patient presenting with Raynaud's phenomenon, the crucial components of the history are to determine the severity of attacks and whether there is an underlying connective tissue disease. Focus on recent changes/deterioration and features that might point to systemic sclerosis or SLE.

1.3.6 Chronic tophaceous gout

Scenario

Mr Jones, a 64-year-old publican with hypertension and renal disease, presented with a long history of pains in his hands, knees, ankles and feet. What is the likely diagnosis?

Introduction

Gout is common, and the cardinal acute inflammatory monoarthropathy. Classic attacks affect the first MTP (podagra), often in the early hours, so this is worth pursuing in the history. Patients with recurrent attacks and persistent hyperuricaemia may develop a polyarthritis with tophi, with symptoms becoming more constant than episodic.

Risk factors to prompt considerations of gout include high alcohol intake, renal disease, medications that predispose to hyperuricaemia (thiazides specifically), obesity and/or metabolic syndromes and psoriasis.

Tophi appear as pea-sized lumps beneath the skin, often on extensor surfaces. Urate crystals collections can frequently be seen just beneath the skin surface; they can produce a brisk inflammatory response (essentially a chemical cellulitis), provoking concerns about superadded infection. Gouty tophi can also erode through the skin and discharge. Tophi may also be apparent on the pinnae of the ears.

Beginning the encounter

Doctor: hello my name is Dr A. I understand you've had problems in your joints for some time now, is that correct?

Doctor: before we get into the details of that, can you tell me if you have any major medical problems? The information I've been given says you have some sort of kidney disease – tell me a bit about that.

Patient: [gives list (with doctor politely but firmly discouraging lengthy detail).]

Doctor: and are you on any tablets or medications? I'm told that you have high blood pressure: are you on anything for that?

Patient: [gives details (and will probably have been asked to produce a written list).]

Now moving onto the problem with the joints …

Doctor: how did this all start, and what's happened since?

Patient: [gives details, often with original monoarthritic attacks as a prelude to more persistent disease.]

Focused history

The remainder of the history should be centred on identifying modifiable risk factors and the patient's experiences of urate-lowering therapeutics. The main risk factors include:

> diet rich in red meat and shellfish

> excess alcohol

> family history of gout

> renal disease of any cause

> psoriasis.

In the past, chemotherapy frequently precipitated attacks of gout as part of the tumour lysis syndrome, but the incidence of this has fallen with the use of prophylactic urate-lowering medication (especially uricase).

Acute attacks of gout (and even chronic disease can have intermittent flares) are managed with NSAIDs, colchicine or steroids, so focus on what has been tried before, and with what outcome.

For chronic disease, allopurinol remains first-line treatment. It can be poorly tolerated if introduced too swiftly and this may become apparent in the history. Allopurinol use is relatively contraindicated in renal disease, which can make management complex.

Focused examination

General features – look for the stigmata of risk factors for gout:

> excess alcohol consumption – ruddy face, palmar erythema and spider naevi

> psoriasis

> obesity.

Footwear – note any special features, eg over-size shoes, incisions over first metatarsophalangeal joints (MTPs), or if they are wearing sandals on a cold day.

Hand examination – check the following:

> Skin and subcutaneous tissues.

>> Subcutaneous tophi – these may be confused with rheumatoid nodules, so look for pale, chalky and subcutaneous lumps; also check for signs of discharge of material of a toothpaste-like consistency. It is also important to note the sites of tophi in the hands, which can include:

>>> around any finger joints, sometimes extending beyond the joints to resemble dactylitis of psoriatic arthritis or reactive arthritis

>>> finger pulps

>>> dorsal or palmar side of the hand

>>>> overlying Heberden's or Bouchard's nodes, particularly in women with gout.

>> Oedema – acute gout is often accompanied by pitting oedema extending well beyond the involved joint.

>> Cutaneous exfoliation can sometimes be seen upon the resolution of an acute attack.

> Joints.

>> Pattern of joints involved – metacarpophalangeal / proximal interphalangeal / distal interphalangeal.

>> Deformity, but note that there is no characteristic pattern of deformity. Patients may develop the swan-neck, boutonniere and flexion deformities seen in rheumatoid arthritis (RA).

>> Swellings – in acute gout there is usually marked erythema: the joints feel hot and they are 'exquisitely' tender.

>> Function – this will be dependent upon the extent of the disease.

> Sensation – check for wrist involvement, or tophi within flexor tendons of the hand and wrist (this is rare), which may cause carpal tunnel syndrome.

Other examination – if you are given the opportunity to extend your examination beyond the hand, then look at/for:

> elbows:

>> olecranon bursae – these are often chronically swollen and may have acute bursitis

>> tophi over elbow / within bursae

> gouty tophi at other sites, particularly:

>> pinnae of the ears

>> first MTPs

>> Achilles tendons

>> prepatellar bursae

> other affected joints: first MTPs, knees and ankles.

> **! Hazard**
> There is no characteristic pattern of deformity in gouty arthritis of the hands. Patients may develop the swan-neck, boutonniere and flexion deformities seen in RA.

Questions from the patient

[On the assumption that the likely diagnosis is chronic tophaceous gout:]

Patient: is there any way we can get rid of these lumps?

Doctor: no, I'm afraid that there isn't … once you've developed lumps, called tophi, like this, then they can be very hard to shift, but we must try to lower your urate level – the thing that causes the lumps – anyway to prevent attacks of arthritis and it's possible that they may improve a bit.

Patient: but my other doctor tried that and it made the arthritis worse, so I stopped taking the tablets. Are you trying a different drug?

Doctor: not necessarily. We can use the same drug in a different way. We'll start at a lower dose, with some anti-inflammatory cover to prevent flares, and increase the dose really slowly until we get to a level that suits you and keeps your urate in the bottom end of the normal range. You can also help the situation by trying to cut back on any alcohol as well, no matter how minimal the amount.

Questions from the examiner

Examiner: what's the mechanism of action of allopurinol?

Doctor: it's a xanthine oxidase inhibitor, which prevents the production of urate at the final stages of purine metabolism.

Examiner: in which patients would you not use allopurinol?

Doctor: I wouldn't use it if a patient had previously had a hypersensitivity reaction, especially Stevens–Johnson syndrome, and its use is relatively contraindicated in those with renal impairment.

Examiner: what is the alternative urate-lowering therapy for patients with renal impairment?

Doctor: febuxostat is another xanthine oxidase inhibitor, which is safer for use in those with reduced glomerular filtration rate (GFR).

Further discussion

In patients presenting with rheumatoid-like deformities in the hands and no tophi elsewhere, it may be difficult to differentiate between RA and gout.

Key point

Differentiating gout and RA

> Rheumatoid factor (RhF) – a negative RhF and lumps over the elbows usually means that the diagnosis is gout because rheumatoid nodules are associated only with seropositive disease.

> Synovial fluid analysis – negatively birefringent needle-shaped crystals indicate gout.

> Radiographs of the hand – erosions are typically periarticular in RA but juxta-articular in gout, with overhanging edges (see Section 2.3.6).

Note that the serum uric acid does *not* differentiate the two: it may be normal in gout or elevated in RA.

Gout is uncommon in young men and premenopausal women, and such cases are likely to be due to an enzyme defect in the purine pathway or a renal tubular defect.

1.3.7 Ankylosing spondylitis

Instruction

Mr Henderson, a 35-year-old man, presented to the rheumatology outpatients clinic with a history of back pain and stiffness. What is the likely diagnosis?

Introduction

Inflammation of the axial skeleton is a cardinal feature of ankylosing spondylitis. Typically this presents as inflammatory back pain, but given the prevalence of back pain in the general population, there is often a considerable delay in diagnosis.

Beginning the encounter

Doctor: hello, my name is Dr A, I understand that you have been suffering from back problems, is that right?

Doctor: before we get into the details of that, can you tell me if you have any major medical problems?

Patient: [gives list (with doctor politely but firmly discouraging lengthy detail).]

Doctor: and are you on any tablets or medications?

Patient: [gives details (and will probably have been asked to produce a written list).]

Focused history

Doctor: now moving onto the problem with your back pain …

The clinician first needs to establish the likelihood of inflammatory as opposed to mechanical back pain. There are certain features that are typically associated with inflammatory back pain and the subsequent focused questions should have this in mind.

Key point

Inflammatory back pain:

> is worse in the morning, with morning stiffness lasting more than half an hour

> may wake the patient in the latter half of the night

> is worse with rest and relieved by use

> is associated with alternating buttock pain

> is responsive to NSAIDs.

Other relevant history – the seronegative spondyloarthropathies have overlapping clinical features and questions should explore the presence of associated pathologies:

> Is there a personal or family history of psoriasis, inflammatory bowel disease or uveitis?

> Are there any rashes? Skin involvement in addition to psoriasis could include circinate balanitis and keratoderma blennorrhagica, which typify reactive arthritis.

> If this is an acute presentation, was it preceded by an infection? So is this a reactive arthritis?

> Is there any evidence of a peripheral arthritis or enthesitis?

Focused examination

General features – some patients with psoriasis will have a spondyloarthropathy, so look for plaques, especially in the scalp, behind the ears, around the umbilicus and in the natal cleft, as well as nail pitting and onycholysis.

Examination of the spine – follow the general principles of inspection, palpation and movement, remembering that it takes a number of years of disease before there is clinically detectable evidence of ankylosing spondylitis. An entirely normal examination is often found in early disease:

> Take a general overview, particularly looking at the shape of the spine. With the patient standing, inspect from the side and from behind. Is there a kyphosis and loss of lumbar lordosis – the typical features of the 'question mark' posture of ankylosing spondylitis?

> Assess movement – cervical spine flexion, extension, rotation and lateral flexion: is there any evidence of fusion?

> Measure the wall to occiput distance – an unaffected individual should be able to put their head against the wall. If they are unable to do so, it may because of fusion of their cervical spine or a thoracic kyphosis.

> Assess lumbar flexion – measure the finger to floor distance (ie the distance from the tips of the fingers to the floor) if a patient is unable to touch their toes.

> Measure their Schober's expansion, which is a more accurate way of determining if there is fusion of the lumbar vertebrae (see Fig 31) and should be from 15–≥20 cm.

> With the patient sitting on the couch, assess thoracic rotation to see if there is fusion.

> Measure chest expansion using a tape measure placed at approximately the level of the nipples: the expansion after inspiration should be ≥3 cm.

Questions from the patient

[On the assumption that the likely diagnosis is ankylosing spondylitis:]

Patient: I've heard that there is a genetic test for ankylosing spondylitis, can you tell me about it?

Doctor: there is a test that can help … it looks for a thing called the *HLA-B27* gene. If you've got it, then this increases the likelihood of ankylosing spondylitis, but it's also found in 10% of the population, so its presence is not diagnostic.

Patient: what treatments are available for back pain in ankylosing spondylitis?

Doctor: treatment initially includes simple analgesia and anti-inflammatory drugs. Physiotherapy is also helpful for the symptoms and to maintain spinal flexibility. If the back pain is severe and not responsive to these measures, either oral or intramuscular steroids can be used in the short term. Otherwise, biological agents including

anti-tumour necrosis factor alpha (TNF-α) medications can be used.

Questions from the examiner

Examiner: how would you investigate this patient?

Doctor: if the history was suggestive of inflammatory back pain and there was circumstantial evidence that would support a diagnosis of ankylosing spondylitis, then I would request imaging and check for elevated serum inflammatory markers such as CRP (C-reactive protein) or ESR (erythrocyte sedimentation rate), and also check for the presence of *HLA-B27*.

Examiner: what imaging would you request?

Doctor: depending on the duration of the symptoms, I would first request an X-ray of the sacroiliac joints. If this was unremarkable and I still suspected ankylosing spondylitis, then I would arrange an MRI of these joints.

Further discussion

The radiographic changes detectable by X-ray are a late sign in ankylosing spondylitis and are consequent to erosive disease. In early disease, inflammation is not detectable by X-rays, but MRI is able to detect early inflammatory lesions.

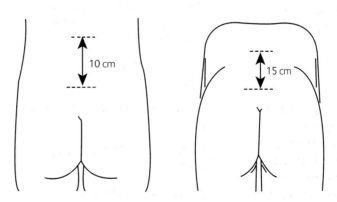

Fig 31 Schober's test to measure lumbar flexion.

1.3.8 Paget's disease of the bone

Instruction

Mr Naismith, a 76-year-old retired electrician, presented to rheumatology outpatients with recent onset bilateral thigh pain on background of a long-standing deformed and painful right tibia. What is the likely diagnosis?

Introduction

Paget's disease is a common disorder of bone that presents in older people and is characterised by focal areas of bone remodelling. It typically affects the spine, femur, tibia and pelvis and is often discovered incidentally on radiographs or due to an elevated alkaline phosphatase. It is often asymptomatic, but typically causes bone pain. It occurs in individuals of European ancestry with a likely genetic component. There is circumstantial evidence that supports a role for viral osteoclast infection in the pathogenesis of the disease.

Beginning the encounter

Doctor: hello, my name is Dr A, I understand that you have been suffering from thigh and leg pain, is that right?

Doctor: before we get into the details of that, can you tell me if you have any major medical problems?

Patient: [gives list (with doctor politely but firmly discouraging lengthy detail).]

Doctor: and are you on any tablets or medications?

Patient: [gives details (and will probably have been asked to produce a written list).]

Focused history

Doctor: now moving onto the problem with your legs …

The clinician first has to determine the cause of the tibial and thigh pain, and in Paget's disease (the obvious consideration here because of the information that the patient has long-standing deformity of the tibia), there are numerous causes to consider.

> Active osteolytic pagetic bone can cause localised pain that can be worse on weight-bearing, is present during the day, and is worse during the night.

> Osteoarthritic joints – the abnormal biomechanics from shortened and deformed bones can contribute to osteoarthritis of nearby joints.

> A sudden increase in swelling and pain of a pagetic bone may be due to an osteosarcoma, a rare complication of Paget's disease, or a fracture of the weakened pagetic bone.

> Neurogenic claudication – pagetic vertebral bodies can cause spinal stenosis and neurogenic claudication. Limb pain that arises after walking or standing that is worse on back extension and relieved by flexion would be suggestive of a spinal stenosis.

Focused examination

General features – look at the posture the patient adopts when standing: is there bowing of the tibia consistent with Paget's disease? Examine his gait. Look for enlargement of the skull and a hearing aid.

Examination of lower limbs – conduct as follows:

> Sit the patient on the couch with their legs straight: again look for any deformity – is there bowing and/or a fixed flexion deformity?

> Assess the patient's skin temperature – is this warm due to increased vascularity of active Paget's disease?

> Palpate the knee to look for tenderness and an effusion (patellar tap / bulge sign).

> Assess full flexion and extension of the knee.

> Ask the patient to flex his hip and test for abduction/adduction and internal and external rotation.

Questions from the patient

[On the assumption that the likely diagnosis is Paget's disease:]

Patient: *what is Paget's disease?*

Doctor: Paget's disease of the bone is a common disorder where abnormal bone is laid down in some areas of the skeleton. The abnormal bone is weak and can cause deformity to the bones and damage the joints.

Patient: *does Paget's disease always cause symptoms?*

Doctor: no, it doesn't … Paget's disease of the bone might not cause any symptoms and is sometimes found by chance when an X-ray or blood test is done. Otherwise, bone pain is the most frequent symptom. Increased blood flow to the abnormal bone may make the area feel warm. Bony enlargement can press on nerves in the spine causing pain in the back and legs, and enlargement of bones in the skull can cause deafness.

Questions from the examiner

Examiner: *what investigations would you request?*

Doctor: a plain radiograph of the symptomatic joint would confirm the diagnosis. The radiograph may also reveal osteoarthritis of nearby joints, fractures of pagetic bone, and – much less likely – radiographic features suggestive of an osteosarcoma. All of these could be a possible cause for bone pain. Serum alkaline phosphatase may be elevated. A radionuclide bone scan would reveal the extent of the disease. MRI of the spine would be indicated in patients with suspected spinal stenosis.

Examiner: *how is Paget's disease treated?*

Doctor: asymptomatic Paget's disease that has been discovered incidentally does not require treatment. Painful Pagetic bone pain can be treated with bisphosphonates. Surgery may be indicated for painful associated osteoarthritic joints, and for complications such as fractures, spinal stenosis and deformity.

Further discussion

X-rays of suspicious areas will reveal the characteristic radiological appearances of Paget's disease. As most lesions are asymptomatic, a radionuclide bone scan will reveal the extent of the disease. The serum alkaline phosphatase concentration gives a good measure of the metabolic activity of the disease and correlates with the extent of skeletal involvement, although a normal serum alkaline phosphatase does not exclude a diagnosis of Paget's. Such individuals are more likely to have limited skeletal involvement, often involving a single bone lesion.

Aminobisphosphonates are the drugs of first choice in the treatment of active Paget's disease of the bone. As well as improving bone pain, bisphosphonates can treat neurological complications of Paget's. Symptomatic response is accompanied with a fall in the serum alkaline phosphatase, reaching a nadir between 3 and 6 months.

1.3.9 Hypermobile joints

Instruction

Mr Taylor, an 18-year-old university student, presented to rheumatology outpatients with joint pains and hypermobile joints. What is the likely diagnosis?

Introduction

The two most likely diagnoses are Marfan syndrome and Ehlers–Danlos syndrome.

Marfan syndrome – an autosomal dominant disorder due to defects in fibrillin. It is best known for musculoskeletal abnormalities as well as extraskeletal involvement of ocular, cardiovascular, pulmonary and skin tissues.

Ehlers–Danlos syndrome – caused by a range of mutations in collagen or related genes. All forms cause skin fragility, unsightly bruising and scarring. The commonest forms (classical form, types I and II, and the hypermobility form, type III) are associated with joint hypermobility. The rarer vascular form (type IV) is the only form associated with risk of arterial, bowel, bladder and uterine rupture, and this is not associated with hypermobility.

Beginning the encounter

Doctor: hello, my name is Dr A, I understand that you have been suffering from joint problems, is that right?

Doctor: before we get into the details of that, can you tell me if you have any major medical problems?

Patient: [gives list (with doctor politely but firmly discouraging lengthy detail).]

Doctor: and are you on any tablets or medications?

Patient: [gives details (and will probably have been asked to produce a written list).]

Focused history

Doctor: now moving onto the problem with your joints … can you tell me about them?

The clinician must first try to determine the cause of the symptoms and if there is a history that is suggestive of hypermobility. Joint pain in hypermobility is mechanical. There may also be a history of joint dislocations. Questions should then be directed to find out whether the patient (or any members of their family) has features that would be compatible with Marfan syndrome or Ehlers–Danlos – inherited disorders that are associated with joint hypermobility.

Regarding Marfan syndrome, important issues to explore include:

> Ocular – is there a history of myopia and lens dislocation (should be apparent by the age of 12 years, but is only present in 50% of patients)?

> Cardiovascular – aortic root dilatation and subsequent aortic dissection is the main cause of early mortality associated with Marfan syndrome; is there a family history of sudden death?

> Respiratory – there may be a history of a restrictive respiratory defect due to scoliosis; another reasonably common respiratory feature is pneumothorax.

Regarding Ehlers–Danlos syndrome, important issues to explore include:

> musculoskeletal – unstable joints that are prone to sprain and dislocation; tearing of tendons or muscles; myalgia

> skin – fragile skin that tears easily; easy bruising; scarring after trauma.

Focused examination

General features – in Marfan syndrome, look for the following.

> Is the patient tall, and does his arm span look greater than his height?

> Fingers – are they long (arachnodactyly)?

> Chest and spine – does he have pectus excavatum / carinatum or kyphoscoliosis?

> Palate – is it high and arched?

> Eyes – lens dislocation (Fig 32) occurs in 50% cases and is usually bilateral.

General features – in Ehlers–Danlos syndrome, look for the following:

> skin – bruising and scarring; look at any operative wounds

> pes planus.

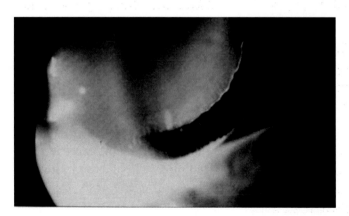

Fig 32 Lens dislocation with stretching of zonules in a patient with Marfan syndrome. (Reproduced from Ho NC, Tran JR, Bektas A. Marfan syndrome. *Lancet* 2005;366:1978–81.)

Other features – (if time permits) screen for cardiac manifestations of Marfan syndrome: mitral valve prolapse and/or aortic incompetence are common.

Key point

Joint examination – to demonstrate hypermobility perform the following manoeuvres, which can be used to calculate the Beighton score:

> Apposition of thumb to flexor aspect of forearm – to be able to do this is abnormal (score 1 point for each hand).

> Hyperextend the little finger at the metacarpophalangeal (MCP) joints – the ability to do this to more than 90° is abnormal (score 1 point for each hand).

> Hyperextend elbows – by >10° is abnormal (score 1 point for each elbow).

> Hyperextend the knees – by >10° is abnormal (score 1 point for each knee).

> Is the patient able to put their hands flat on the floor with their knees extended? (score 1 point).

A score of 4 or more (out of 9) indicates that the patient has a joint hypermobility syndrome.

Questions from the patient

[In the circumstance that the patient gives a positive family history of Marfan syndrome in their brother, but has no signs themselves other than joint hypermobility:]

Patient: do I have Marfan syndrome?

Doctor: at the moment I'm not sure. Your brother has Marfan syndrome. You have got hypermobile joints, but you don't have any other features. I think we need to do some more tests to look for other features of Marfan syndrome

… they should hopefully tell us whether you have it or not.

Patient: is there a cure for Marfan syndrome?

Doctor: no, it isn't something that can be cured, but there are treatments that can alleviate and prevent complications. This treatment is tailored to the individual patient and depends on which systems are affected.

Questions from the examiner

Examiner: how could you investigate a possible diagnosis of Marfan syndrome?

Doctor: this is a matter of looking for key diagnostic criteria including: thoracic echocardiography to detect aortic root dissection or aneurysm; slit-lamp examination of the lens to look for ectopia lentis; CT or MRI scan for lumbar dural ectasia; and X-rays for hip acetabular protrusion. Finally, *FBN1* genetic testing, especially if there is a family history of a known mutation.

Examiner: how is aortic disease managed?

Doctor: aortic disease can lead to life-threatening aortic dissection. Management relies on early detection through screening by echocardiography to identify at-risk individuals and initiation of therapy, typically beta-blockers and/or angiotensin-converting enzyme (ACE) inhibitors, to prevent dissection. If severe, aortic root disease can be managed surgically.

Further discussion

Marfan syndrome

This is an inherited autosomal dominant multisystem disorder of connective tissue caused by mutations in the extracellular matrix protein, fibrillin 1. The main burden of the disease predominantly affects the cardiovascular system (mitral valve prolapse and dilated aortic root with risk of

dissection), eyes (ectopia lentis and severe myopia) and the skeleton (kyphoscoliosis, pectus deformities, high-arched palate and arachnodactyly). The Ghent criteria (recently revised in 2010) have been developed so that the diagnosis of Marfan syndrome is based on defined clinical criteria – aortic root aneurysm and ectopia lentis are cardinal features.

Cardiovascular disease was responsible for the poor life expectancy of individuals with Marfan syndrome, who often succumbed to aortic disease, either regurgitation or dissection. Life expectancy has since improved with the use of beta-blockers and angiotensin receptor blockers and prophylactic aortic surgery.

1.3.10 Foot drop and weight loss in a patient with rheumatoid arthritis

Letter of referral to the rheumatology outpatient clinic

Dear Doctor,
Re: Mr Michael Jennings, aged 63 years

This man with long-standing seropositive rheumatoid arthritis (RA) has felt non-specifically unwell for the past 3 months and has lost over 10 kg in weight. His arthritis, which has been inactive recently, has been treated in the past with disease-modifying treatments, including gold and corticosteroids. His weight loss has been extensively investigated by the gastroenterologists without an underlying cause being identified. Over the past week he has noticed that his left foot is flopping, leading to difficulty in walking. What is the most likely explanation for his foot drop?

Yours sincerely,

Introduction

Foot drop is a rare complication of RA and tends to occur in patients with long-standing disease on a background of previous steroid treatment and smoking. Although his joint disease appears to be quiescent, the combination of foot drop and unexplained weight loss raises the possibility of rheumatoid vasculitis.

The severity of RA and associated extra-articular disease, including vasculitis, has declined with the widespread adoption of disease-modifying treatments. The current annual incidence of rheumatoid vasculitis is estimated at 3–4 per million.

Beginning the encounter

Doctor: hello, my name is Dr A. I understand that you have long-standing RA and have felt unwell for the past few months, with difficulty in walking over the past week. Is that right?

Doctor: before we get into the details of that, can you tell me if you have any major medical problems?

Patient: [gives list (with doctor politely but firmly discouraging lengthy detail).]

Doctor: and are you on any tablets or medications?

Patient: [gives details (and will probably have been asked to produce a written list).]

Focused history

Doctor: now moving onto the problem with your rheumatoid arthritis … can you tell me about this?

Patient: yes, I've had arthritis for a long time but it's my left foot that now seems to be weak and floppy.

Doctor: before looking into the problems with your foot, could you tell me about your RA. When was it diagnosed and what treatments have you had up to now?

Patient: I've had RA for over 15 years and been treated with various medications including steroid tablets and gold injections.

These introductory questions will provide useful background information relating to the behaviour of the patient's RA until the onset of foot drop.

Key point

Consider systemic rheumatoid vasculitis in RA in the presence of:

> persistent fever, fatigue and unexplained weight loss (present in 95% of cases)

> painful red eye – scleritis and 'corneal melt' syndrome

> nailfold infarcts, splinter haemorrhages, chronic leg and sacral ulcers, and digital gangrene (Figs 20, 33 and 34)

> mononeuritis multiplex (in 50% of cases)

> glomerulonephritis (in <5% of cases).

Focused history

Doctor: tell me about your foot drop. Did it appear suddenly or did it develop over the past few weeks?

Patient: it appears to have crept up on me over the past 2 weeks, though I've been losing weight for the past few months. I've had lots of tests but no explanation has been found for my weight loss.

Specific questions to explore the cause of foot drop should include:

> In the context of possible vasculitis, ask specifically about the features of rheumatoid vasculitis as detailed in the 'key point' box – painful red eyes, leg ulcers, digital ischaemia and other skin lesions.

> In addition to the pattern of onset and severity of foot drop, ask about patchy alteration in sensation and focal weakness that might suggest a more widespread mononeuritis multiplex, which would be suggestive of vasculitis.

> Do not exclude the possibility that the foot drop might reflect more mundane pathology such as a lumbar disc prolapse: so does the patient have a history of back pain?

Doctor: apart from the problems with your foot, have you noticed any problems with weakness or numbness of any other part of your body? (screening for evidence of eg mononeuritis multiplex)

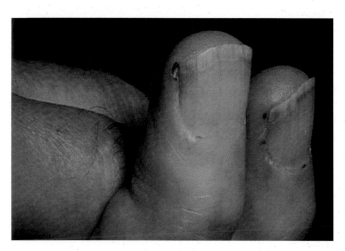

Fig 33 Nailfold digital infarcts in rheumatoid vasculitis. (Reproduced with permission from Dieppe PA, Kirwan J, Cooper C. *Arthritis and rheumatism in practice*. London: Gower Medical Publishing, 1991.)

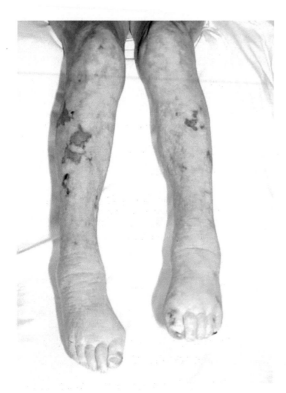

Fig 34 Vasculitic skin rash in RA.

Focused examination

The history should help clarify whether the patient's neurological problems are confined to foot drop or are a part of a wider mononeuritis multiplex picture in association with rheumatoid vasculitis.

General – look for nailfold infarcts, splinter haemorrhages, digital gangrene and leg ulcers.

Neurological, the foot and leg – look for muscle wasting and sensory loss in the affected leg and assess strength and reflexes. Common peroneal (or fibular) nerve palsy causes the following signs:

> motor – foot drop with loss of ankle and toe dorsiflexion, and ankle eversion

> sensory – numbness over the lateral aspect of the lower leg and dorsum of the foot.

Neurological, other – be prepared to widen your examination if the history suggests mononeuritis multiplex

(the examiner is likely to tell you if this is unnecessary).

Questions from the patient

[On the assumption that the history and examination suggest isolated foot drop in a patient with RA:]

Patient: *why does my left foot drop on walking?*

Doctor: I think it's most likely that inflammation of blood vessels supplying the nerves to your leg has resulted in weakness of your ankle muscles.

Patient: *can this be treated?*

Doctor: yes it can … to try to prevent further nerve damage, we will need to use drugs which act rapidly to suppress the inflammatory process in the blood vessels supplying the affected nerves. This is best achieved by steroid injections, combined with other drugs that act by dampening the activity of the immune system.

Questions from the examiner

Examiner: *how do you differentiate between foot drop due to lumbar disc prolapse and that due to mononeuritis multiplex?*

Doctor: this would be done on the basis of the history, supplemented with findings on clinical examination. Foot drop due to lumbar disc prolapse would be suggested by a preceding history of sudden backache and examination findings confined to nerve root compression. In contrast, foot drop that is part of a wider picture of mononeuritis multiplex would be associated with systemic ill health and characteristic findings suggestive of vasculitis (see focused examination). Imaging of the spine would provide confirmatory evidence in the case of disc prolapse.

Examiner: *how on examination would you distinguish between a common peroneal nerve lesion and an L5 root lesion?*

Doctor: a common peroneal nerve lesion will cause weakness of ankle dorsiflexion and eversion, but will not affect inversion, whereas a root lesion will affect inversion.

Examiner: *if you were the medical registrar in outpatients, how would you confirm a diagnosis of rheumatoid vasculitis?*

Doctor: rheumatoid vasculitis is typically a clinical diagnosis based on a constellation of clinical features. I'd attempt to obtain histological confirmation of vasculitis by undertaking a sural nerve biopsy, in addition to electrophysiological studies to document the extent and type of neuropathy. Other tests that would yield useful information would be acute phase indices (C-reactive protein (CRP), erythrocyte sedimentation rate (ESR)), renal function and urine dipstick testing for proteinuria and haematuria. I'd expect a patient's CRP and ESR to

Table 20 Comparison of systemic rheumatoid vasculitis and polyarteritis nodosa (PAN)

Feature	Systemic rheumatoid vasculitis	PAN
Joints	Almost always occurs on a background of seropositive, nodular RA	Arthralgia in 50% of cases
Skin, purpura and digital infarcts	Seen in both conditions	Frank non-deforming arthritis in 20% of cases
Mononeuritis multiplex	Seen in both conditions	Seen in both conditions
Glomerulonephritis	In <5% of cases	Rare in classic PAN
Angiography	Not useful	Diagnostically useful investigation revealing aneurysms of visceral arteries
Hepatitis B surface antigen	No association	Positive in 20% of cases
Complement (C3 and C4)	Normal or ↓	Normal or ↓
ANCA	p-ANCA in 10–20%	Negative in classic PAN

ANCA, antineutrophil cytoplasmic antibody; RA, rheumatoid arthritis.

be elevated in rheumatoid vasculitis, and proteinuria and haematuria with impaired renal function would raise the possibility of renal vasculitis.

Further discussion

Although many of the features of rheumatoid vasculitis may also occur in other systemic vasculitides such as polyarteritis nodosa (PAN), in practice there is little difficulty in differentiating between the two (Table 20).

1.3.11 A swollen neck and dry mouth

Scenario

Mr Lawrence Ashworth, a 65-year-old man, is well in himself but has developed painless progressive swelling of his neck over the past 12 months, associated with a dry mouth. The only significant finding on routine blood tests is a markedly elevated erythrocyte sedimentation rate (ESR) (110 mm/h) (normal threshold <20 mm/1st h). His full blood count, renal and liver function tests are all normal.

What is the likely diagnosis?

Introduction

The differential diagnosis here is wide. The neck swelling has not been described in detail but could be due to enlargement of lymph nodes, thyroid gland, salivary or parotid glands, or other structures within the neck. The causes of such swelling could be malignant, infiltrative or inflammatory, but the fact that the patient is said to be well, and the fact that the condition has been progressing for a year or so, argue strongly against a malignant process. The presence of a dry mouth would not be an expected feature in a case of thyroid enlargement, so – although thyroid cases are common in PACES – this would not seem to be likely in this instance.

Beginning the encounter

Doctor: hello, my name is Dr A. I understand that your neck has been progressively swelling over the past 12 months, and that you've got a dry mouth. Is that right?

Doctor: before we get into the details of those things, can you tell me if you have any major medical problems?

Patient: [gives list (with doctor politely but firmly discouraging lengthy detail).]

Doctor: and are you on any tablets or medications?

Patient: [gives details (and will probably have been asked to produce a written list).]

These introductory questions will provide useful clinical context and may immediately give a clue to the likely diagnosis, eg evidence of a multisystem inflammatory disease.

Focused history

Doctor: tell me about the neck swelling … when did you first notice it? What's happened since then? How does it affect you – any difficulty with swallowing, or when you take a deep breath (does this make a funny sound)?

Doctor: tell me about the dry mouth … when did you first notice it? What's happened since then? Are your eyes dry or gritty?

Doctor: have you had any other symptoms that are troubling you?

Specific questions about symptoms that would be helpful in this case are:

> systemic symptoms – sweats/fevers, weight loss or enlarged glands elsewhere (would increase suspicion of a lymphoproliferative disorder)

> symptoms suggestive of thyroid over- or under-activity.

Focused examination

General inspection – aside from observing the general state of the patient's health (said to be good), look quickly at the eyes for signs of thyroid disease (unlikely to be present).

Mouth – look carefully at teeth, tongue and fauces.

Neck – inspect carefully for obvious swelling and scars; palpate all lymph node areas, glands (salivary, parotid) and thyroid carefully.

Other – palpate other lymph node areas and check for hepatosplenomegaly.

Questions from the patient

[On the assumption that the patient looks well and has swollen submandibular salivary glands with associated lymph node enlargement:]

Patient: *do you know why my neck glands are swollen?*

Doctor: I'm not sure, but I think it's most likely that there's an inflammatory condition affecting the glands, but need to carry out additional tests for confirmation.

Patient: *am I likely to have cancer?*

Doctor: no, I think that is very unlikely. You're in good health and have had the problem for quite a long time. We need to do tests to find out what's going on, but I think that the chances of this being due to cancer are very small.

Questions from the examiner

Examiner: *how would you investigate to find out what's going on?*

Doctor: the key investigations would be blood tests to look for evidence of autoimmune rheumatic disorders –

autoantibody screen (antinuclear antibody (ANA), rheumatoid factor), immunoglobulins, C-reactive protein (CRP); a chest X-ray to look for evidence of lymphadenopathy or pulmonary infiltrate; a biopsy of one of the enlarged glands; and, depending on the findings, it would probably be appropriate to organise a CT scan of the neck, thorax and abdomen.

Examiner: *what is your differential diagnosis?*

Doctor: the main possibilities are an inflammatory condition such as Sjögren's syndrome or IgG4-related disease (IgG4-RD), or a slowly progressive lymphoproliferative disorder.

Examiner: *supposing the blood tests revealed a polyclonal increase in serum immunoglobulins and a low CRP, but the autoantibody screen was negative: what would that suggest by way of diagnosis?*

Doctor: I think that would mean that IgG4-RD was most likely. Sjögren's syndrome is usually associated with a positive ANA and antibodies to extractable nuclear antigens (ENA). A predominant increase in IgG4 as opposed to an increase in all subclasses would favour IgG4-RD. The histopathological examination would help differentiate between lymphoma and IgG4-RD.

Examiner: *how would you explain the discordance between this patient's markedly elevated ESR (>100 mm/h) and the normal CRP?*

Doctor: although both the CRP and the ESR are markers of the acute phase response, the ESR is largely driven by changes in plasma proteins and red cells, whereas changes in CRP are mainly driven by pro-inflammatory

cytokines (interleukin (IL)-1, IL-6, tumour necrosis factor (TNF)). Rises in CRP and ESR generally go together, but a discordant rise in ESR in the context of a constitutionally well patient would be explained by hypergammaglobulinaemia.

Examiner: *is an elevated IgG4 specific for the diagnosis of IgG4-RD?*

Doctor: no, it isn't. About 50% of patients with histologically confirmed IgG4-RD have normal serum IgG4 levels at presentation. An elevated IgG4 is also a feature of other inflammatory, autoimmune and allergic disorders.

Further discussion

IgG4-RD is a recently recognised distinct clinical entity of unknown aetiology characterised by systemic or localised fibro-inflammatory swelling and histological evidence of IgG4-associated lymphoplasmacytic infiltration. Patients with IgG4-RD are not acutely ill and may present with single or multiorgan involvement. Table 21 compares the features of IgG4-RD and Sjögren's syndrome.

Key point

Consider IgG4-RD in any clinical context characterised by unexplained fibro-inflammatory disease presenting as:

> autoimmune pancreatitis

> lymphadenopathy

> salivary or lacrimal gland enlargement

> upper airways obstruction

> retroperitoneal fibrosis

> inflammatory aortitis

> tubulo-interstitial nephritis.

Table 21 Comparative analysis of the key features of IgG4-RD and Sjögren's syndrome

Feature	IgG4-RD	Sjögren's syndrome
Gender distribution	Male:female ratio 3:1	Male:female ratio 1:10
Lymphadenopathy and or organomegaly	Yes	Unusual with uncomplicated disease
Pancreatic involvement	Yes, approximately 30% of cases	Uncommon
Histopathology	Lymphoplasmacytic infiltration and storiform fibrosis with abundant IgG4-positive plasma cells	Focal lymphocytic infiltration not associated with IgG4 expression
Polyclonal hypergammaglobulinaemia	Yes, with predominant rise in IgG4	Yes, diffuse elevation in all IgG subclasses
Treatment	Steroids Pancreatic enzyme replacement for patients with pancreatitis	Symptomatic treatment of sicca symptoms Steroids and immunosuppressive drugs are of little value

IgG, immunoglobulin G; IgG4-RD, IqG4-related disease.

1.3.12 Recurrent red eyes and oral ulcers

Scenario

Mr Hassan Topal, a 19-year-old Turkish man, has presented to the rheumatology outpatient clinic with gradual onset of malaise, arthralgia and mouth ulcers. In the past couple of weeks his joints have become more painful, and both of his eyes have become red and inflamed. What is the likely diagnosis?

Introduction

Mouth ulceration and red eyes in a young man from a country along the Silk Route must always raise the possibility of Behçet's disease, which is regarded as an auto-inflammatory syndrome characterised by predominant venous vasculitis. Diagnosis is based on internationally agreed criteria (Table 22). Episodic relapses are probably triggered non-specifically by intercurrent infection or commensal organisms. Untreated episodes can lead to blindness due to uveitis and retinal vasculitis. Almost any organ can be involved.

Beginning the encounter

Doctor: hello, my name is Dr A, I understand that you've been feeling unwell, with joint pains, headaches and mouth ulcers, is that right?

Doctor: before we get into details, can you tell me if you have any major medical problems?

Patient: [gives answer (with doctor politely but firmly discouraging lengthy detail).]

Doctor: are you on any tablets or medications?

Patient: [gives details (and will probably have been asked to produce a written list).]

A young patient is less likely to have a significant past medical history or long list of comorbidities, or to be on many medications, but it is appropriate to check before beginning to take a detailed history as any history of eg autoimmune rheumatic disorder would clearly be of relevance.

Focused history

Doctor: tell me about how these problems began [work through malaise, arthralgia, headaches, mouth ulcers and red eyes systematically].

Doctor: has anything like this ever happened before ... have you had bad mouth ulcers or red eyes before this?

History taking should focus on ascertaining whether the patient meets the International Study Group criteria for Behçet's disease (Table 22):

Table 22 International Study Group criteria for Behçet's disease (1990)

Oral ulcers at least three times a year	And two of the following:
	Genital ulcers
	Skin lesions: acne (outside adolescent age group), erythema nodosum or pustular lesions
	Uveitis (anterior or posterior/retinitis)
	Pathergy (pustules forming at site of sterile trauma)

> Genital ulcers – have you had any ulcers or problems on your penis or anus or around your private parts?

> Skin lesions – have you had any unusual spots or rashes on your skin?

> Eyes – apart from redness, have you had any other problems with your eyes or vision? Do you have pain in your eyes? Is your vision normal (with reading glasses)? Do you have any 'floaters' (floating black specks)?

> Pathergy – have you ever had spots or problems on your skin where you've had blood taken, or had a scratch or cut yourself, or had some other damage to the skin?

Hazard

In a patient with Behçet's, loss of visual acuity, pain or vitreous opacities are 'red flag' symptoms suggesting need for urgent action to prevent possible uveitis-related permanent loss of vision.

Questions related to additional possible complications and the main differential diagnoses (Table 23) of Behçet's disease:

> Systemic – fatigue is almost universal, but significant fever is unusual.

> Rheumatological – 'I know that your joints are painful, but do they swell? What time of day or night is worst? Which joints are affected?' Inflammatory arthritis of Behçet's typically affects knees, ankles and wrists, and is worst in the mornings.

> Venous thromboembolism – find out if there is a history of deep vein thrombosis ('Have you ever had a blood clot causing a swollen arm or leg?') or superficial thrombophlebitis ('Have you ever had a painful, hard vein?').

> Neurological complications – find out if there is a history of cerebral venous sinus thrombosis or, less commonly,

Table 23 Differential diagnosis of Behçet's disease

Symptoms	Differential diagnosis	Distinguishing test(s)
Mouth ulcers	Herpes simplex	Viral swab for herpes simplex PCR
Mouth ulcers, malaise, diarrhoea	Coeliac disease	tTG antibodies, duodenal villous atrophy on biopsy HLA-DQ2 or -DQ8
Mouth ulcers, arthralgia or arthritis	Systemic lupus erythematosus	Antinuclear, double-stranded DNA and anti-ENA antibodies
Mouth ulcers, arthritis, ocular inflammation (episcleritis, scleritis)	Rheumatoid disease	CCP antibodies
Diarrhoea, abdominal pain, arthritis, ocular inflammation (conjunctivitis)	Inflammatory bowel disease	Intestinal biopsy showing granulomata (Crohn's) or typical colonic ulceration. Sacroiliac involvement on X-ray or MRI HLA-B27 (HLA-B27 disease)
Fever, arthritis, oral ulceration	Autoinflammatory syndrome (hyper IgD syndrome, PFAPA syndrome)	Family history, high fever Presence of amyloid Diagnostic genetic mutation
Erythema nodosum, uveitis, malaise	Sarcoidosis	Raised serum ACE level Chest X-ray showing hilar lymphadenopathy
Fever, erythema nodosum	Tuberculosis	Chest X-ray Interferon-γ release assay Ziehl–Neelsen stain and cultures
Acne, synovitis	SAPHO syndrome	Presence of chondritis and osteitis
Orogenital ulcers	MAGIC syndrome	Presence of chondritis
Oral ulcers, ocular involvement, vascular involvement	ANCA-associated vasculitis	Presence of ANCAs and or biopsy evidence of small vessel vasculitis

Also consider syphilis and HIV, which can present with a wide range of symptoms and signs that overlap with those caused by Behçet's disease.

ACE, angiotensin-converting enzyme; ANCA, antineutrophil cytoplasmic antibody; CCP, cyclic citrullinated peptide; ENA, extractable nuclear antigens; HLA, human leukocyte antigen; IgD, immunoglobulin D; MAGIC, mouth and genital ulcers with inflamed cartilage; PCR, polymerase chain reaction; PFAPA, periodic fevers with aphthous stomatitis, pharyngitis and adenitis; SAPHO, synovitis, acne, pustulosis, hyperostosis and osteitis; tTG, tissue transglutaminase.

stroke ('Have you ever had a blood clot in the brain?' 'Have you had problems with eye or facial movements or sensation, or swallowing?'). Meningism or lymphocytic meningitis may occur with severe exacerbations.

> Other complications – find out if there are arterial aneurysms (particularly affecting pulmonary arteries), or inflammatory bowel disease, sometimes with fistulation (histology is non-specific).

> Ethnic origin – this is given in the scenario, but otherwise ask 'where is your family from?'

Focused examination

Skin – look for acneiform or other pustular lesions (relevant particularly in post-adolescents), erythema nodosum, superficial thrombophlebitis or signs of pathergy.

Mouth – examine the oral cavity for ulcers, typically aphthous on an erythematous background. May be minor (<10 mm), major (>10 mm) or herpetiform.

Eyes – look for anterior uveitis (erythema, hypopyon), check acuity and visual fields, and perform fundoscopy to check for retinitis (exudates, haemorrhages). Diagnosis of anterior uveitis often requires slit-lamp examination.

Genitals – in routine clinical practice you would, with assistance of a chaperone, carefully examine the genitals for signs of ulceration. In PACES you should explain to the examiner that this is would be your intention (and they will tell you that you do not need to do so in the exam).

Other – check joints (arthritis), meninges (neck stiffness, Kernig's sign) and neurological examination (particularly cranial nerves).

Questions from the patient

Patient: what do you think is causing all these problems?

Doctor: I'm not sure at the moment, but I think it's most likely that you have got a problem called Behçet's disease

Patient: can this be treated? Can it be cured?

Doctor: Behçet's disease is a condition that has exacerbations or 'flare-ups', and remissions, times when you are well. I am afraid that there isn't any treatment that will cure it completely, but symptoms can be controlled, and there are medications that will help to prevent exacerbations and to prevent permanent damage.

Patient: why have I got Behçet's disease?

Doctor: that's a good question, and I'm afraid that I can't give you a good answer. It seems to be an autoimmune disease, where white cells in the body that should react against infection seem to react against the body itself, and it's often found in people from Turkey and neighbouring countries.

Questions from the examiner

Examiner: what is your main differential diagnosis?

Doctor: apart from Behçet's disease, we need to do be aware of other differential diagnoses such as infection, other vasculitides or autoimmune disease [Table 23].

Examiner: how would you confirm the diagnosis?

Doctor: there are no confirmatory tests for Behçet's. The diagnosis is based on a comprehensive history and examination, and investigations are largely to assess risk of complications and to exclude differential diagnoses.

Examiner: if you'd just seen this patient in clinic, would you be asking for any specialist help?

Doctor: yes, in view of his red eyes, my most immediate concern would be his vision. I would request an urgent

ophthalmological opinion. Anterior uveitis and retinitis are typical of Behçet's, whereas conjunctivitis or scleritis would be more in keeping with human leukocyte antigen (HLA)-B27 disease or rheumatoid disease, respectively.

Examiner: what investigations would you arrange?

Doctor: on routine bloods, I would expect a mild neutrophilia and a moderately raised C-reactive protein (CRP). I would request urine analysis and serum antinuclear antibody (ANA) and antineutrophil cytoplasmic antibody (ANCA) to exclude other vasculitic disorders. I'd ask for a chest X-ray, looking for hilar lymphadenopathy (sarcoid or less likely infection such as tuberculosis). I would send viral swabs from the mouth ulcers and check syphilis serology. It would be reasonable to check HLA type – HLA-B51 positivity is associated with Behçet's in this ethnic group, but this is not diagnostic and not immediately essential.

Examiner: how would you treat this patient?

Doctor: I'd ask for specialist advice before I started anything, but if it's agreed that the diagnosis is Behçet's, and if the patient has significant eye involvement, then prompt treatment with high-dose steroids such as intravenous methyl prednisolone is essential to preserve sight, followed by a reducing dose of oral prednisolone over the subsequent weeks once control is achieved. Longer-term disease-modifying agents, such as azathioprine, would usually be started early, as soon as diagnosis is confirmed, for disease of this severity. Tumour necrosis factor (TNF) antagonists such as infliximab, or interferon-α could be considered as alternatives. Meticulous oral hygiene, antiseptic mouthwashes and topical steroid for ulcers are important. Oral colchicine is helpful for mucosal disease or arthritis.

Key point

Behçet's is a rare relapsing-remitting vasculitic disorder. Features include severe orogenital ulceration, pustular/inflammatory skin lesions and uveitis. There is no specific diagnostic marker. Control of symptoms is with high-dose corticosteroids or tumour necrosis factor (TNF) inhibitors. Long-term treatment is with topical measures, oral colchicine, immunosuppressives or biologicals, depending on disease severity.

1.4 Acute scenarios

1.4.1 Fulminant septicaemia in an asplenic

Case history

A 50-year-old asplenic woman presents to the emergency department with a 2-day history of fever and confusion. Her observations on admission confirm fever (of 39°C), tachycardia (150/min) and hypotension (blood pressure 80/40 mmHg). She carries a splenectomy card stating that she underwent splenectomy 7 years ago for refractory immune thrombocytopenic purpura.

As a junior medical doctor on duty, you suspect – given her asplenia – that she is septicaemic and initiate immediate treatment with broad-spectrum antibiotics.

Introduction

Asplenic patients are prone to overwhelming infection, particularly with encapsulated bacteria, because of their impaired ability to produce antibodies against capsular polysaccharide antigens of *Streptococcus pneumoniae*, *Haemophilus influenzae* and *Neisseria meningitidis*. This is a direct consequence of the loss of splenic marginal zone B-lymphocytes. In addition, the loss of approximately a quarter of the body's total macrophage population renders patients susceptible to certain other blood-borne bacteria and some intraerythrocytic protozoa (Table 24).

Causes of hyposplenism are shown in Table 25.

History of presenting problem

Is there a history of dog bite or travel abroad?

This is important to ascertain because asplenic patients are at particular risk of infection with *Capnocytophaga canimorsus* (a Gram-negative bacillus found in canine saliva) and protozoal infections such as *Plasmodium* species.

Other relevant history

What measures were or could have been taken to reduce the infective risks associated with asplenia before or after splenectomy?

Was the patient immunised with 23-valent pneumococcal polysaccharide (Pneumovax), *Haemophilus* conjugate

Table 24	Organisms causing overwhelming infection in asplenic patients	
Bacteria		**Parasites**
Streptococcus pneumoniae *Streptococcus suis* (from pigs and farm animals)		Malaria
Haemophilus influenzae		*Babesia* spp (from tick bites)
Neisseria meningitidis		
Staphylococcus aureus		
Klebsiella pneumoniae		
Salmonella enteritidis		
Capnocytophaga canimorsus (DF-2) (from dog bites)		

Table 25	Causes of hyposplenism	
Splenectomy		**Functional hyposplenism**
Trauma Haematological autoimmunity Haematological malignancy		Sickle-cell anaemia Essential thrombocythaemia Lymphoproliferative disease Coeliac disease Inflammatory bowel disease

and meningococcal type C conjugate vaccines before splenectomy? Current guidelines from the British Committee for Standards in Haematology recommend that vaccination be performed at least 2 weeks before elective splenectomy or as soon as possible after emergency splenectomy.

Examination

Key point

In any patient with overwhelming sepsis, consider hyposplenism.

This woman's profound hypotension indicates that she is extremely ill. Aside from repeating her vital signs, note the following to establish a baseline from which you can judge whether she is improving or deteriorating over the next 30 minutes or so:

> Peripheral perfusion – are her peripheries hot or cold, and if cold, how far proximally does this extend?

> Respiration – is she cyanosed? Does she look exhausted? If either of these symptoms are present, then call for assistance from the intensive care unit (ICU) sooner rather than later. Can she speak in sentences or only a few words at a time? Do not be falsely reassured by a normal respiratory rate (12–16/min), if the patient looks tired and can hardly speak it means that they are tiring and may arrest soon. Check pulse oximetry, but note that it may not be possible to get a proper reading in a patient who is peripherally shut down.

> She is confused – check the Glasgow Coma Score. Is there meningism?

> Are there any clues that the patient may have a particular cause of septicaemia? Some patients with meningococcal septicaemia, in particular, may present with signs of disseminated intravascular coagulation (DIC), including skin

purpura and digital gangrene. Examine the lungs: is there consolidation to indicate that the underlying condition is almost certainly pneumonia?

Investigation

To establish the diagnosis

In view of the high probability of septicaemia, send blood cultures before starting immediate antimicrobial therapy. The patient will require urethral catheterisation to monitor their urine output. Send urine for culture, and also swabs/specimens from any other sites that might be infected. In selected cases, other specific tests will be required, eg thick and thin films for malaria.

Organise a chest radiograph to look for lobar consolidation that is likely to be due to pneumococcal pneumonia in this context, and also for features suggesting acute respiratory distress syndrome.

To establish a baseline / presence of complications

Check electrolytes and renal, liver and bone function; FBC; clotting screen (possibility of DIC); and check inflammatory markers (C-reactive protein and erythrocyte sedimentation rate) to assess severity of tissue damage.

Check arterial blood gases to assess oxygenation, ventilation and for acidosis.

Management

This woman clearly requires resuscitation. Full details of how to approach a very ill patient can be found in the *Acute medicine* Medical Masterclass book, but key issues are:

> Oxygenation – give high-flow oxygen via a reservoir bag, aiming to keep oxygen saturation at >92%.

> Fluid resuscitation – give colloid or 0.9% saline rapidly (as fast as the cannulae will allow) to raise the jugular venous pressure (JVP) to about 8–10 cm, but reassess clinically after every litre of fluid has been given to check for pulmonary oedema. Stop rapid infusion if breathing deteriorates

in any way. The insertion of a central venous line to monitor central venous pressure (CVP) may be helpful, but note that the first priority is to give fluid to an obviously hypotensive patient, not to try to insert a CVP line. The presence of hypotension that is refractory to fluid challenge or hypotension in association with pulmonary oedema indicates that the patient is *in extremis*: call for urgent help from the ICU.

> Antimicrobials – as septicaemia is suspected.

> Support of failing systems – if this woman does not respond to the treatments indicated above, then she may require one or more of the following: mechanical ventilation, inotropic support or haematological support (fresh frozen plasma or platelet transfusion).

What principles should guide your choice of antimicrobials?

Until the results of blood cultures are available, you should choose a broad-spectrum antimicrobial with bactericidal activity against the pathogens that are most likely to cause septicaemia in an asplenic host (Table 24). Most hospitals will have their own 'antibiotic policy', but unless there are unusual features to the case – such as recent foreign travel or a dog bite – then a third-generation cephalosporin in conjunction with an aminoglycoside would be appropriate until the results of the cultures are available.

Further comments

The risk of serious infection following splenectomy is related to the age at surgery and the presence of underlying disease. The infection rate is particularly high in children under the age of 5 years (>10%). Although the period of greatest risk in all asplenic patients is the first 2 years following surgery, delayed infection may occur more than 20 years later, thus underlining the need for constant vigilance.

Table 26	Vaccination recommendations for hyposplenic adults	
Vaccine	Revaccination schedule	Comments
23 valent Pneumovax (pneumococcal polysaccharide)	5 years	Consider monitoring antibody levels. If Prevnar (pneumococcal conjugate) vaccine is given then consider an early booster dose to cover additional serotypes
13 valent Prevnar (pneumococcal conjugate)	Not known	Consider using prior to pneumococcal polysaccharide vaccine, as it is likely to give long-term protection
Haemophilus conjugate	Not routinely recommended	Use if previously unvaccinated
Quadrivalent meningococcal conjugate (MenACWY)	Every 3–5 years depending on age at last dose	Use if previously unvaccinated
Meningococcal group B vaccine	Prior to travel to high-risk area	Use if previously unvaccinated
Influenza vaccine	Annual	

What measures would you adopt to minimise a recurrence of septicaemia in the future?

If and when the patient recovers, ensure that she is optimally protected against further episodes of sepsis due to encapsulated bacteria by vaccinating her with the relevant vaccines (Table 26). Although no formal evidence is available, it is likely that asplenic patients will derive additional protection from immunisation with the newly introduced pneumococcal conjugate vaccine by virtue of its greater immunogenicity. The need for booster immunisations should be dictated by antibody levels and reviewed at 5-yearly intervals. It is also prudent to offer patients annual influenza immunisation to minimise the risk of secondary bacterial infection following influenza.

Lifelong antibiotic prophylaxis using oral penicillin is recommended by the Chief Medical Officer in the UK, although the evidence for its efficacy is unclear.

All patients should carry a splenectomy card and a Medic-Alert bracelet stating their asplenic status, and should be educated regarding the risks associated with animal bites and travel to malarious areas.

How can splenic function be assessed?
The assessment of functional hyposplenism in patients with intact spleens is a difficult area since the traditional marker, Howell–Jolly bodies (Fig 35), may be insufficiently sensitive in many early cases. Alternative methods of assessing splenic function include quantification of the circulating pitted red cell count by image contrast microscopy (Fig 36), which reflects the physiological function of phagocytosing effete red cells in the spleen, and radionuclide imaging to assess splenic uptake of isotopes. There are no reliable methods for directly assessing the important immunological functions of the spleen.

1.4.2 Collapse during a restaurant meal

Case history

A 19-year-old medical student is admitted to the emergency department with facial swelling, difficulty in breathing and a generalised urticarial rash. Her symptoms began minutes after starting a meal with friends in a local restaurant. You are called to see her urgently.

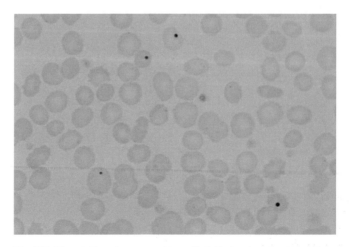

Fig 35 Blood film depicting Howell–Jolly bodies (intraerythrocytic nuclear fragments) in a patient after splenectomy for immune thrombocytopenic purpura. (Courtesy of Dr D Swirsky, Leeds General Infirmary.)

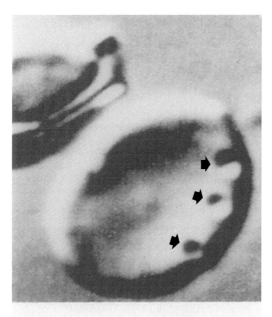

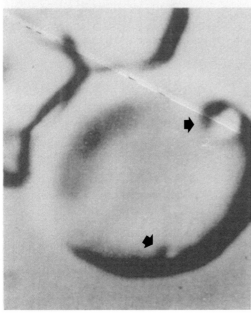

Fig 36 Interference phase-contrast microscopy showing red cells with surface indentations or 'pocks' in an asplenic patient. 'Pocks' (arrows in both panels) occur in more than 12% of the red cells of patients with asplenia. (Reproduced with permission from Feder HM, Pearson HA. Assessment of splenic function in familial asplenia. *N Engl J Med* 1999;341:211, copyright © 1999 Massachusetts Medical Society.)

Introduction

Anaphylaxis occurs when there is systemic mast cell degranulation as a result of immunoglobulin E (IgE)-mediated binding to an allergen. Symptoms usually start within a few minutes of contact with the allergen

and progress rapidly. Common features include the following:

> more common after ingestion of an oral allergen:

> > angio-oedema

> > laryngeal obstruction

> wheeze

> colicky abdominal pain with vomiting or diarrhoea

> more common after intravenous exposure to allergen:

> > hypotension

> cutaneous features occur in almost every episode of anaphylaxis:

> > urticaria

> > flushing.

History of the presenting problem

In all cases of possible anaphylaxis the history is crucial, both to make the diagnosis and to prevent future episodes.

 Key point

Anaphylactic reactions usually occur within minutes of encountering the allergen: life-threatening reactions virtually never occur more than 30 minutes after contact.

The priority in this case is clearly to get on with treatment and you should not delay while you are seeking a detailed history, but you need to know what she ate to prevent recurrence. Get her friends to contact the chef at the restaurant she was at to obtain a list of all the ingredients from her meal as soon as possible, but note that any food she ate more than an hour prior to the anaphylaxis is most unlikely to be the cause. Beware of hidden allergens: nuts, nut oils and spices are very common allergens that may be overlooked. Contact with latex and insect stings is unlikely to be relevant here, but should be considered in other cases.

Other relevant history

Previous episodes

Has the patient had any previous episodes, perhaps less severe? Does she have any known allergies? Atopic people (with eczema, asthma or hay fever) have a greater risk of anaphylaxis.

Drug history

The following drugs make treatment of anaphylaxis difficult or dangerous and should be avoided in the future:

> Epinephrine will cause severe hypertension if given to patients on beta-blockers due to unopposed stimulation of α-adrenergic receptors.

> Tricyclic antidepressants, monoamine oxidase inhibitors and cocaine potentiate epinephrine and increase the risk of arrhythmias and hypertension.

Other medical conditions

A history of heart disease or hypertension, unlikely in this case, would increase the risks of epinephrine treatment – but faced with life-threatening anaphylaxis, the balance of benefits and risks very clearly favours treatment.

Examination

 Key point

Although this case scenario is described here in the traditional format, with management following on from history, examination and investigation, in practice the clinical urgency of the situation means that immediate acute management of anaphylaxis takes precedence.

This is a medical emergency: your patient has typical features of anaphylaxis and without prompt treatment she may die from respiratory tract obstruction, bronchoconstriction or hypotension. If she looks as though she is about to arrest, then call the cardiac resuscitation team immediately – do not wait for her heart to stop!

When the patient is *in extremis* you should take no more than a few seconds for a brief assessment. Aside from noting vital signs, the key issue is to look for evidence of upper and/or lower airway obstruction:

> Can the patient speak?

> Can she swallow?

> Is she cyanosed?

> Is she using her accessory muscles to support breathing?

> Look in her mouth, but do not force this open because this may occlude a critically compromised airway – note the degree of facial, tongue and pharyngeal swelling.

> Stridor or wheeze – remembering that absence of these may indicate very poor air entry and incipient respiratory arrest.

> Count her respiratory rate, but note that a normal value is not always reassuring (see Section 1.4.1).

> Chest movement – does her chest seem to be expanding normally? Is there indrawing of the intercostal muscles?

> Check pulse oximetry.

Other features to note include erythema, urticaria, rhinitis, vomiting or diarrhoea. Does she have a Medic-Alert bracelet?

Immediate management

While you are conducting the assessment, give high-flow oxygen via a reservoir bag and have emergency drugs prepared. If airway obstruction is the dominant problem, the patient will be most comfortable sitting; if it is

hypotension, then lying flat will be best. Then:

> Give epinephrine 0.5 mg (0.5 mL of 1:1000) intramuscularly – most patients with anaphylaxis or anaphylactoid reactions respond promptly to this treatment, but repeat after 5 minutes if there is no response or if symptoms recur.

> Establish intravenous access, and if the patient is hypotensive, give 1–2 L of physiological (0.9%) saline.

> Give an antihistamine, such as chlorpheniramine 10–20 mg and hydrocortisone 100–500 mg (each by intramuscular or slow intravenous injection), to help minimise later reactions.

> Recheck the patient's blood pressure and listen to her chest – nebulised salbutamol (5 mg) will help any residual bronchoconstriction; intravenous salbutamol may be necessary if the patient has recently taken a beta-blocker.

Investigation

The diagnosis in this case is almost certainly anaphylaxis, but sometimes all is not what it appears to be and a case that seems to start off as a 'straightforward case of anaphylaxis' becomes much less straightforward with time. There are other causes of facial and laryngeal swelling (see Table 27), and panic attacks can be dramatic. Do not forget C1 inhibitor deficiency, especially if the response to epinephrine is poor.

Table 27	Differential diagnosis of facial and laryngeal swelling
Common	Allergy, including anaphylaxis
	Anaphylactoid reactions (usually to drugs)
	Idiopathic and angiotensin-converting enzyme inhibitor-induced angio-oedema
	Salicylate hypersensitivity
	Infection: erysipelas, dental infections, parotitis and quinsy
	Trauma, including burns
Must consider	C1 inhibitor deficiency

Key point

Consider panic attacks – these may cause dramatic breathlessness, with loud upper airway noises and occasionally erythema, but without the other features of anaphylaxis.

Measurement of serum mast cell tryptase is useful in demonstrating that the presenting episode was associated with demonstrable mast cell degranulation, ie was anaphylactic or anaphylactoid. Serial samples should be taken, ideally at 1 and 4 hours after onset with a further sample at 24 hours, by which time raised tryptase levels should have returned to baseline. Even a single measurement can be invaluable if the diagnosis is later questioned.

Specific IgE can be estimated for suspect allergens, as dictated by the clinical history, but note that tests may occasionally be negative immediately after an episode of anaphylaxis. If in doubt, repeat at a later date. Skin-prick tests may be performed at a later date in clinic.

Further management

After resuscitation the patient is likely to be well, but she should be kept under observation for at least 12 hours – biphasic anaphylactic reactions occasionally occur. During this time:

> ensure that asthma management, if required, is optimal

> prescribe self-injectable epinephrine and train her in its use (Fig 37)

> advise her to avoid likely allergens, including hidden allergens such as nuts, pending results of further assessment (see Section 1.2.1)

> refer her to an allergy clinic, making sure that her history and details of possible allergens are documented.

Further comments

Key point

Asthma and food allergy

In patients with food allergy, poorly controlled asthma is an important risk factor for fatal anaphylaxis, underlining the need for optimal asthma control in these patients.

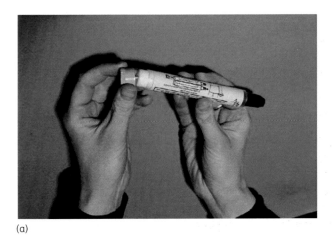

(a)

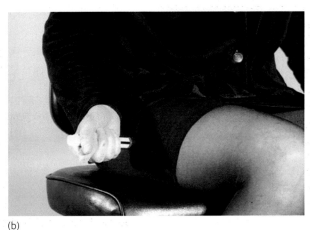

(b)

Fig 37 Use of EpiPen. **(a)** Take cap off the back of the EpiPen. **(b)** Holding the pen as shown, press firmly to the lateral part of the thigh, through clothes if necessary. A click will be felt as the epinephrine is injected. Hold for 10 seconds. After epinephrine self-administration, patients should seek urgent medical attention because the benefit may be temporary. A second 'back-up' epinephrine dose should be provided for use if symptoms do not improve or for if they recur en route to the hospital.

1.4.3 Systemic lupus erythematosus and confusion

Case history

A 35-year-old woman of African-Caribbean origin presents with an acute confusional state.

She first came to medical attention 2 years ago when she presented with joint pains and oedema. A diagnosis of systemic lupus erythematosus (SLE) was made; renal biopsy revealed grade IV glomerulonephritis; and she was initially treated with intravenous pulses of methylprednisolone (followed by oral prednisolone) and cyclophosphamide. Since then her lupus has been active and difficult to control at times. For the past 6 months she has been on prednisolone 15 mg daily and mycophenolate 1 g bd. She has now developed an acute confusional state, the cause of which is not clear and her condition is deteriorating.

On examination her vital signs are not grossly abnormal: temperature 37.4°C, pulse 80 beats per minute, respiration 14 breaths per minute, blood pressure 132/82 mmHg. Her peripheral circulation is normal and her pulse oximetry shows an oxygen saturation of 98% on air. Her Glasgow Coma Score is 13/15 and her Abbreviated Mental Test score is 6/10. Neurological examination is difficult, but there are no clear focal signs and no meningism.

Introduction

Neurological symptoms in a patient with SLE merit urgent investigation. Your aim is to distinguish between the following:

> neuropsychiatric SLE

> central nervous system (CNS; or other) infection in an immunocompromised individual

> a side effect of drug, eg prednisolone, treatment

> unrelated neurological/psychiatric illness.

This can be a very difficult differential diagnosis, but crucially important because the treatment of these conditions is radically different.

History of the presenting problem

Is the lupus active?

Neurological involvement in lupus usually occurs on a background of active systemic disease, but may occasionally occur anew. You should therefore ask relevant questions to assess whether the patient's lupus is active (eg malar rash, mouth ulcers, alopecia, Raynaud's, fatigue, inflammatory arthritis or pleurisy). If the patient is incapable of coherent conversation, ask a relative or partner.

Is this neuropsychiatric lupus?

Neuropsychiatric SLE may present with diffuse or focal symptoms. Ask about the following:

> headache

> seizures

> problems with vision

> limb weakness and numbness

> psychotic symptoms.

How much immunosuppressive treatment has the patient received?

A patient such as this, who has been given pulsed methylprednisolone, cyclophosphamide and other 'aggressive' treatments, is clearly prone to immunosuppression-related infection. By contrast, someone who has received only a modest dose of steroids, perhaps with azathioprine, is at much lower risk.

Has the patient been taking their medications?

It is important to check drug compliance: failure to take medications in a patient with a background of active SLE will predispose the individual to develop a flare.

What features would support a diagnosis of infection?

Pyrexia with obvious evidence of meningism or septicaemia should raise the possibility of meningitis. However, be aware that many of the usual clinical manifestations of sepsis such as fever may be absent in the patient who is immunosuppressed.

Key point

Opportunistic infection may masquerade as neuropsychiatric SLE in patients on prolonged immunosuppressive therapy, and a recent increase in steroid dosage may suggest steroid-induced psychosis.

Other relevant history

Has anything like this happened before, and if so, what was the diagnosis? Does this patient have any history of psychiatric disorders?

Examination

Look carefully for evidence of lupus activity, eg rash, inflammatory arthritis or pericardial/pleural rubs. Given the presentation with confusion, particular emphasis on the neurological examination is required, so look carefully for the following:

> Meningism – if present this would suggest an infective cause.

> Fundi for papilloedema and/or exudates – papilloedema, signifying an increase in intracranial pressure, is unusual in neuropsychiatric SLE and would point to one of the alternative diagnoses. Retinal exudates may occur with both lupus and opportunistic infections such as toxoplasmosis.

> Cranial and peripheral nerves for mononeuritis multiplex, which would suggest active lupus vasculitis.

> Evidence of transverse myelitis in the limbs/trunk/thorax – isolated transverse myelitis is a recognised complication of lupus and would characteristically manifest as a paraparesis with a sensory level.

Investigation

This will be dictated by the nature of the presentation. The differential diagnosis of an acute confusional state is very wide. If the patient looks as though she has a sepsis syndrome, eg cool or warm peripheries, hypotension and a high fever (not present in this case), then she should be treated accordingly, acknowledging that the differential diagnosis will be wider than usual in someone who is immunosuppressed. Neuropsychiatric SLE does not cause circulatory compromise.

Immunological

Key point

Neuropsychiatric SLE is primarily a clinical diagnosis. There is no single reliable laboratory or radiological marker of the condition. A good clinician assessing appropriate serum, cerebrospinal fluid (CSF) and imaging studies has the best chance of coming to the correct conclusion.

Urgent serology is required to assess lupus activity. Check antinuclear antibodies, antibodies to double-stranded DNA, complement C3 and C4 levels, erythrocyte sedimentation rate (ESR) and C-reactive protein (CRP). Antineuronal antibodies directed against the N-methyl-D-aspartate glutamate receptor (anti-NR2) and antiribosomal P antibodies

have been promoted as markers of neuropsychiatric SLE, but are rarely used in practice because of a combination of methodological difficulties and poor sensitivity. Although many cases of neuropsychiatric SLE are associated with worsening serology, exceptional cases may occur with stable serology. A raised CRP is unusual in lupus itself (see Section 3.1.1) and should raise suspicions of infection.

Antiphospholipid antibodies (anticardiolipin and lupus anticoagulant) are useful in delineating patients with the antiphospholipid syndrome, who may present with confusion secondary to thrombotic disease.

Other tests

The following will be required:

> Dipstick urine for protein and blood: if positive for protein, quantitate the urinary albumin to creatinine ratio; if positive for blood, use microscopy to analyse the urine for red cell casts. If these tests are significantly more abnormal than they were at the patient's last routine review, then they suggest that she might have active lupus nephritis, which would make neuropsychiatric SLE more likely.

> Check FBC, electrolytes, renal/liver/bone function tests, blood cultures and urine cultures.

> Brain imaging: a gadolinium-enhanced MRI would be the preferred test, but if one is not readily available, then proceed to a contrast-enhanced CT scan.

> Lumbar puncture: perform as soon as imaging has excluded raised intracranial pressure / mass effect.

Key point

Investigation of suspected neuropsychiatric lupus

It is urgent that you perform brain imaging to exclude space-occupying lesions. A gadolinium-enhanced MRI is the imaging modality of choice, but note that a negative scan does not rule out CNS lupus.

Lumbar puncture – examination of CSF is essential to exclude opportunistic infection; a non-specific cellular pleocytosis, rise in protein and CSF oligoclonal bands occur in 30% of cases of neuropsychiatric lupus.

Management

Urgent specialist advice is required for management of this patient, but the important general message is that neuropsychiatric SLE requires aggressive immunosuppressive therapy – usually using parenteral steroids and cyclophosphamide – with concomitant antimicrobial therapy if infection cannot be excluded. Opportunistic CNS infection should be treated appropriately.

Further comments

The heterogeneity of neuropsychiatric SLE suggests that multiple aetiological factors, ranging from vascular injury to intracranial vessels to antineuronal and antiphospholipid antibodies, are responsible for driving the diverse clinical manifestations of the condition. Cerebral lupus is a diagnosis of exclusion because of the lack of a diagnostic marker and the real difficulties in differentiating between neuropsychiatric lupus and infection of the CNS.

1.4.4 Acute hot joints

Case histories

Case A

A 73-year-old woman presents with a 24-hour history of a painful, swollen and hot right knee. She feels generally unwell and has a temperature of 38.1°C. She has had minor pain and stiffness in both knees for many years.

Case B

A 42-year-old man presents with a hot swollen left elbow. He gives a history of two attacks of severe pain and redness of the big toes over the past 2 years. He is overweight and drinks four or five pints of beer several nights a week.

Case C

A 21-year-old man develops a painful swollen right knee 1 week after returning from a holiday in Spain. He subsequently develops pain and swelling in the left midfoot. He denies any recent episodes of diarrhoea or genitourinary symptoms.

Introduction

What are the differential diagnoses for each case?

> Case A – septic arthritis, pseudogout (pyrophosphate arthritis), gout and haemarthrosis

> Case B – septic arthritis and gout

> Case C – septic arthritis and reactive arthritis.

Which diagnosis should be considered in all of these cases?

Septic arthritis is the primary concern in the assessment of the acute hot joint. This is not the commonest cause of an acute monoarthritis (Table 28), but it is the most serious and has serious potential for severe joint damage and life-threatening septicaemia. If sepsis has been considered and excluded, the main differential diagnosis is between a crystal arthritis and a post-infective reactive arthritis. The history and examination may give pointers towards the correct diagnosis, but sepsis can never be completely excluded on this basis alone. The most important tool in the assessment of the acute hot joint is aspiration of synovial fluid for microscopy, including crystals and culture.

Key point
The hot joint

> The best diagnostic tool is synovial fluid aspiration.

> Always consider the possible diagnosis of septic arthritis.

History of the presenting problem

The history of joint swelling is usually straightforward but helps little with the differential diagnosis. A history of trauma may point to haemarthrosis. Rapid onset of pain and systemic malaise can occur in all the common causes, but severe systemic symptoms and a focus of infection should increase the suspicion of sepsis. A slow, subacute onset makes pyogenic bacterial sepsis less likely, but the possibility of tuberculosis (TB) should be considered. The differential diagnosis is influenced by age: crystal arthritis is the most common cause in older people, whereas reactive arthritis tends to occur in sexually active young adults. Gout and reactive arthritis are more common in men.

Other relevant history

Consider the diagnoses listed in Table 28 – which of these fits the picture best?

Risk factors for sepsis

Is there a history of penetrating injury (either near the joint or elsewhere), which might have acted as a portal of entry? Don't forget intravenous drug abuse. Is there a history of immunosuppression (especially corticosteroid treatment)? Is the patient diabetic?

Table 28	Differential diagnosis of acute hot joints
Frequency of disorder	Examples
Common	Crystal arthritis > Gout (Case B) > Pseudogout (Case A) > Reactive arthritis (Case C) Non-gonococcal septic arthritis caused by pyogenic bacteria > *Staphylococcus aureus* (70%) > Other Gram-positive cocci (20%) > Gram-negative bacilli (10%)
Rare	Haemarthrosis Other spondyloarthritides Other infections > Gonococcal arthritis (becoming more common but still rare in the UK, more common in the USA and Australasia) > Lyme disease > Tuberculosis Palindromic RA Monoarticular presentation of RA Osteonecrosis (especially involving the hip)

RA, rheumatoid arthritis.

Previous similar episodes

Episodic, severe, flitting monoarthritis raises particular suspicions of gout, especially if the first metatarsophalangeal joint has been involved. Palindromic rheumatoid arthritis (RA) may produce a similar picture.

Chronic rheumatological disease

A history suggestive of pre-existing osteoarthritis in the hot joint may point to pseudogout. Patients with RA have an increased risk of sepsis (independent of treatment, but steroid therapy increases the risk further).

Risk factors for gout

Gout is far more common in men, particularly those who are obese, those who drink heavily and those with a family history of the condition. Diuretics (especially thiazides and furosemide (frusemide)) are a common predisposing factor, especially in older people. Gout hardly ever occurs in women, except in the context of diuretic usage or renal impairment.

Infection

Is there any evidence of infection that might have triggered a reactive arthritis? Rheumatologists reserve the term 'reactive arthritis' for a specific syndrome of acute non-infectious monoarthritis or oligoarthritis with a predilection for the large joints of the legs, which occurs after bacterial gastrointestinal infection (*Salmonella*, *Shigella*, *Campylobacter* or *Yersinia* spp) or sexually acquired chlamydial infection. Arthritis can occur alone or together with ocular and mucocutaneous disease. Ask the patient about any recent travel, diarrhoeal illness and genitourinary symptoms, such as penile or vaginal discharge.

Key point

Taking a sexual history

It may be necessary to take a sexual history, but this should be sensitively handled because patients are usually unaware of any possible link between their painful knee and their sex life. This discussion should therefore be left to the end of the consultation, after the rest of the history and examination have been performed, and the topic should be introduced carefully, with explanation, perhaps as follows:

'I need to ask one or two more questions to try to work out why your knee is giving you trouble …'

'There are many reasons why it might be …'

'Some infections can cause the problem …'

'In particular, some genital infections can do this …'

'Are you at risk of any of these …?'

'Have you had any problems in that department?'

'Have you had any discharge or ulceration on your penis/vagina?'

'Have you had sex with any new partners recently?'

Examination: general features

A sick febrile patient should always be considered to have sepsis until proven otherwise (check their temperature, pulse and blood pressure) but remember that sepsis can be present in a patient who initially appears clinically well, especially if they are older or immunosuppressed.

Examination: specific features

> Confirm that the swelling is articular rather than periarticular or subcutaneous. Is an effusion present? Erythema around the joint can occur in gout but should raise a very strong suspicion of sepsis.

> Are the other joints normal, or is there evidence of a more widespread acute inflammatory arthropathy? Are there features of a chronic arthritis preceding the acute illness?

> Look for features suggestive of reactive arthritis / Reiter's syndrome – conjunctivitis/uveitis; scaly rashes on the palms and soles; balanitis; and urethral discharge.

> Look for tophi, which can occur on any pressure point.

Investigation

Key point

Aspiration of synovial fluid is vital for accurate diagnosis. Techniques are not difficult, but if you are not confident then ask someone else. On call, these skills are most likely to be found among the orthopaedic team. Do not defer aspiration because you lack this skill (see Section 3.5).

Joint aspiration

A few drops of fluid are sufficient for microscopy and culture (Fig 38). The macroscopic appearance of synovial fluid may give some clues:

> grossly purulent fluid suggests sepsis

> blood-stained fluid may suggest haemarthrosis, but also occurs in pseudogout.

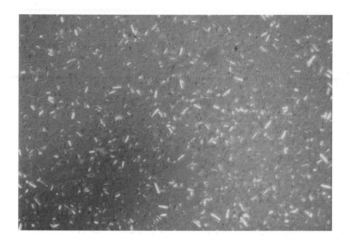

Fig 38 Monosodium urate crystals in synovial fluid from acute gout observed by polarised light microscopy.

Fluid should be sent for urgent:

> polarised light microscopy for crystals

> Gram stain for organisms

> culture.

Gout only rarely coexists with sepsis (unless there is an ulcerating tophus) but pseudogout can coexist with sepsis, hence it may be best to wait 24 hours for culture results before concluding that pseudogout is the primary diagnosis.

Other tests
Blood cultures are mandatory when sepsis is suspected. Other tests provide less useful information:

> FBC – the white cell count, particularly the neutrophil count, is typically raised in acute sepsis, but it may be normal.

> Serum urate often drops in an acute attack of gout so may be unhelpful.

> Inflammatory markers, particularly the C-reactive protein, are rarely diagnostically helpful, but are useful in measuring the subsequent response to therapy.

> Autoantibody testing is hardly ever helpful in this context.

> A clotting screen should be performed in those with haemarthrosis.

> Joint radiographs are largely unhelpful as they show evidence of chronic

joint disease only, although chondrocalcinosis may be seen in a patient with pseudogout.

Management
Immediate management should be admission to hospital if there is a strong suspicion of sepsis or mobility is severely restricted (and appropriate support at home cannot be arranged). If sepsis is unlikely, the patient may be managed as an outpatient with early follow-up.

Start empirical antibiotic therapy if sepsis is clinically likely, ie the patient looks ill or there is purulent synovial fluid / organisms on their Gram stain. In adults, use high-dose flucloxacillin plus a third-generation cephalosporin initially. Antibiotics can be withdrawn if cultures are negative at 24 hours. The minimum period of antibiotic treatment for joint sepsis is 6 weeks (usually including 2 weeks where drugs are given intravenously).

> **Hazard**
> Beware prior antibiotic treatment masking the diagnosis of sepsis.

Further comments
Orthopaedic assessment is useful: arthrotomy / joint wash-out may be

indicated. Orthopaedic surgeons should always deal with suspected sepsis in a prosthetic joint.

NSAIDs may give useful symptom control, but avoid them if possible in the presence of renal impairment (often present in this context). Also beware of past or current history suggestive of peptic ulceration, reflux or NSAID intolerance.

Treatment of non-septic arthritides with intra-articular steroids may be indicated. In most patients, do this only after negative culture, although some may be injected at the time of initial assessment (eg recurrent gout). If in doubt, wait.

Consider unusual infections (eg TB and fungal) in patients with immunosuppression or a history of foreign travel.

Avoid weight bearing on a severely inflamed joint, but splintage is not usually necessary. Arrange for early mobilisation as inflammation subsides; physiotherapy input will be required.

Do not forget longer-term issues: screening for chlamydial infection in sexually active patients with non-crystal, non-septic arthritis; gout prophylaxis; and gout as a surrogate marker for diabetes, hypertension and hyperlipidaemia.

1.4.5 A crush fracture

> **Case history**
> A 65-year-old woman develops severe low thoracic back pain and right flank pain while gardening. She has a history of thyrotoxicosis and smokes 10 cigarettes per day. She is reviewed in the emergency department by the urologists for suspected renal colic, but investigation of her urinary tract is normal and she is referred to the physicians. You are asked to see her.

Introduction

A genitourinary cause for her symptoms has been excluded – the remaining differential diagnoses are:

> vertebral collapse due to osteoporosis

> vertebral collapse due to other causes, eg malignancy

> mechanical thoracic back pain and radiculopathy

> gastrointestinal disease, eg pancreatitis

> aortic aneurysm.

The most likely cause of a vertebral crush fracture in a woman of 65 years is osteoporosis, but trauma (not likely to be relevant in this case) and local vertebral pathology (especially secondary tumours or myeloma) should be considered. The most common sites for osteoporotic vertebral fractures are mid-dorsal and the thoracolumbar junction, giving potential for confusion with other causes of chest and flank pain.

Important considerations if the diagnosis is osteoporotic collapse are the cause (postmenopausal, corticosteroid-induced, myeloma, etc) and the severity, which is predictive of the risk of further fractures.

Key point

The risk of osteoporotic fracture is influenced heavily by the risk of falling. This risk should be assessed and treatable causes addressed.

History of the presenting problem

Osteoporotic fracture

The diagnosis of possible osteoporotic fracture will often have been made before referral to you, but the condition should be considered in spinal pain with the following characteristics:

> sudden onset

> provoked by movement

> ameliorated by rest

> present especially in postmenopausal women and others at increased risk of osteoporosis

> associated with nerve root irritation or entrapment, which may produce referred pain or paraesthesia with dermatomal distribution.

Other causes of the fracture

Are there any clues to a malignant process? Think about the possibilities as you take the history. Check whether the patient has had any of the following symptoms recently:

> malaise or weight loss

> difficulty breathing or a productive cough – these might indicate respiratory pathology (lung cancer) or anaemia (gastrointestinal (GI) bleeding, bone marrow secondaries or myeloma) in this context

> indigestion or change in her bowels (GI malignancy)

> bone pain elsewhere (secondaries or myeloma).

Other relevant history

Osteoporosis

A history of femoral neck fracture, Colles' fracture or clinical/radiological evidence of a previous vertebral fracture (Fig 39) are the best surrogate markers of the severity of bone loss and future fracture risk.

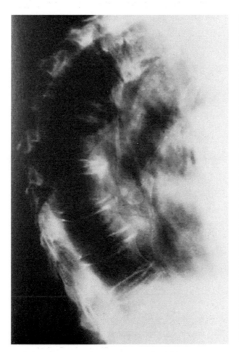
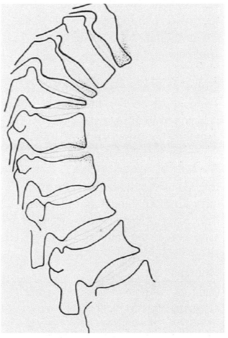

Fig 39 Multiple osteoporotic fractures in the thoracic spine. (Courtesy of Dr M Pattrick.)

Causes of osteoporosis

Ask about the following:

> menstrual history – at the age of 65 years she will certainly be postmenopausal, but what was her age at menopause, and has she had a hysterectomy/oophorectomy or prolonged amenorrhoea at any time, eg due to anorexia nervosa?

> steroid treatment – risk depends on the dose and duration of treatment

> frequency of exercise

> dietary history – in particular, does she have an adequate calcium intake?

> family history.

Risk of falls

Ask about the following:

> previous falls

> pre-existing neurological or locomotor disease

> postural dizziness

> alcohol use

> use of psychotropic drugs.

Other causes of vertebral fracture

Does she have a history of malignancy or 'problems with the blood'?

Examination: general features

Does the patient look as though she might have a malignancy? Take particular care to look for the following: weight loss / cachexia; pallor; lymphadenopathy; breast lump; and abnormal chest, abdominal or rectal signs.

Could the patient have a secondary cause for osteoporosis? Is there evidence of thyrotoxicosis, hypogonadism (in a man) or Cushing's disease?

Examination: specific features

The level of the vertebral fracture may be marked by a palpable step. Look for diffuse dorsal kyphosis as a marker of long-standing severe bone loss.

Look for the following to assess the risk of falling:

> visible unsteadiness/frailty

> postural drop in blood pressure

> neurological signs – in particular, is there a sensory level, sphincter disturbance and/or weakness in the legs as pointers towards possible cord compression?

Investigations

These will obviously be dictated by the findings on history and examination.

Consideration of secondary causes

The need to pursue secondary causes of osteoporosis varies depending on the patient's age, other risk factors, ill-health and clinical suspicion. The following tests should be considered: FBC; renal and liver function; bone biochemistry (raised alkaline phosphatase may suggest osteomalacia or secondaries; hypercalcaemia may suggest malignancy, especially myeloma); immunoglobulins and serum and urine electrophoresis (to exclude myeloma in older people); thyroid function; testosterone (in men); chest radiograph; and investigations for Cushing's syndrome.

Diagnosis of osteoporosis

The gold standard for the diagnosis and planning of treatment is bone densitometry at two sites, usually the hip and the lumbar spine. The presence of a fracture consistent with osteoporosis in the presence of risk factors is often enough to make the diagnosis. Histology is rarely useful and even more rarely obtained.

Management

Pain control – pain may be severe and require opiates. Consider supplementary approaches such as TENS (transcutaneous electrical nerve stimulation) machines and epidural analgesia. Calcitonin will improve acute pain.

Avoid immobility – this will increase the risk of bronchopneumonia and venous thromboembolism (consider prophylactic heparin).

Treat secondary causes of osteoporosis if any are identified, but most symptomatic osteoporosis will be postmenopausal and managed by the following:

> lifestyle modification – avoid falls, but encourage safe exercise

> optimisation of calcium intake

> bisphosphonates, which are now the standard treatment for osteoporosis. It is important to explain to the patient how bisphosphonates should be taken (eg if taking alendronate or risedronate, the patient must take the drug on an empty stomach and remain upright for a further 30 minutes before further eating or drinking).

There are alternative treatments if the patient cannot tolerate or has contraindications to bisphosphonates. These include:

> raloxifene, a selective oestrogen receptor modulator (SERM) that has oestrogenic actions on bone

> strontium ranelate, which increases bone formation and inhibits resorption

> teriparatide, a parathyroid hormone analogue that stimulates osteoblasts and inhibits bone resorption

> denosumab, a humanised monoclonal antibody that binds and inhibits RANKL (receptor activator of *nuclear factor kappa B* (NFκB) ligand), thereby blocking osteoclast survival and function.

Rheumatology and clinical immunology: Section 2

2 Diseases and treatments

2.1 Immunodeficiency

2.1.1 Primary antibody deficiency

Aetiology/pathophysiology/pathology

Common variable immunodeficiency (CVID) comprises a group of heterogeneous acquired primary antibody deficiency syndromes characterised by hypogammaglobulinaemia. While B-cells are present in most patients they fail to produce immunoglobulin G (IgG), immunoglobulin A (IgA) and sometimes immunoglobulin M (IgM) (Fig 40). Some variants are associated with sarcoid-like granulomas. Autoimmunity (organ specific and haematological) is common. There may be coexistent T-cell defects. Most cases are polygenic in origin but a number of monogenic forms have been described (Table 29).

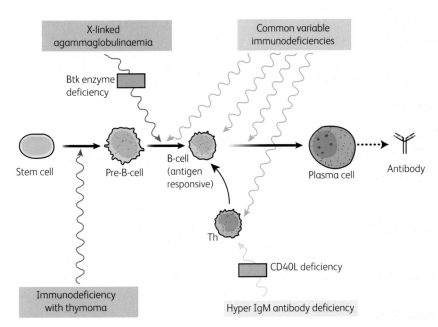

Fig 40 Overview of the steps in B-cell maturation and the levels at which more common defects in antibody production may occur. (Reproduced with permission from Chapel H, Haeney M, Misbah S, Snowden N. *Essentials of clinical immunology*, 4th edn. Oxford: Blackwell Science, 1999.)

Table 29	Selected monogenic CVID-like immunodeficiencies	
Gene	**Clinical features**	**Autoimmunity**
CTLA-4	Autosomal dominant, respiratory infections, diarrhoea, lymphoid organ infiltration	Yes – multiple
ICOS	Recurrent respiratory and GI infections	Yes
LRBA	Recurrent respiratory infections, enteropathy	Yes
NFKB2	Autosomal dominant, recurrent respiratory infections, meningococcal meningitis, adrenal insufficiency	Yes - ITP
PIK3CD	Autosomal dominant, recurrent respiratory infections, severe herpes virus infections, lymphoma	No

ITA, idiopathic thrombocytopenic purpura.
Adapted with permission from: Bonilla F, Barlan I, Chapel H *et al.* International Consensus Document (ICON): Common Variable Immunodeficiency Disorders. *Journal of Allergy and Clinical Immunology: In Practice* 2016;4:38–59.

Key point

Evidence against an intrinsic B-cell defect in common variable immunodeficiency

> B-cells in CVID are capable of secreting immunoglobulins *in vitro* with appropriate stimulation.

> Infection with viruses (HIV, hepatitis C virus) can sometimes reverse hypogammaglobulinaemia in CVID.

Epidemiology

The incidence is estimated at one in 10,000 to one in 50,000. It may be sporadic or inherited in an autosomal dominant manner with variable phenotype; affected family members may have autoimmunity alone, IgA or IgG subclass deficiencies, or CVID. Ninety-five per cent of patients present in adulthood.

Clinical presentation

Common

Complications of antibody deficiency

Complications include bacterial infections, especially of the respiratory and gastrointestinal tracts, and the skin (Fig 41).

Autoimmunity

Organ-specific (especially thyroid disease and pernicious anaemia):

> haematological: anaemia, neutropenia and thrombocytopenia

> arthritis: reactive or septic; consider the possibility of *Mycoplasma* spp if cultures are negative.

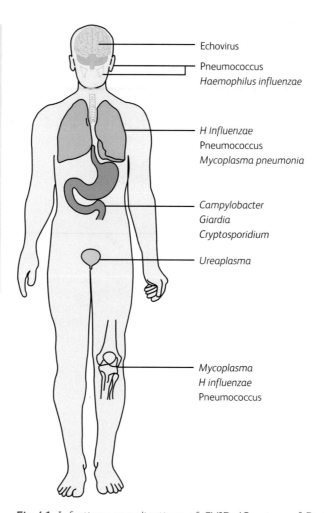

Echovirus
Pneumococcus
Haemophilus influenzae

H Influenzae
Pneumococcus
Mycoplasma pneumonia

Campylobacter
Giardia
Cryptosporidium

Ureaplasma

Mycoplasma
H influenzae
Pneumococcus

Fig 41 Infectious complications of CVID. (Courtesy of Dr ADB Webster.)

Key point

B-cells in CVID exhibit a curious paradox

Despite their inability to mount antibody responses to exogenous antigens, patients with CVID do mount antibody responses to self-antigens, resulting in autoimmune disease.

Granulomas

These include lung infiltrates and hepatosplenomegaly (Fig 42).

Uncommon

> coeliac-like enteropathy

> diseases associated with T-cell deficiencies such as herpes zoster.

Rare

> nodular lymphoid hyperplasia

> thymoma.

Physical signs

Common physical signs

> signs of bronchiectasis

> lymphadenopathy and hepatosplenomegaly

> arthritis

> thyroid enlargement.

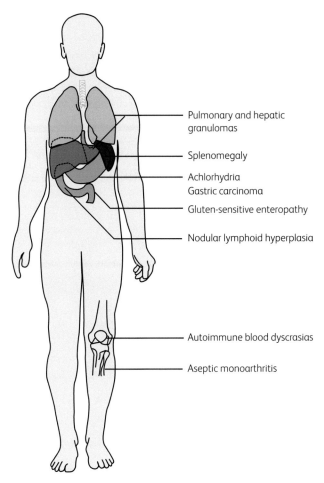

Pulmonary and hepatic granulomas

Splenomegaly

Achlorhydria
Gastric carcinoma

Gluten-sensitive enteropathy

Nodular lymphoid hyperplasia

Autoimmune blood dyscrasias

Aseptic monoarthritis

Fig 42 Non-infectious complications of CVID. (Courtesy of Dr ADB Webster.)

Uncommon physical sign

> wasting.

Investigation

> Serum IgG, IgA and IgM. IgG subclasses are of limited value. Assess the severity of antibody deficiency by measuring antibodies to past immunisations (tetanus and diphtheria) and common pathogens (*Streptococcus pneumoniae* and *Haemophilus influenzae* type b). If baseline antibody levels are low, proceed to test immunisation and measure antibody levels in 4 weeks.

> CD3, CD4, CD8 and CD19 lymphocyte markers (to quantify total, helper and cytotoxic T-cell and B-cell

numbers, respectively). Most patients with CVID have normal numbers of circulating B-cells; a minority have no B-cells and clinically resemble X-linked agammaglobulinaemia (XLA).

> Quantification of circulating class-switched memory B-cells (CD27+, IgM-, IgD-) is useful in defining subpopulations of patients with granulomatous disease, splenomegaly, bronchiectasis and autoimmunity.

> Blood count and differential.

Differential diagnosis

> Secondary antibody deficiencies: the result of drugs (anti-B-cell biologics, gold, penicillamine, cytotoxics and antiepileptics); associated with

lymphoproliferative disease (particularly chronic lymphocytic leukaemia, myeloma or lymphoma); and post-bone marrow transplantation.

> Bruton's XLA: peak age of presentation 4 months to 2 years of age. Presents with absent B-cells, absent lymphoid tissue, and no granulomas or autoimmune disease.

> Combined immunodeficiencies: T-cell-associated infections are more prominent (see Section 2.1.2) and usually present in early childhood.

Hyper-IgM syndromes

These are characterised as follows:

> CD40 ligand deficiency is the best characterised.

> They are X-linked.

> IgG levels are low, while levels of IgM are high or normal.

> T-cell numbers are normal but functionally defective, with a high risk of long-term opportunistic infection, particularly *Pneumocystis* pneumonia or cryptosporidial sclerosing cholangitis.

> Bone marrow transplantation should be considered.

> Other causes of hyper-IgM syndromes include uracil-*N*-glycosylase deficiency, CD40 deficiency (features and management as for CD40 ligand deficiency) and activation-induced cytidine deaminase deficiency (less severe, T-cell function normal and managed as for CVID).

X-linked lymphoproliferative disease (Duncan's syndrome)

This disease, a defect in SAP (a signalling lymphocyte-activating, molecule-associated protein), usually presents with overwhelming Epstein–Barr virus infection or lymphoma, but occasionally with a CVID-like picture. Bone marrow transplantation may be considered.

Treatment

Emergency
Prompt treatment of all infections, with an appropriate course of antibiotics.

Long term
Regular subcutaneous or intravenous immunoglobulin therapy at 1 or 3 weekly intervals, respectively (see Section 3.7). Aim to achieve trough serum IgG levels well within the normal range.

Key point

Trough serum IgG levels maintained at >5 g/L prevent deterioration in lung function.

Complications

Common

> bronchiectasis secondary to recurrent infection

> anaemia, thrombocytopenia and neutropenia (haematological autoimmunity, splenomegaly and vitamin deficiencies resulting from malabsorption).

Uncommon

> increased risk of lymphoma (23–100-fold)

> gastric carcinoma (50-fold increase).

Key point

Difficulties in the diagnosis of lymphoma in CVID

Lymph-node biopsies in patients with CVID may reveal a bizarre histology mimicking lymphoma. Biopsies should therefore be reported by a histopathologist experienced in examining tissue from patients with immune deficiency.

Rare

> severe opportunistic infections caused by T-cell deficiency such as *Pneumocystis* pneumonia.

Prognosis

Morbidity

> Of those with CVID, 75% suffer frequent or chronic infections.

> 14% have structural damage, such as bronchiectasis.

Mortality
The mean age at death for all patients who have antibody deficiencies is 40.5 years, but the range is wide. The main causes of death are sepsis, chronic lung disease, lymphoma and other malignancies.

Prevention
The mean delay in diagnosis of 7.5 years accounts for a great deal of the cases that result in morbidity and mortality. Serum immunoglobulins should be checked in anyone with unusually severe, prolonged or recurrent bacterial infections, or granulomatous disease.

2.1.2 Combined T-cell and B-cell defects

Aetiology/pathophysiology/pathology
Inherited genetic defects result in the failure of the normal development or maturation of T-lymphocytes and B-lymphocytes, or the build-up of metabolites toxic to developing lymphocytes (Table 30). Without T-cell help, the production of antibodies by B-cells is severely limited. To date, at least 18 distinct molecular defects associated with severe combined immunodeficiency (SCID) have been identified, with eight of the more common defects listed in Table 30.

Epidemiology
These defects are a heterogeneous group of conditions. They usually have autosomal recessive or sex-linked inheritance. The incidence of SCID is estimated to be between one in 50,000 and one in 100,000 live births in France.

Clinical presentation

Common

> presents in infancy

> recurrent infections, sometimes with unusual 'opportunistic' organisms, and a slow response to treatment

> pneumonia, skin infections, eczema and persistent diarrhoea

> failure to thrive

> absent thymic shadow on chest X-ray

> features of associated syndromes.

Key point

Persistent lymphopenia in an ill baby is an important clue pointing towards SCID.

Uncommon

> graft-versus-host disease (GVHD) from immunocompetent maternal cells or transfused blood

> invasive disease from Bacillus Calmette–Guérin (BCG) given at birth.

Rare

> adult presentation: this usually means a milder phenotype

> papilloma viruses: warts, or cervical or anal intraepithelial neoplasia

Table 30 Combined immunodeficiency disorders

Time of presentation	Disorder	Key features
Presenting as SCID during infancy	ADA deficiency[1]	Marked T- and B-cell lymphopenia, and reduced serum immunoglobulin Autosomal recessive
	Common cytokine receptor γ-chain deficiency (γ chain shared by IL-2, IL-4, IL-7, IL-9 and IL-15)	Marked T-cell lymphopenia, reduced serum immunoglobulin, normal or increased B-cell numbers and X-linked
	IL-7 receptor α-chain deficiency	T-cell lymphopenia and reduced serum immunoglobulins
	Janus kinase 3 deficiency	As for cytokine receptor γ-chain deficiency Autosomal recessive
	Recombinase activating gene 1/2 deficiency	Marked T- and B-cell lymphopenia, and reduced serum immunoglobulin
	Omenn syndrome	Increased serum IgE, eosinophilia, reduced serum immunoglobulin and B-cell numbers normal or reduced
	IL-2 receptor α-chain deficiency	T-cell lymphopenia, serum immunoglobulin and B-cell numbers normal
	Purine nucleoside[1] and phosphorylase deficiency	T-cell lymphopenia, reduced serum urate and serum immunoglobulin normal or reduced
Presenting in later life, including adulthood	X-linked hyper-IgM (CD40 ligand deficiency)	Reduced serum IgG and IgA, with increased or normal IgM

1 Milder forms of SCID may present in adulthood, eg ADA deficiency.
ADA, adenosine deaminase; IgA, immunoglobulin A; IgE, immunoglobulin E; IgG, immunoglobulin G; IgM, immunoglobulin M; IL, interleukin; SCID, severe combined immunodeficiency.

> herpes viruses: herpes simplex 1 and 2, severe varicella zoster virus and Epstein–Barr virus-associated disease

> lymphoproliferation and lymphomas

> John Cunningham (JC) virus: associated with progressive encephalopathy

> bacterial infections, especially respiratory tract and intracellular bacteria such as *Salmonella* spp

> mycobacterial disease, including tuberculosis

> fungal infections: mucocutaneous *Candida* infection, *Pneumocystis* pneumonia (Fig 43) and invasive cryptococci

> protozoal disease: cryptosporidial diarrhoea and cholangitis, and toxoplasma cerebral abscess.

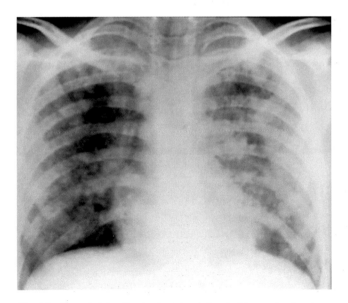

Fig 43 Chest radiograph showing bilateral lung shadowing caused by *Pneumocystis carinii* pneumonia.

Physical signs

Common signs are:

> poor growth and structural organ damage from repeated infections

> active infections often present.

Investigations

Babies with clinical features suggestive of SCID and lymphopenia (lymphocytes $<1.5 \times 10^9$ in a newborn) should be referred urgently to a regional centre (see Section 3.3).

Differential diagnosis

Secondary immunodeficiency, such as HIV or lymphoid malignancy.

Treatment

Short term

> avoid live vaccines

> irradiate blood products

> active diagnosis and early, aggressive treatment of infections.

> **! Hazard**

> To avoid graft versus host disease (GVHD), blood products should be irradiated before transfusion in patients with suspected cellular immune defects.

Long term

Prophylaxis of infection

Intravenous immunoglobulin and an antibiotic (co-trimoxazole), which provides cover against *Pneumocystis* and bacterial infections.

Correction of defect

In some cases, enzyme replacement (eg in adenosine deaminase (ADA) deficiency) may be possible, but success is limited. Alternatively:

> Consider haemopoietic stem cell transplantation (HSCT) if a human leukocyte antigen (HLA) match is available. Currently, HSCT from an HLA-matched sibling donor offers an 80% chance of cure for babies with SCID, while a fully HLA-matched unrelated transplant offers a 70% chance of cure.

> In the absence of a matched bone marrow donor, gene therapy has been successful in some children with ADA and some with common γ-chain deficiency. A new generation of self-inactivating lentiviral vectors has been successfully used to date in common γ-chain SCID to reduce the previously observed risk of insertional mutagenesis.

Complications

Structural damage from recurrent infections:

> malignancy, especially lymphoma

> vasculitis resulting from immune dysregulation.

Prognosis

Morbidity

Morbidity is severe, due to recurrent infections.

Mortality

Most affected individuals die in infancy or early childhood. For those surviving until adulthood, their prognosis is poor if prior bone marrow transplantation has not been carried out. Death occurs from uncontrolled infection or malignancy.

Prevention

Prenatal diagnosis is often possible. Neonatal screening for SCID using PCR (polymerase chain reaction)-based analysis of T-cell receptor excision circles (TRECS – a measure of thymic T-cell output) on Guthrie card blood spots has recently been introduced in the USA.

Disease associations

Combined immunodeficiencies often occur in association with other congenital diseases, particularly cardiac, haematological, neurological (including learning difficulties) or skeletal (including dysmorphic facies).

2.1.3 Chronic granulomatous disease

Aetiology/pathophysiology/pathology

Chronic granulomatous disease (CGD) is due to an inherited defect in one of four *phox* genes, which encode subunits of nicotinamide adenine dinucleotide phosphate (NADPH) oxidase, the enzyme that catalyses the phagocyte respiratory burst (Fig 44), resulting in the defective killing of engulfed organisms.

Epidemiology

> Rare – incidence is one in 250,000.

> Most cases (67%) present in infancy, but diagnosis is occasionally delayed until early adulthood.

> 65% are X-linked and 35% have autosomal recessive inheritance.

Clinical presentation

Common

Infections

Pneumonia, lymphadenitis, skin infections, hepatic abscesses, osteomyelitis, perianal suppuration and enteric infections. Organisms are usually catalase positive (Table 31).

Granulomas

As chemotaxis and phagocytosis are unimpaired, ineffective killing by phagocytes results in the formation of granulomas; these manifest as lymphadenopathy, hepatosplenomegaly, Crohn's disease-like enteropathy with diarrhoea, dermatitis or obstructive hydronephrosis.

Miscellaneous

> anaemia of chronic disease

> gingivitis

> asymptomatic chorioretinopathy.

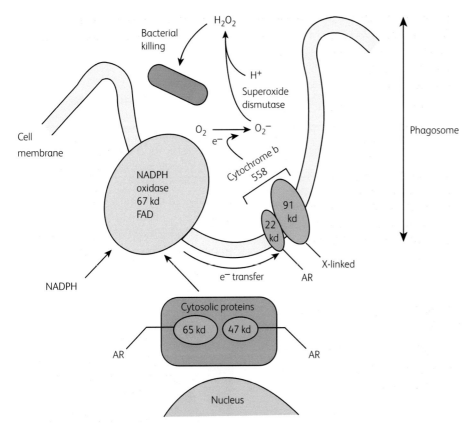

Fig 44 Diagrammatic representation of components of the NADPH oxidase system within a phagosome, depicting bacterial killing and the site of abnormalities in chronic granulomatous disease (CGD). AR, autosomal recessive; FAD, flavin adenine dinucleotide. (Modified with permission from Gallin JI, Malech HL. Update on chronic granulomatous diseases of childhood: immunotherapy and potential for gene therapy. *JAMA* 1990;263:1533–7.)

Table 31	Common pathogens in CGD
Bacteria	**Fungi**
Staphylococcus spp	*Aspergillus* spp
Escherichia coli	*Candida* spp
Salmonella spp	
Klebsiella spp	
Serratia spp	
Burkholderia spp	

Investigations

Screen with the nitroblue tetrazolium (NBT) test (see Fig 5) or the dihydrorhodamine fluorescence test (see Section 1.1.4). If the screening test is abnormal, check for the presence of NADPH oxidase subunits and associated gene defects.

Key point

The NBT screening test may be misleadingly normal in some patients with CGD. Proceed to flow cytometric evaluation of the respiratory burst and genetic studies in case of diagnostic doubt.

Differential diagnosis

> idiopathic abscesses without obvious immunodeficiency

> Crohn's disease

> neutrophil glucose-6-dehydrogenase, myeloperoxidase or glutathione peroxidase deficiency.

Key point

Other neutrophil defects

Common

> Neutropenia: usually secondary to medication or disease. Treat/withdraw the causative agent. Consider granulocyte colony-stimulating factor (GCSF).

Rare

> Cyclical neutropenia: 3-weekly cycle of neutropenia, associated with infection. Neutrophil count may be normal or high by the time the patient presents. Check their neutrophil count three times weekly for 1 month. Treat with antibiotic prophylaxis (co-trimoxazole) or exceptionally with GCSF, to cover the predicted times of neutropenia.

> Leukocyte adhesion molecule deficiencies (CD18/CD11 and CD15): marked neutrophilia (even during infection-free intervals) caused by defective leukocyte–endothelial interaction, impaired pus formation and poor wound healing. Severe phenotypes present in childhood and require bone marrow transplantation.

Treatment

Emergency

This requires early, empirical treatment of the suspected infection with broad-spectrum antimicrobials.

Short term

> Aggressive search for source and organism; cultures of blood and a sample from the possible site(s) of infection. Drain large abscesses. Take biopsies; an excision biopsy of inflammatory masses and lymph nodes is preferable because of the risk of fistula formation.

> Initiate early empirical parenteral antibiotic treatment. Consider adjunctive interferon-γ (IFN-γ). Prolonged treatment is usually required.

> Granulomas may be troublesome. Steroids (prednisolone 0.5 mg/kg, reducing after a few weeks) can help, but take care that any infections are controlled with antibiotics.

Long term

> Antimicrobial prophylaxis with co-trimoxazole and itraconazole.

> Consider IFN-γ 0.05 mg/kg three times weekly, which reduces infections despite the persistence of defective respiratory burst.

> Bone marrow transplantation is curative, but requires expert risk–benefit evaluation as the risks outweigh the benefits for many patients.

> Gene therapy offers a promising future treatment.

Complications

> chronic suppurative perianal disease

> anaemia of chronic disease

> structural damage caused by abscesses or granulomas.

Prognosis

Morbidity

Morbidity from infections and granulomas is significant.

Mortality

Of patients with CGD, 30–50% historically survived to adulthood. Prognosis has improved significantly with better prophylaxis and treatment.

Prevention

Primary

Prenatal diagnosis is possible.

Secondary

> avoidance of fungal spores (composts, rotting hay, humidifiers and marijuana)

> no smoking

> immediate cleaning of all abrasions and rinsing with 2% hydrogen peroxide

> meticulous perianal hygiene and avoidance of constipation

> careful dental cleaning, flossing and use of mouthwash.

Disease associations

McLeod's syndrome

This is a mild haemolytic anaemia caused by poor expression of erythrocyte Kell antigens. Patients with McLeod's syndrome require Kell-negative products if transfusion is required.

2.1.4 Cytokine and cytokine-receptor deficiencies

Aetiology/pathophysiology/pathology

Mutations in the genes for the interleukin (IL)-12, IL-12 receptor, IL-12 signalling pathway and the interferon-γ (IFN-γ) receptor (Fig 45) are associated with defective macrophage and T-helper (Th) 1-cell function, which lead to failure to eradicate mycobacteria. At least seven autosomal mutations and two X-linked mutations confer susceptibility to non-tuberculous mycobacteria (Fig 45). In addition, functional defects of the IL-12–IFN-γ pathways can present in adulthood. These may be idiopathic or caused by IFN-γ antibodies.

Key point

Other cytokine and cytokine receptor deficiencies

Mutations in the common γ chain of IL-2, IL-4, IL-7, IL-9 and IL-15 receptors and IL-2 or IL-7 deficiency result in severe combined immunodeficiency.

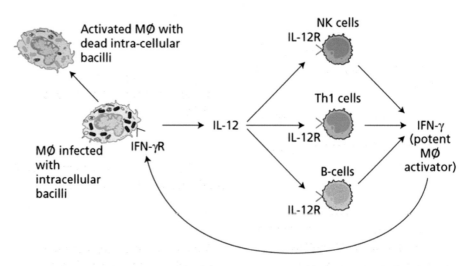

Fig 45 Role of the IL-12–IFN-γ pathway in protective immunity. IL-12R, interleukin-12 receptor; IFN-γ, interferon-γ; MØ, macrophage; IFN-γR, interferon-γ receptor; NK, natural killer; Th1, T helper 1.

Epidemiology

These are rare inherited autosomal dominant or recessive or X-linked recessive disorders, although instances of disease presenting in middle age may be acquired.

Clinical presentation

Common

> disseminated disease as a result of environmental mycobacteria of low virulence, or after BCG immunisation.

Uncommon

> recurrent *Salmonella* infection.

Physical signs

The signs are similar to those for mycobacterial disease in immunocompetent individuals.

Investigation

IFN-γ production by activated lymphocytes is reduced in IL-12, IL-12 receptor and IFN-γ receptor deficiencies. Routine immunological investigations are normal or non-specific, but clinical features will suggest the need for further investigation.

Differential diagnosis

Consider other primary or secondary T-cell defects, particularly late-stage HIV infection.

Tumour necrosis factor (TNF) or IL-12 inhibitors may be associated with disseminated tuberculosis or atypical mycobacteria.

Treatment

> antibiotic treatment of mycobacterial disease: prolonged treatment with multiple agents is likely to be required

> IFN-γ supplementation

> acquired IFN-γ antibodies may require rituximab treatment

> bone marrow transplantation – although results are poor in the presence of active mycobacterial infection.

> **Hazard**
> Atypical mycobacteria are resistant to some conventional antituberculous drugs, such as isoniazid, rifabutin, ethambutol, azithromycin and ciprofloxacin. Some second-line antituberculous drugs may be useful despite apparent resistance *in vitro*. Expert advice is required.

Complications

Complications are those of uncontrolled mycobacterial disease.

Prognosis

Morbidity

There is considerable morbidity from mycobacterial disease and its treatment.

Mortality

> very high

> long-term control of disease is possible in variants that respond to IFN-γ.

Prevention

Avoid BCG in close family members until the defect has been excluded.

Disease associations

> Some individuals have increased susceptibility to *Salmonella* spp.

> There is occasional association with CD4 lymphopenia.

> There is occasional association with chronic mucocutaneous candidiasis and organ-specific autoimmunity (IFN-γ antibodies).

2.1.5 Terminal pathway complement deficiency

Aetiology/pathophysiology/pathology

> inherited deletion of the terminal complement (C5–C9) gene

> lack of complement-mediated lysis results in inefficient clearance of neisserial infections.

Epidemiology

Autosomal recessive inheritance.

Clinical presentation

Common

> recurrent invasive meningococcal disease

> asymptomatic relative.

> **Key point**
> **Primary complement deficiency with meningococcal infection**
>
> The following are pointers towards primary complement deficiency in patients with meningococcal infection:
>
> > unusual meningococcal serotype
>
> > recurrent disease
>
> > a family history of meningococcal disease.

Uncommon

> disseminated gonococcal disease.

Physical signs

There are usually no physical signs specifically associated with complement deficiency.

Investigations

Assess the integrity of the complement pathway by checking haemolytic complement activity (classical pathway CH50 and alternative pathway AP50). The absence or marked reduction of both CH50 and AP50 suggests deficiency of terminal complement proteins C5–C9 (see Fig 46 and Table 1).

Key point

> Complement proteins are labile.
> Samples for haemolytic complement activity should therefore be sent to the laboratory immediately.

Differential diagnosis

> consider external connection to subarachnoid space: head injury, erosive sinus disease and post-pituitary surgery

> properdin or factor D deficiency (AP50 will be absent and CH50 will be normal)

> other immunodeficiency.

Treatment

Emergency

This involves the prompt treatment of neisserial infection.

Short term

> chemoprophylaxis of household contacts.

Long term

> prophylactic antibiotics

> meningococcal immunisation

> annual influenza immunisation.

Complications

The complications are those of neisserial disease.

Prognosis

Meningococcal disease may not be as severe in the presence of complement deficiency. However, there is a significant risk of permanent disability or death.

Key point

Meningococcal disease tends to be less severe in complement-deficient patients, presumably reflecting the requirement for an intact complement pathway to cause bacterial endotoxin release.

Prevention

Primary

Primary prevention is by genetic counselling and screening of relatives at risk.

Key point

Other complement deficiencies

> C1q, C2 or C4 deficiency: C1q deficiency is strongly associated with systemic lupus erythematosus, followed in turn by homozygous C4 and C2 deficiency. Individuals with such deficiencies may be antinuclear antibody negative, but are more likely to be Ro positive.

> Mannan-binding ligand deficiency is common and results in a mild predisposition to bacterial infections. However, this is usually evident only if another immunodeficiency is present.

> C3 deficiency causes glomerulonephritis and a predisposition to bacterial infections.

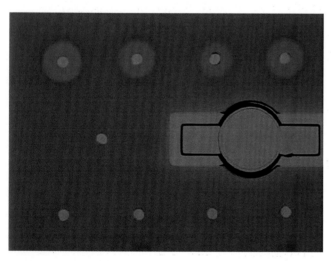

Fig 46 Haemolytic complement screening test for complement deficiency. This test measures the ability of complement in the patient's serum to lyse antibody-coated erythrocytes via the classical pathway. The coated erythrocytes are embedded in a gel. Control and test sera are placed in wells and left overnight. Normal sera containing complement components C1–C9 lyse the erythrocytes – seen as a ring around the well (top wells). Sera that are completely deficient in one or more complement components do not cause lysis (middle and bottom rows).

2.1.6 Hyposplenism

Aetiology/pathophysiology/pathology

The spleen is the major lymphoid organ for blood-borne antigens. Splenic macrophages remove bacteria, immune complexes and abnormal erythrocytes from the circulation. Anatomically, the spleen is organised into distinct T- and B-cell zones (Fig 47). The splenic marginal zone, which borders the white pulp, is an important repository of B-cells critical for the production of antibodies to polysaccharide antigens.

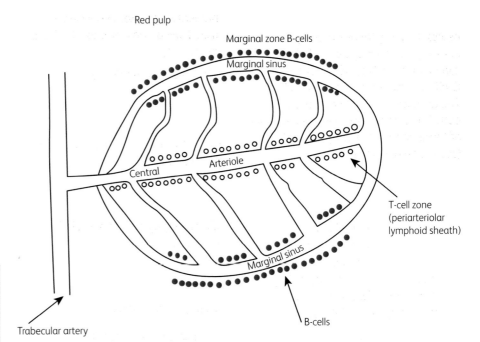

Fig 47 Schematic representation of spleen depicting T- and B-cells zones.

Key point

Immunological consequences of asplenia

> removal of a large reservoir of polysaccharide-responsive B-cells

> impaired clearance of encapsulated bacteria and intracellular protozoans (*Plasmodium* and *Babesia* spp)

> necessity for higher antibody levels for macrophages to clear encapsulated bacteria

> reduction in immunoglobulin M (IgM) memory B-cells leading to impaired response to polysaccharide antigens.

Clinical presentation

Common

> asymptomatic: known because of underlying condition

> fulminant septicaemia.

Uncommon

> Howell–Jolly bodies noted on blood film.

Rare

> congenital asplenia, with cardiac abnormalities and biliary atresia.

Physical signs

There are usually no physical signs except for a splenectomy scar.

Investigations

> If a blood film shows Howell–Jolly bodies (see Fig 35) this suggests functional hyposplenism. However, the absence of Howell–Jolly bodies does not reliably exclude hyposplenism. Proceed to functional studies of splenic function (pitted red cell count and radioisotope uptake) in cases of diagnostic uncertainty.

> Ultrasonography to confirm anatomical absence.

> Pneumococcal, *Haemophilus influenza* type b and meningococcal antibodies – higher antibody levels are required for protection in asplenic individuals.

Treatment

Emergency

Any febrile illness should be urgently investigated and empirical treatment started immediately.

Long term

> pneumococcal, *Haemophilus* and meningococcal immunisation (see Section 1.4.1 for recommendations on immunisation)

> annual influenza vaccination

> lifelong penicillin prophylaxis.

Complications

Common

> fulminant septicaemia, especially with encapsulated organisms (pneumococci, *Haemophilus influenzae* type b and meningococci).

Uncommon

> severe malaria.

Rare

> babesiosis

> infection with *Capnocytophaga canimorsus* (from dog bite).

Prognosis

Mortality

There is a significant lifelong risk of death from overwhelming infection.

Disease associations

> haemoglobinopathies

> coeliac disease

> inflammatory bowel disease

> bone marrow transplantation.

2.2 Allergy

2.2.1 Anaphylaxis

Aetiology/pathophysiology/pathology

The mechanisms of allergy (Fig 48) involve sensitisation (exposure to allergen and specific immunoglobulin E (IgE) production); followed by mast cell degranulation (re-exposure to allergen binds preformed IgE on the mast cell surface, inducing the release of histamines and other vasoactive mediators).

Epidemiology

There are very few data on overall incidence of anaphylaxis, which is estimated at one in 10,000 of the population each year. Common allergens include foods, drugs, insect venoms or latex.

Clinical presentation

Key point

Definition of anaphylaxis

One or more of these symptoms:

> laryngeal oedema

> bronchoconstriction

> hypotension.

Anaphylaxis is caused by IgE-mediated mast cell degranulation. Abdominal cramps with severe vomiting and diarrhoea may occur. Anaphylactoid reactions are caused by non-IgE-mediated mast cell degranulation but are otherwise identical.

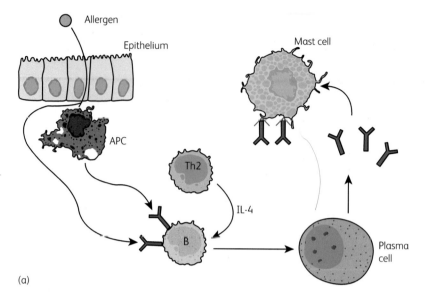

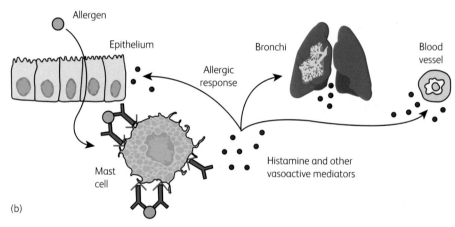

Fig 48 Mechanism of allergy. **(a)** Sensitisation: exposure to allergen results in activation of the B-cell, which becomes an IgE-secreting plasma cell. Secreted IgE binds to IgE receptors on mast cells. **(b)** Re-exposure to the same allergen results in cross-linking of preformed allergen-specific IgE on the mast cell surface. This causes the mast cell to degranulate. The release of histamine and other vasoactive substances from the granules causes the clinical manifestations of allergy or, if severe, anaphylaxis. APC, antigen-presenting cell; IL, interleukin; Th2, T-helper cell type 2.

Common

> facial, tongue or throat swelling

> wheeze

> syncope

> feeling of impending doom.

Uncommon

> abdominal cramps

> diarrhoea and vomiting.

Physical signs

Common

> urticaria, angio-oedema, skin erythema or extreme pallor

> stridor or wheeze

> hypotension.

Investigations

> mast cell tryptase (within 6 hours) as a marker of mast cell degranulation in cases of diagnostic uncertainty

> skin-prick testing of suspect allergens, with positive and negative controls (Figs 49 and 50)

> IgE: total and specific to suspect allergens (radioallergosorbent test).

Key point

Tryptase

Tryptase levels are a marker of mast cell degranulation:

> Elevated serum β-tryptase levels are useful in differentiating anaphylactic/anaphylactoid reactions from other disorders with similar clinical manifestations.

> As β-tryptase is stable, stored serum or serum obtained post-mortem should be assayed if anaphylaxis is suspected.

Differential diagnosis

> panic attack

> asthma

> syncope

> angio-oedema: idiopathic, angiotensin-converting enzyme (ACE) inhibitor-related or C1 inhibitor deficiency

> mastocytosis

> ruptured hydatid cyst (rare).

Treatment

See Fig 51.

Emergency

Administer:

> intramuscular epinephrine

> oxygen

> intravenous crystalloid.

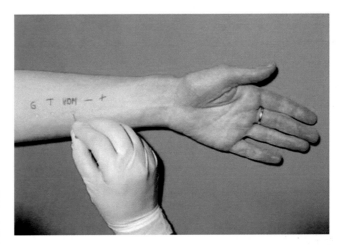

Fig 49 Skin-prick testing: a drop of a standardised extract of the suspect allergen is put on the skin. The superficial layer of the skin is lifted with a needle tip (or pricked with a lancet) through the drop. Positive (histamine) and negative (diluent) controls are included.

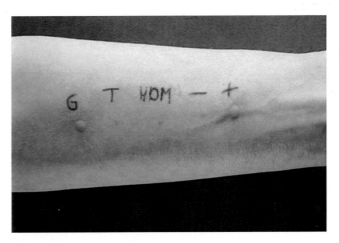

Fig 50 Skin-prick test reactions are read at 15 minutes. The mean diameter of the wheal (not the flare) is recorded. Reactions more than 3 mm greater than the negative control are significant.

Key point

Epinephrine is the drug of choice because it immediately counteracts the vasodilatation and bronchoconstriction of anaphylaxis.

Hazard

Anaphylaxis in individuals on pre-existing beta-blockers may prove to be refractory to epinephrine. Consider the use of cardiac inotropes in such cases.

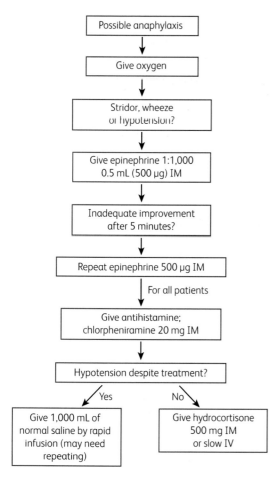

Start: **Possible anaphylaxis**

↓

Give oxygen

↓

Stridor, wheeze or hypotension?

↓

Give epinephrine 1:1,000 0.5 mL (500 μg) IM

↓

Inadequate improvement after 5 minutes?

↓

Repeat epinephrine 500 μg IM

For all patients

↓

Give antihistamine; chlorpheniramine 20 mg IM

↓

Hypotension despite treatment?

Yes → **Give 1,000 mL of normal saline by rapid infusion (may need repeating)**

No → **Give hydrocortisone 500 mg IM or slow IV**

Fig 51 Algorithm for the treatment of anaphylaxis. (Adapted with permission from Consensus Guidelines of the Project Team of the Resuscitation Council, UK.)

Short term
Administer:

> antihistamines

> corticosteroids

> consider salbutamol (IV or nebulised).

Long term

> identification and avoidance of allergen

> desensitisation immunotherapy: bee or wasp venoms and, in rare cases, drugs

> patients should have a Medic-Alert bracelet and carry epinephrine in an easily injectable form (eg Epi-Pen or Ana-Kit) (see Fig 37).

Prognosis

Mortality

Significant numbers of deaths occur. Previously healthy young adults are often the victims.

Disease associations

Atopy (predisposition to asthma, eczema or hay fever).

Occupational aspects

> beekeepers (due to bee stings)

> medical personnel (due to latex).

2.2.2 Mastocytosis

Aetiology/pathophysiology/pathology

Mastocytosis encompasses a spectrum of disorders characterised by mast cell proliferation. This may be confined to the skin as in cutaneous mastocytosis, or can affect other organs (eg bone marrow, gut and bones) as in systemic mastocytosis (SM).

The demonstration of gain-of-function mutations (Asp816→Val) in the gene encoding the mast cell c-kit tyrosine kinase receptor (CD117) in the majority of patients with SM lends support to the view that SM is a clonal haematopoietic neoplasm. The Asp816→Val mutation results in ligand-independent activation of the c-kit receptor, resulting in uncontrolled mast cell proliferation. By contrast, cutaneous mastocytosis is not associated with the c-kit mutation.

Epidemiology

The precise prevalence is unknown. The estimated frequency of cutaneous mastocytosis is said to be one in 1,000 to one in 8,000 of dermatology outpatient visits.

Clinical presentation

This presentation depends on which organs are affected. Cutaneous mastocytosis is characterised by urticaria, the fixed reddish-brown maculopapules of urticaria pigmentosa (see Section 1.1.5) and dermographism. SM typically presents with episodic flushing, diarrhoea and palpitations caused by the release of mast cell mediators. However, testing for c-kit mutations has led to the diagnosis of mastocytosis in some patients with recurrent idiopathic or perioperative anaphylaxis. Organ infiltration may result in hepatosplenomegaly, lymphadenopathy and bone pain.

Physical signs

> These are mainly confined to urticaria and the pigmented plaques of urticaria pigmentosa.

> Dermographism and Darier's sign may be present.

Investigation

The key investigations are to demonstrate mast cell proliferation on skin and bone marrow trephine biopsies (Figs 52 and 53), coupled with biochemical evidence of elevated mast cell mediators – plasma tryptase and urinary methylhistamine.

Key point

Establish the presence of mast cells in SM – immunophenotyping using monoclonal antibodies to CD117 and mast cell tryptase is useful in distinguishing atypical mast cells from basophils.

Following an episode of anaphylaxis, failure of basal tryptase levels to return to normal raises the likelihood of mastocytosis.

Differential diagnosis

See Table 4.

Treatment

The principles of management of SM are based on:

> inhibition of mast cell mediator release using a combined H_1- and H_2-receptor blockade to alleviate cutaneous symptoms and reduce gastric acid production, respectively. This approach will suffice for patients with mild symptoms

> use of cytoreductive therapy such as interferon-α in patients with aggressive disease associated with organ infiltration.

Imatinib, a tyrosine kinase inhibitor which inhibits c-kit, shows promise in the minority of patients with SM who do not have the Asp816→Val mutation.

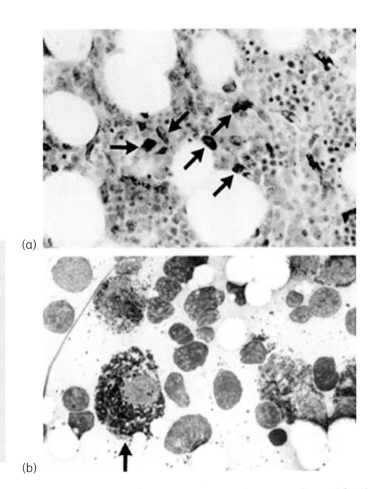

(a)

(b)

Fig 52 Bone marrow biopsy specimen with staining for acid-fast bacilli. **(a)** Mast cells (arrows) on a bone marrow aspirate (×400). **(b)** Typical normal-appearing mast cell (arrow) (×1000). (Reproduced with permission, from Sawalha *et al. N Engl J Med* 2003;349:2255–6, copyright © 2003 Massachusetts Medical Society.)

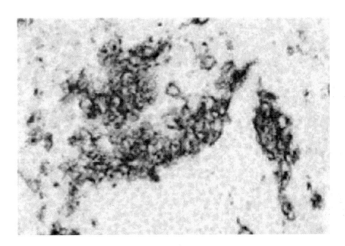

Fig 53 Bone marrow biopsy specimen with immunohistochemical staining for CD117 (to detect c-kit) showing numerous mast cells. (Reproduced with permission, from Sawalha *et al. N Engl J Med* 2003;349:2255–6, copyright © 2003 Massachusetts Medical Society.)

Prognosis

In general, SM progresses very slowly. For the small minority of sufferers who develop an associated myeloproliferative or lymphoproliferative disorder, the prognosis depends on the haematological disorder.

2.2.3 Nut allergy

Aetiology/pathophysiology/pathology

Nut allergy is due to immunoglobulin E (IgE)-mediated mast cell degranulation precipitated by contact with peanuts (strictly speaking these are pulses not nuts) or tree nuts (Brazil, almond, walnut or hazelnut) (see Fig 48). T-cell clones from patients with nut allergy overproduce interleukin-4 while underproducing interferon-γ, consistent with a T-helper 2-like cytokine profile.

Epidemiology

Nut allergy is more common in atopic individuals. It follows sensitisation to nut(s), usually in early childhood.

Clinical presentation

Common

Symptoms typically occur within minutes of contact with the nut:

> lip tingling, swelling, angio-oedema and urticaria

> anaphylaxis, with laryngeal oedema or bronchoconstriction.

Rare

> anaphylaxis with hypotension.

Investigations

> detailed dietary history

> skin-prick testing or specific serum IgE measurements

> specific IgE testing to nut components to stratify risk

> oral challenge if diagnosis remains uncertain.

Hazard

Skin-prick and challenge testing should take place where there are facilities for resuscitation, ideally in an allergy clinic.

Key point

Specific IgE to nut storage proteins (eg Ara h 2 for peanut) is associated with high risk of anaphylaxis.

Pollen-food syndrome

Specific IgE to proteins present in common aeroallergens, such as PR10, suggest cross-reactivity with proteins in the nut and lower the risk of anaphylaxis. Pollen-food syndromes are common in this situation.

Also known as oral allergy syndrome, pollen-food syndrome occurs in people sensitised to components of tree, grass or weed pollen which are similar to proteins found in many fresh fruits or vegetables. Symptoms of oral itching or swelling occur within minutes of contact with raw fruits or vegetables, usually in a patient with hay fever. Cooked food is tolerated. Throat symptoms, nausea and vomiting can occur, but anaphylaxis is rare.

Differential diagnosis

> pollen-food syndrome

> allergy to other foods

> idiopathic angio-oedema, with or without urticaria.

Treatment

Emergency

If anaphylaxis occurs, the emergency treatment is as follows:

> intramuscular epinephrine (see Section 2.2.1)

> antihistamines

> corticosteroids.

Long term

Avoidance of allergen is the cornerstone of treatment as allergen immunotherapy is not an option at present. Sublingual immunotherapy has shown promise in patients with hazelnut and peanut allergy, but requires validation in larger randomised trials. Humanised monoclonal anti-IqE (omalizumab, Fig 54) is beneficial in patients with severe peanut allergy but the need for regular injections and its prohibitive cost makes it unlikely that this treatment will be widely used at present. Recent evidence suggests that early dietary exposure to peanut appears to reduce the risk of development of peanut allergy.

Prognosis

Mortality

This is unknown, but there are several deaths from nut allergy each year in the UK.

Prevention

Primary

> avoidance of contact with nuts in infancy and childhood, especially if there is a family history of atopy. Peanut products may be hidden in processed foods or creams and ointments (such as arachis oil)

> good control of asthma.

Secondary

> constant avoidance – detailed dietary advice is required. Most patients do not 'outgrow' peanut allergy, underlining the need for indefinite vigilance.

> self-injectable epinephrine (see Fig 37).

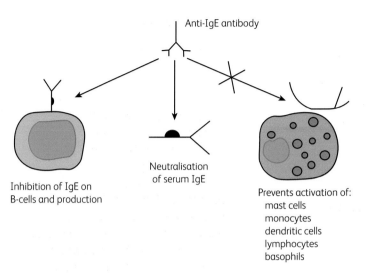

Anti-IgE antibody

Inhibition of IgE on
B-cells and production

Neutralisation
of serum IgE

Prevents activation of:
  mast cells
  monocytes
  dendritic cells
  lymphocytes
  basophils

Fig 54 Mechanism of action of anti-IgE antibodies as a treatment for allergic disease. The anti-IgE antibody binds to the section of the IgE molecule that associates with high affinity Fcε receptor. (Reproduced with permission from the BMJ Publishing Group; from Holgate ST. Science, medicine, and the future: allergic disorders. *BMJ* 2000;320:231–4.)

Disease associations

> asthma

> hay fever

> eczema.

Key point

Patients with a food allergy and poorly controlled asthma are at particular risk of anaphylaxis.

Further allergies

Other allergies may include the following:

> tree nuts (common even if main allergy is to peanuts)

> other foods (such as eggs, milk and fresh fruit)

> common airborne allergens (pollen, house dust mite, animal dander and moulds)

> pulses (peas, lentils and beans).

2.2.4 Drug allergy

Aetiology/pathophysiology/pathology

Immunological reactions to drugs can be classified according to the four subtypes of hypersensitivity (see Table 32). However, the immunological mechanisms underlying many drug reactions, particularly those affecting the skin, remain unclear. In practice, the line between immunological and non-immunological reactions to drugs is often blurred.

Susceptibility to drug reactions is poorly understood, but genetic factors have been identified for some drug-induced syndromes, eg genetically determined slow acetylation of the triggering drug is associated with drug-induced lupus and with co-trimoxazole sensitivity in HIV. Some immunological diseases are also associated with an increased risk of adverse drug reactions, particularly HIV infection and systemic lupus erythematosus (SLE). Pharmacogenomic testing to predict hypersensitivity has been proven to be effective for abacavir (human leukocyte antigen (HLA)-B 5701) and for carbamazepine-induced Stevens–Johnson syndrome (HLA-B 1502 in Asians).

Table 32	Immunological classification of drug hypersensitivity		
Type	**Mechanism**	**Clinical picture**	**Examples**
I	Immediate hypersensitivity	Anaphylaxis Urticaria and angio-oedema Bronchospasm	Penicillins
II	Cytotoxic antibodies	Haematological cytopenias	Penicillins Heparin
III	Immune complex	Drug-induced lupus Vasculitis Serum sickness	Minocycline Carbimazole
IV	T-cell mediated	Contact dermatitis Interstitial nephritis	Topical antibiotics NSAIDs Halothane Hepatitis

Epidemiology

Incidence figures vary enormously from drug to drug. Crude estimates suggest that between 1% and 10% of prescriptions are complicated by some form of allergic adverse reaction.

Clinical presentation

Drug hypersensitivity can affect any system of the body and mimic many other forms of disease (Table 33).

Investigations

The diagnosis of drug allergy is based largely on the history and the recognition of typical patterns of drug reaction, eg acute interstitial nephritis and toxic erythema of the skin are highly suggestive of drug reactions.

When there is a mild reaction to a therapeutically important drug, drug challenge is sometimes justified, but this must always be used cautiously. Skin tests (a local form of challenge testing) can be useful in immediate hypersensitivity (anaphylaxis) and contact dermatitis induced by topical medication.

Key point

Skin testing
Skin testing in suspected drug allergy is useful for the following agents:

> antibiotics: penicillins and cephalosporins

> anaesthetic drugs: neuromuscular blocking agents (muscle relaxants) and thiopental (thiopentone sodium)

> enzymes: streptokinase and chymopapain

> chemotherapeutic agents: cisplatin

> others: insulin and latex.

Note that false-positive and false-negative reactions may occur.

Detection of drug-specific immunoglobulin E (IgE) has been described in some types of drug-induced anaphylaxis, particularly to the penicillins, but is unreliable. No other clinically useful blood tests for drug allergy have been described.

Key point

A negative skin test to both the major and the minor determinants of penicillin followed by tolerance of an oral challenge with amoxicillin (as a representative member of the penicillin family) excludes IgE-mediated allergy to β-lactam antibiotics.

Differential diagnosis

Beware of drug reactions that mimic idiopathic systemic diseases, eg SLE (see Table 33).

Treatment

> supportive care depending on organ system involved

> treatment of immediate hypersensitivity: antihistamine and epinephrine

> other forms of hypersensitivity: consider corticosteroids

> the overwhelming majority of reactions will resolve on drug withdrawal.

2.3 Rheumatology

2.3.1 Carpal tunnel syndrome

Key point

This is the most common entrapment neuropathy; it presents commonly in rheumatology clinics.

Table 33 Drug reactions that mimic other syndromes

Syndrome	Examples of triggering drugs
Systemic lupus	Minocycline Hydralazine
Myasthenia gravis	D-Penicillamine
Pemphigus	D-Penicillamine
Pulmonary fibrosis	Amiodarone Nitrofurantoin Some cytotoxics
Pulmonary eosinophilia	NSAIDs Antibiotics
Vasculitis	Antibiotics Thiazides Carbimazole
Immune haemolytic anaemia	Methyldopa Penicillin
Neutropenia	Carbimazole
Thrombocytopenia	Gold salts Diuretics Heparin

Aetiology/pathophysiology/pathology

The median nerve is easily compromised in the tight space of the carpal tunnel. Pathological processes that limit the space in the carpal tunnel have the potential to cause a median neuropathy. The following mnemonic covers important causes:

C – crystal arthritis: Colles' and other fractures

R – rheumatoid arthritis

A – amyloidosis: acromegaly (rare)

M – myxoedema (rare)

P – pregnancy

E – elusive: no cause identified

D – diabetes: drugs.

Clinical presentation

The median nerve receives sensory input from the radial three-and-a-half fingers (Fig 55). However, symptoms are often more diffuse than this. The patient often describes paraesthesia in the whole hand or even extending up the arm, which is usually uncomfortable and often painful (the pain may also be the result of the underlying cause). The symptoms are often intermittent and can be provoked by certain activities. They are usually worse at night and early in the morning, and a history of nocturnal paraesthesia alone should suggest the carpal tunnel syndrome. Patients often describe shaking their hand(s) to improve the symptoms. Paraesthesia is frequently accompanied by wrist pain that can radiate distally into the fingers and also proximally up the forearm. Individuals with carpal tunnel syndrome often complain of hand clumsiness, which is probably caused by sensory dysfunction and pain instead of true muscle weakness (although this can also occur). Autonomic dysfunction can also occur, with loss of sweating in the innervated digits.

Physical signs

It should be emphasised that examination may be entirely normal if the symptoms are intermittent (usually nocturnal). A sensory discrepancy on the radial and ulnar side of the ring finger is highly suggestive of a median nerve lesion. Fixed sensory changes, weakness of thumb abduction and wasting of the thenar eminence are usually only found in severe cases and (in the presence of wasting) long-standing, median nerve compression.

Two provocation tests are often used:

> percussion over the median nerve (Tinel's test)

> maintenance of fixed flexion of the wrist (Phalen's test).

These tests are positive if they produce transient sensory disturbance with a similar quality to the original symptoms. If positive, they are of good predictive value.

Investigations

A definitive diagnosis can be made using nerve conduction studies, although these may sometimes be normal in very mild intermittent compression. Electrophysiology is not obligatory in every case. Use only where the diagnosis is uncertain, or where the result will affect your management. Many surgeons require electrophysiological confirmation before carpal tunnel decompression.

Key point

Consider also an investigation of underlying cause, although these patients may have underlying thyroid disease and thus will have a very low threshold for thyroid function testing.

Differential diagnosis

Cervical root compression and peripheral neuropathy are the main differential diagnoses. Although a C6/7 nerve root lesion may give similar sensory symptoms, it would not cause motor symptoms in the hand (supplied by T1). Ulnar nerve lesions are easy to distinguish by the pattern of sensory disturbance.

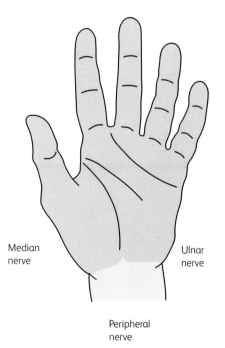

Median nerve

Ulnar nerve

Peripheral nerve

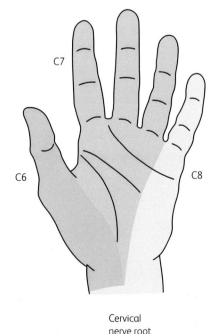

C7

C6

C8

Cervical nerve root

Fig 55 Sensory innervation of the palmar surface of the hand.

Treatment

This is dictated by the severity of the symptoms. Many mild cases with occasional symptoms need no treatment. Conversely, intervention will be needed in most patients with severe unremitting symptoms. Most cases lie somewhere in between. Treatment options are as follows.

> Night-time splintage of the wrists is often used in mild compression, although there is little evidence that this is effective.

> Injection of corticosteroids into the carpal tunnel is a simple outpatient treatment that may produce prolonged relief of symptoms, particularly in cases of recent onset or with an underlying inflammatory cause.

> Surgical decompression is the definitive treatment and is highly effective unless permanent nerve damage has occurred, which is usually in severe, long-standing cases (possibly predictable from electrophysiology).

2.3.2 Osteoarthritis

Aetiology/pathophysiology/pathology

Key point

Osteoarthritis is a process of joint failure rather than a disease. It can occur as a primary disorder or secondary to other insults to the joint.

The usual description of 'wear and tear' is misleading. Osteoarthritis (OA) is best considered as the result of an inadequate attempt by cartilage and periarticular bone to repair itself after injury. The following are the cardinal pathological features (Fig 56):

> progressive disruption and loss of articular cartilage

> remodelling of periarticular bone, usually leading to new bone formation (osteophytes in hypertrophic OA) but sometimes to bone destruction (atrophic or erosive OA)

> secondary changes in synovial membrane and other soft tissues

> genetic factors are important: there is usually a strong family history in generalised nodal osteoarthritis (GNOA). The underlying genetic defects are not yet identified. OA associated with calcium pyrophosphate crystal deposition is a common feature of hereditary haemochromatosis.

Other aetiological factors include the following:

> obesity

> trauma or other disruptions to joint anatomy (such as a previous fracture or congenital hip dysplasia)

> acquired hip disease (eg Perthes' or slipped femoral epiphysis)

> occupation

> inflammatory joint disease.

Epidemiology

OA is very common. It can be detected radiologically in 25% of 45 year olds and virtually everyone over the age of 65 (Fig 57). Severe disease and hand involvement are more common in women.

Clinical presentation

OA usually presents with pain and functional impairment, but it may be asymptomatic, particularly in the cervical and lumbar spine. Clinical features depend on the joint involved. The most common pattern of polyarticular OA is GNOA, which is characterised by the following:

> distal and proximal interphalangeal joint (PIP) involvement

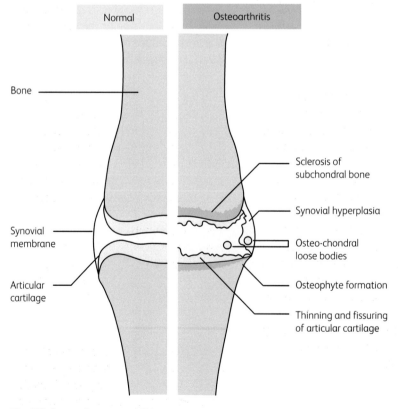

Fig 56 Joint changes in OA.

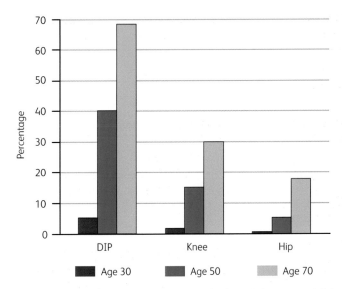

Fig 57 Percentage prevalence of radiological changes of OA at three different sites and at three different ages in white people living in Western Europe. DIP, distal interphalangeal joint.

> involvement of the base of the thumb (first carpometacarpal joint (CMC))

> hip, knee, cervical and lumbar spine involvement

> perimenopausal onset.

Physical signs

Tenderness, bony swelling (reflecting osteophyte formation), painful restriction of movement and crepitus are the usual findings. The formation of Heberden's and Bouchard's nodes in the distal interphalangeal joints (DIPs) and PIPs, respectively, is pathognomonic. The base of the thumb often has a square appearance (see Fig 24). Note also the muscle wasting around affected joints and the evidence of nerve or nerve root entrapment (most commonly carpal tunnel syndrome and cervical or lumbar root entrapment; more rarely, but more seriously, spinal cord compression).

Investigations / differential diagnosis

See Section 1.3.2.

Treatment/prognosis

A definitive, curative medical treatment for OA remains a remote prospect. The overall outcome depends as much on muscle strength and overall fitness as on joint damage.

Osteoarthritis of the hand

Outcome in OA of the hand is usually good, with long-term function usually preserved despite pain. Pain is often worse at onset, as osteophytes grow, and tends to settle with time. Severe changes at the base of the thumb may be associated with a worse functional outcome. Localised intra-articular injections, especially to the first CMC, can provide symptomatic relief. Surgery may be helpful in relieving pain, but is less useful in improving hand function.

Osteoarthritis of the hip and knee

Hip and knee OA is progressive only in a minority, but it may cause severe pain and disability in this subgroup. Severely impaired mobility and rest pain are the main indications for joint replacement.

The outcomes from hip and knee replacement are excellent. Arthroplasty of other joints is less widely used, but the outcomes from shoulder and elbow replacement are improving.

If there is OA in an atypical joint distribution (see Section 1.3.2), consider the secondary causes of OA:

> congenital:

>> leg hypermobility

>> leg length discrepancies

>> hip dislocation

>> dysplasias

> metabolic disorders:

>> haemochromatosis

>> ochronosis

>> storage disorders, eg Gaucher's disease

>> haemoglobinopathies

> endocrine disorders:

>> acromegaly

> neuropathic joints (Charcot's)

> other:

>> chronic inflammatory/septic arthritis

>> osteonecrosis.

2.3.3 Rheumatoid arthritis

Rheumatoid arthritis (RA) is the cardinal distal symmetrical deforming polyarthropathy. Although it affects the small joints of the hands and feet most frequently, any synovial joint can ultimately become involved, and extra-articular manifestations are not uncommon. Patients presenting with a new complaint on a background of RA pose an interesting clinical problem – the best approach is often to ask yourself: 'Is this the disease, a result of a drug used to treat the disease, or something completely new?'.

Aetiology

The aetiology is unknown, but current evidence supports a combination of genetic and environmental factors acting in concert. Genetic and environmental factors have both been implicated in the susceptibility of an individual to, and determination of the severity of, RA. Strong evidence for a genetic contribution comes from twin studies with human leukocyte antigens (HLA), which are thought to explain about half of the genetic predisposition. There is a strong association with particular HLA antigens: HLA-DR4 and HLA-DR1 ('rheumatoid epitope' or 'shared epitope', respectively). Over 70% of patients with erosive, seropositive disease are likely to be HLA-DR4-positive (compared with 25% of the normal population). The most powerful environmental factor is cigarette smoking, especially in those with the shared epitope and the cyclic citrullinated peptide (CCP) antibody. Other environmental factors include hormonal and reproductive factors, socioeconomic factors, diet and infection.

Epidemiology

RA affects 1% of the population worldwide and occurs in all ethnic groups. Like many autoimmune conditions, it is more common in women. The peak incidence of onset is in the sixth decade.

Pathology

In health, the synovial joint lining is only a few stromal cells thick. As RA develops, the synovium proliferates and becomes heavily infiltrated by lymphocytes, macrophages and plasma cells; in some individuals these B-cells group together to form lymphoid aggregates. Rheumatoid nodules (Fig 58) have a characteristic histological appearance with central fibrinoid necrosis surrounded by fibroblasts. Advances in

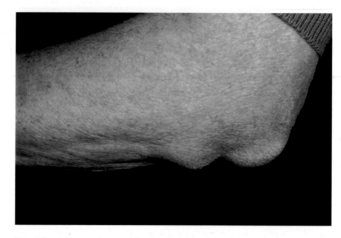

Fig 58 Subcutaneous rheumatoid nodules in a patient with seropositive RA.

our understanding of RA biology have led to the development of biologic treatments (monoclonal antibodies or fusion proteins that target key pathogenic cells or cytokines), which have transformed RA treatment over the past decade. Although several lines of evidence suggest that T-cells and macrophages play a key role in RA, recent evidence attesting to the efficacy of rituximab (monoclonal anti-CD20) has reignited interest in the role of B-cells in the pathogenesis of RA.

Clinical presentation

Common

The pattern of joint involvement is typically symmetrical, and predominantly affects the hands and feet, but characteristically spares the distal interphalangeal joints. Several distinct patterns of onset are recognised (see Sections 1.1.14 and 1.3.3). There is no diagnostic test for RA, but the following European League Against Rheumatism (EULAR) / American College of Rheumatology (ACR) classification criteria (which have superseded the 1987 ACR criteria) are useful in identifying those with inflammatory arthritis who are likely to develop established rheumatoid disease. They are used both in diagnosis and in clinical trials.

Key point

Classification criteria for rheumatoid arthritis (2010 EULAR/ACR criteria)

A score of ≥6 is definite RA

Joint distribution	(0–5)
1 large joint	0
2–10 large joints	1
1–3 small joints	2
4–10 small joints	3
>10 small joints	5
Serology	**(0–3)**
Negative RhF and negative ACPA	0
Low-positive RhF or low-positive ACPA	2
High-positive RhF or high-positive ACPA	3
Symptom duration	**(0–1)**
<6 weeks	0
>6 weeks	1
Acute phase reactants	**(0–1)**
Normal CRP and normal ESR	0
Abnormal CRP or abnormal ESR	1

ACPA, anticitrullinated peptide antibody; CRP, C-reactive protein; ESR, erythrocyte sedimentation rate; RhF, rheumatoid factor.

Physical signs

Common

Acute synovitis of an involved joint leads to pain, swelling, stiffness and loss of function. Chronic active disease leads to joint damage and the characteristic deformities of RA (Fig 30 and Section 1.3.3). Rheumatoid nodules are seen only in patients with positive RhF (Fig 58).

Uncommon

Extra-articular manifestations (see Table 19).

Investigations

The diagnosis of RA is based on a collection of clinical features, rather than on a specific pathognomonic abnormality. Investigations are helpful in assessing disease severity and prognosis.

Blood count

Red cell count

Many patients with active disease are anaemic. Aetiology of anaemia is multifactorial.

Key point

Causes of anaemia in rheumatoid arthritis

> normochromic normocytic anaemia caused by chronic disease itself

> hypochromic microcytic anaemia secondary to iron deficiency (gastrointestinal (GI) bleeding caused by NSAIDs)

> macrocytic anaemia resulting from folate deficiency (sulfasalazine and methotrexate) or vitamin B_{12} deficiency (associated pernicious anaemia)

> haemolysis (drug induced by sulfasalazine)

> bone marrow suppression (drug induced by methotrexate, sulfasalazine and leflunomide)

> hypersplenism as in Felty's syndrome.

White cell count

This may be normal. It is elevated in patients with severe disease, infection or in those who are on steroid therapy. Leukopenia may be drug induced or secondary to peripheral consumption, as in Felty's syndrome.

Platelet count

This is usually normal. Thrombocytosis is a feature of active disease whereas thrombocytopenia may be caused by drug-induced marrow suppression or Felty's syndrome.

Acute phase indices

Both the ESR and the CRP are elevated in active disease and correlate with disease severity.

Autoantibodies: rheumatoid factor and anti-citrullinated peptide antibody

Rheumatoid factor (RhF) is a self IgG or IgM and is positive in 70% of patients with definite RA. High titres are usually associated with severe RA, particularly with extra-articular features. Antibodies to cyclic citrullinated peptides (ACPA) have been shown to have greater sensitivity and (crucially) greater specificity for the diagnosis of RA. Intriguingly, they can be positive up to a decade before the advent of clinically apparent disease, indicating a pre-symptomatic immune tolerance breach, and raising the possibility of very early intervention.

Radiology

Small joints of the hands and feet are affected early in the disease. Typical changes include the following:

> soft tissue swelling

> periarticular osteoporosis

> loss of joint space

> marginal erosions regarded as a characteristic feature of RA.

Synovial fluid analysis

See Sections 1.1.14 and 3.5.

Synovial biopsy

Synovial histology is rarely necessary and is not pathognomonic. It is sometimes useful in excluding tuberculosis (TB) in a patient with monoarticular disease.

Differential diagnosis

See Section 1.1.14.

Treatment

The following are the aims of any treatment:

> relief of inflammatory joint pain and swelling

> suppression of active disease and arrest of disease progression

> restoration of function to affected joints.

To achieve these aims, a multidisciplinary team approach is vital, encompassing rheumatologists, occupational therapists, physiotherapists, nurses, social workers and orthopaedic surgeons. Patient education is equally crucial. Patients must understand the chronicity of disease, with its periods of exacerbations and (hopefully) remissions.

Drug treatment

The historical approach to drug therapy, in which NSAIDs were used as first-line agents with the late introduction of disease-modifying antirheumatic drugs (DMARDs), is no longer appropriate. Early aggressive use of combination DMARD has been shown to be most effective at establishing and maintaining remission, reducing joint damage and maintaining functional ability. This is now standard practice. Modifications to treatment are guided by a treat-to-target principle according to the patient's disease activity score (see 'key point' box below). This is particularly relevant with the use of biologic therapies.

Key point

The disease activity score (DAS28) is based on the identification of tenderness and swelling in 28 standard joints (shoulders, elbows, wrists, metacarpophalangeal joints (MCPs), proximal interphalangeal joints (PIPs) and knees), the acute phase, and a patient's own assessment of disease activity using a visual analogue score of 0–100. The swollen joint count (SJC), tender joint count (TJC), ESR/CRP and a visual analogue scale (VAS) are fed into an algorithm available online or on a 'DAS calculator' to determine disease severity. A score of <2.6 indicates remission; a score of >5.1 indicates severe disease activity.

Disease-modifying antirheumatic drugs

Disease-modifying antirheumatic drugs (DMARDs) are divided into the conventional synthetic DMARDs, such as methotrexate, sulfasalazine, hydroxychloroquine and leflunomide, and biologic DMARDs, such as anti-tumour necrosis factor alpha (TNF-α) agents (see below). Older DMARDs such as gold and penicillamine are now rarely used.

Conventional synthetic DMARDs

Methotrexate is the first-line DMARD provided there are no contraindications such as pregnancy. Used increasingly early in disease, DMARDs are orally bioavailable slow-acting drugs that

inhibit cytokine-mediated inflammatory damage, thereby preventing joint destruction and preserving joint function. Regular monitoring is required to prevent toxicity (Table 34).

Biologic DMARDs

Biologic therapies are monoclonal antibodies that target key cells or cytokines implicated in disease. Being cellular products and complex proteins, they are expensive to manufacture and must be given either subcutaneously or intravenously. In RA there are currently four biologics that are licensed and National Institute for Health and Care Excellence (NICE)-approved for use in severe RA (ie DAS >5.1 despite treatment with at least two conventional synthetic DMARDs, of which one must be methotrexate). These are agents that are anti-TNF-α, anti-B-cell, anti-T-cell and anti-interleukin (IL)-6. Anti-TNF-α is often chosen as a first-line agent; anti-B-cell treatment is only NICE-approved as a second-line agent in seropositive individuals if another biologic has failed.

> TNF-α inhibition – this is achieved either by a use of a monoclonal antibody directed against the TNF-α molecule itself (eg infliximab, adalimumab) or a fusion protein (IgG bound to a soluble TNF-α

receptor, eg etanercept). These agents are generally well tolerated and effective. The main risk associated with their use is the reactivation of latent TB, so all patients must be screened for this prior to use. Other contraindications include demyelinating disease, recent malignancy and severe congestive cardiac failure.

> B-cell targeting – rituximab is an anti-CD20 monoclonal antibody that specifically targets a subsection of B-cells (immature and plasma cell populations are preserved).

> T-cell targeting – abatacept is a CTLA-4–IgG fusion protein which blocks the second signal in T-cell co-stimulation.

> IL-6 receptor targeting – tocilizumab targets the IL-6 receptor, preventing cytokine binding.

As these drugs come off patent, so-called 'biosimilars' (ie copies of the original product) are being generated. Such competition is likely to reduce the cost of these drugs, thereby increasing their availability, but some residual concerns remain around their effectiveness and immunogenicity.

Other anti-inflammatories

Non-steroidal anti-inflammatories (NSAIDs) only provide symptomatic

Table 34	Side effects of conventional synthetic DMARDs	
Drug	**Side effects**
Methotrexate	Nausea, vomiting, mouth ulcers, hepatotoxicity, bone marrow suppression and pneumonitis
Sulfasalazine	Nausea, vomiting, rash, mouth ulcers, hepatotoxicity, bone marrow suppression and transient azoospermia
Hydroxychloroquine	Retinopathy ('Bulls-eye maculopathy')
Leflunomide	Diarrhoea, hypertension, hepatotoxicity and bone marrow suppression

relief by suppressing inflammation; they do not influence the underlying disease process. Steroids are used via either the intra-articular or the intramuscular route to provide temporary relief during acute exacerbations of disease, or as a bridge before DMARDs start acting. Oral steroids are rarely justified, although intravenous steroid pulses may be useful as a short-term adjunct for very severe extra-articular manifestations (eg rheumatoid vasculitis), when use of cyclophosphamide should also be considered.

Surgery

Joint replacement is indicated once irreversible joint damage has occurred. The overall outcome after knee, hip and MCP replacements is favourable, with promising results also being seen with elbow and shoulder replacement.

Prognosis

The advent of treat-to-target strategies and biologic therapies has vastly improved the prognosis in RA. Secondary amyloidosis is now rarely seen. Multi-drug resistant severe disabling disease occurs in <5–10% of all cases of RA. The major cause of death is increased comorbidity (especially accelerated atheroma and cardiovascular disease) and infection.

Key point

Poor prognostic factors in rheumatoid arthritis

> female patients or young male patients

> severe disease and/or erosions at presentation

> extra-articular disease

> high concentration of RhF and/or antibodies to cyclic citrullinated peptides (ACPA).

2.3.4 Seronegative spondyloarthropathies

Key point

Definition of seronegative spondyloarthritis

This is a generic term for a group of rheumatological disorders characterised by:

> sacroiliitis

> peripheral arthritis (usually affecting large joints, predominantly the lower limbs)

> mucocutaneous inflammation

> significant familial aggregation.

Rheumatoid factor is absent (hence seronegative).

These disorders include the following:

> ankylosing spondylitis (AS) (features of which may occur in all the other syndromes)

> psoriatic arthritis

> reactive arthritis

> enteropathic arthritis (associated with inflammatory bowel disease).

Considerable overlap may occur between these syndromes and, in some

patients, the generic label seronegative spondyloarthropathy may be more appropriate than any of the above.

Aetiology/pathophysiology/pathology

Genetic factors are important, with human leukocyte antigen (HLA)-B27 being the most clearly defined association (Table 35). Infectious agents (mucosal or skin) are thought to be the most important environmental trigger. This is best defined for reactive arthritis, with infectious agents including the following:

> *Chlamydia trachomatis*

> *Salmonella* spp

> *Shigella* spp

> *Campylobacter jejuni*

> *Yersinia enterocolitica*.

The inflammatory process probably results from an immune response against non-viable bacterial antigens sequestered in musculoskeletal tissues, perhaps leading to a secondary autoimmune response. Several lines of evidence point to overactivity of the interleukin (IL)-23 / IL-17 pathway playing a key role in driving inflammation in axial spondyloarthropathy. The cardinal pathological feature is enthesitis; an enthesis being the junctional tissue between the muscle/ligament/tendon

Table 35	Prevalence of HLA-B27
Disease	Percentage prevalence
UK controls	5–10%
AS	95%
Reactive arthritis	80%
Psoriatic arthritis (total)	20%
Psoriatic spondylitis	50%

AS, ankylosing spondylitis.

and bone. Enthesitis is responsible for spinal inflammation in AS and localised problems, such as plantar fasciitis and Achilles tendonitis. Enthesitis is also probably the first pathological change in joint inflammation in these disorders.

Epidemiology
All these disorders show either a male preponderance or equal gender distribution, in contrast with most chronic immunological rheumatic diseases.

Ankylosing spondylitis
Ankylosing spondylitis (AS) has a prevalence of 0.1–0.2% in Caucasian populations. It is strongly associated with HLA-B27, although only around 2% of individuals who are HLA-B27 positive develop AS. It is rare in African-Caribbean populations, reflecting their low prevalence of HLA-B27. The male to female ratio is around 4:1, with the peak onset in late adolescence or early adulthood.

Reactive arthritis
Reactive arthritis is typically a disorder of young adults. Most patients report a positive family history. The frequency of reactive arthritis after having an enteric infection caused by *Salmonella*, *Shigella* or *Campylobacter* has been reported in the order of 1–4%, with HLA-B27 predisposing to a more chronic and more severe disease.

Psoriatic arthritis
Rates of psoriatic arthritis have been estimated between 0.04% and 0.1%. The male:female ratio is 1:1, with the mean age of onset between 30 and 50 years. There is an increased prevalence in HIV-positive populations.

Clinical presentation

Key point

Common features that may occur in all spondyloarthropathies:

> insidious onset of spinal pain and restriction

> localised enthesitis, eg plantar fasciitis and Achilles tendonitis

> large-joint synovitis

> acute uveitis (painful red eye).

Ankylosing spondylitis
Axial spinal symptoms predominate, look for:

> involvement of whole spine (Fig 59)

> the patient may have large joint oligoarthritis in lower limbs, especially the hips.

Reactive arthritis
This often begins acutely: severe systemic disturbance may be present and mimic sepsis (which should be actively excluded). Common features include:

> A history of diarrhoea or urethritis up to a month before the articular disease. However, these features are often absent, particularly in post-chlamydial reactive arthritis. A triggering infection can be reliably identified only in about 50% of patients.

> The spectrum of the disease ranges from purely articular to multisystem disease.

> The most common presentation is acute in lower limb, large joint monoarthritis or oligoarthritis in a young male.

> Patients often present with enthesitis (inflammation of the insertion of tendon into bone), such as Achilles tendinitis or plantar fasciitis.

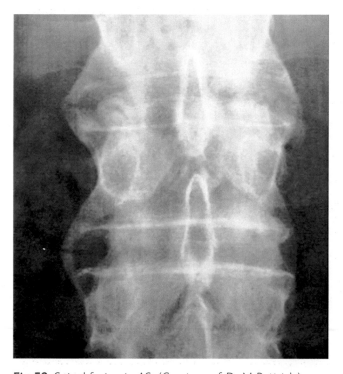

Fig 59 Spinal fusion in AS. (Courtesy of Dr M Pattrick.)

> There may be a scaly psoriasis-like eruption on the hands/feet (keratoderma blennorrhagica).

> The glans penis may have an eroded appearance (circinate balanitis).

> Conjunctivitis is more common than uveitis.

> **!** **Hazard**
> Chlamydial genitourinary infections are often clinically silent and need to be actively excluded in reactive arthritis.

Psoriatic arthritis

There are several patterns, which may overlap (percentages are of total psoriatic arthritis population):

> distal interphalangeal joint (7–17% of cases) (see Fig 27)

> asymmetrical oligoarthritis (30–55% of cases)

> symmetrical polyarthritis, similar to rheumatoid arthritis (20–40% of cases)

> arthritis mutilans (not unlike rheumatoid, but grossly destructive and often with telescoping digits) (2–15% of cases)

> sacroiliitis and spondylitis (5–30% of cases).

Dactylitis (sausage-like finger or toe swelling, usually affecting only one or two digits) is a distinctive feature, occurring in around 25% of patients.

The severities of the skin and joint disease are not correlated. Aggressive arthritis can be accompanied by very mild psoriasis and vice versa. Some patients may have joint disease that is highly suggestive of psoriatic arthritis, but no obvious skin disease. Skin disease may appear many years later.

Enteropathic arthritis

There are two patterns (again they may overlap):

> large-joint, lower-limb oligoarthritis or monoarthritis (activity tends to mirror the severity of bowel inflammation)

> ankylosing spondylitis (AS).

Uncommon features

> aortitis, which may lead to aortic incompetence

> pulmonary fibrosis (in AS)

> spinal discitis, which may lead to instability and spinal cord and nerve root compression

> amyloid (as in all chronic inflammatory disease).

Physical signs

It is necessary to assess spinal disease in AS, as follows.

Lumbar spine

Restricted movement is almost always found, usually more so than in mechanical back pain and usually in all directions. The modified Schober's test is used for serial measurement: the increase in distance following forward flexion of two points 15 cm apart, one 5 cm below and one 10 cm above a line drawn between the dimples of Venus (see Fig 31).

Thoracic spine

Dorsal kyphosis often develops as disease progresses. Chest expansion is the best index: <5 cm is abnormal.

Cervical spine

This is globally restricted, with the neck being forced into a flexed position by dorsal kyphosis. When standing with their back to a wall, can the patient touch the wall with their occiput? If not, measure the occiput to wall distance.

Investigations

Synovial fluid

Microscopy and culture are essential to exclude sepsis and crystal arthritis.

Blood tests

Measures of the acute phase response are useful:

> to distinguish inflammatory from non-inflammatory back pain

> to assess disease activity / response to treatment.

Ascertainment of HLA-B27 status is of limited diagnostic value because it is present in around 5–10% of population, but it may be of limited use in completing the diagnostic jigsaw.

Identifying a triggering cause

Looking for a triggering cause in reactive arthritis:

> *Chlamydia* spp are the most common triggering cause, and may be clinically silent. Chlamydia serology is of little use. Diagnosis can be made only by detection of the organism in the genital tract (antigen detection or polymerase chain reaction). Referral to a genitourinary physician may be required.

> Diagnosis of *Campylobacter/Shigella/Salmonella* infection may be possible by culture if the patient has recently had diarrhoea, but this is unlikely to be successful if the gastrointestinal symptoms have settled.

> In practice, the clinical picture is often suggestive of reactive arthritis, but no triggering organism is identified.

 Key point

Think about HIV
Remember that florid reactive arthritis and psoriatic arthropathy may be presenting features of HIV infection.

Radiology

Sacroiliitis

This may be asymptomatic. It is worth looking for in unexplained monoarthritis and oligoarthritis because the presence of bilateral sacroiliitis makes the diagnosis of a spondyloarthropathy very likely. Beware of unilateral sacroiliitis: this may be due to sepsis, so consider aspiration or biopsy.

Spinal radiographs

These are indicated in back pain of an inflammatory pattern. Sacroiliitis and vertebral changes may be diagnostic long before the classic bamboo spine develops.

MRI

There is increasing evidence that MRI is able to detect acute spinal lesions even in the early stages of sacroiliitis/AS. This tool is being used in research to monitor disease progression and responsiveness to therapy.

Peripheral joint disease

Look for erosions and use to assess the progress of damage.

Occult inflammatory bowel disease

Consider small bowel radiology / large bowel endoscopy in:

> 'reactive arthritis' with persistent bowel symptoms

> erythema nodosum

> persistent monoarthritis/oligoarthritis with an acute phase response or anaemia that seems out of proportion to the articular disease.

Differential diagnosis

> spinal disease: beware infective or neoplastic spinal pathology, especially in an older patient. Mechanical back pain may sometimes give a very inflammatory picture

> monoarthritis: consider sepsis and crystal arthritis (see Section 1.4.4)

> oligoarthritis: consider crystal arthritis, rheumatic fever in a younger patient or Lyme disease if the patient has travelled / is resident in an endemic area. Dactylitis is also a feature of sarcoid arthropathy

> polyarthritis: parvovirus arthritis and other postviral arthritides, also rheumatoid disease

> joint and mucocutaneous disease: systemic lupus erythematosus and Behçet's disease

> joint and gut disease: vasculitis, Whipple's disease and coeliac disease.

Treatment

Short term

> exclude sepsis, symptomatic NSAIDs for pain and stiffness, and intra-articular corticosteroid injections

> treat any associated sexually transmitted infection in reactive arthritis (this has little or no influence on the joint disease)

> control inflammatory bowel disease.

Long term

> A lifelong daily exercise plan from physiotherapists can be beneficial for spinal disease.

> Sulfasalazine and methotrexate are useful in peripheral joint disease, but have little or no impact on spinal disease.

> Methotrexate is particularly useful in cases of psoriatic arthritis.

> Anti-tumour necrosis factor therapy is now licensed for severe AS and psoriatic arthritis. More recently, secukinumab, an anti-IL-17A monoclonal antibody has been licensed for both these indications, while ustekinumab (anti-IL-12 / anti-IL-23) has been licensed for psoriatic arthritis.

Prognosis

Ankylosing spondylitis

Many patients do well, with only a minority having severely disabling disease. Joint replacement is necessary in 15% of cases (most often for hips).

Key point

Poor prognostic features in ankylosing spondylitis

> onset in adolescence

> high acute phase response

> extraspinal joint disease.

Reactive arthritis

> Remission occurs in more than 70% of patients at 1 year and 85% at 2 years, but relapse can occur in 30–50% of patients, perhaps provoked by recurrent exposure to a triggering infection.

> This is a persistent long-term disease in 10–30% of patients.

> Persistence and recurrence are more likely if HLA-B27 is present.

Psoriatic arthritis

The outcome of psoriatic arthritis depends on the pattern. Asymmetrical oligoarthritis has a good long-term outcome but arthritis mutilans is associated with considerable disability.

2.3.5 Idiopathic inflammatory myopathies

Aetiology/pathophysiology/pathology

Key point

Usual classification

> primary idiopathic polymyositis (PM)

> primary idiopathic dermatomyositis (DM)

> PM or DM with malignancy

> juvenile DM (not discussed here)

> PM or DM with another connective tissue disease (CTD)

> inclusion body myositis

> necrotising autoimmune myopathy

> rare forms of idiopathic myositis, eg eosinophilic myositis, focal myositis and orbital myositis.

These myopathies are usually considered to be autoimmune disorders. They are paraneoplastic in 10% of cases. The immunological mechanism of muscle damage is largely via T-cells in PM, and antibody and complement in DM. Striated muscle involvement predominates, although cardiac and smooth muscle can be involved. Skeletal muscle pathology usually shows lymphocytic infiltration and fibre damage.

Statin-associated necrotising autoimmune myopathy accompanied by antibodies directed against the pharmacological target of statins (3-hydroxyl-3-methylglutaryl-coenzyme A reductase (HMGCR)) has emerged as a distinct entity, though it is unclear whether the association is causal or coincidental.

Epidemiology

These are rare disorders, with an incidence of around five per 10 million per year. The female:male ratio is about 2:1, although the sexes are equally affected by paraneoplastic myositis.

Clinical presentation

Muscle

This is usually affected by proximal weakness rather than pain. The assessment of the patient with proximal weakness is discussed in Section 1.1.11. Non-skeletal involvement may produce cardiac failure, respiratory failure and oropharyngeal dysfunction.

Skin

The following are important features:

> nailfold capillary dilatation, usually visible to the naked eye

> the development of scaly rashes on light-exposed skin, eg metacarpophalangeal joints (Gottron's papules)

> heliotrope rash (lilac-coloured rash on the eyelids)

> angio-oedematous changes, particularly on the face.

Lung

Intercostal and diaphragmatic weakness occurs in severe cases, which can lead to respiratory failure. The vital capacity should be monitored in inpatients. Interstitial lung disease, clinically indistinguishable from cryptogenic fibrosing alveolitis / idiopathic pulmonary fibrosis, occurs in around one-fifth of cases. The lung disease may be the presenting feature, initially with mild muscle changes. It is often associated with the presence of the anti-Jo-1 antibody, which is discussed further in Section 3.2.1.

Investigations

An assay of creatine kinase (CK) is the best marker of muscle inflammation, although it is not specific to myositis (see Section 1.1.11). CK is also a useful marker of response to treatment.

PM and DM may occasionally present with a normal CK. Screening for malignancy, use of muscle biopsy, electromyography and muscle imaging are discussed under Section 1.1.11. A raised alanine aminotransferase (ALT) may occasionally be due to myositis; CK should therefore be included in the screen for causes of a raised ALT.

Key point

Autoantibodies in inflammatory myositis:

> Anti-histidyl-transfer RNA synthetase (anti-Jo-1) – this is associated with interstitial lung disease, Raynaud's phenomenon and non-erosive arthritis (anti-synthetase syndrome).

> Anti-3-hydroxyl-3-methylglutaryl-coenzyme A reductase (anti-HMGCR) – this is the pharmacological target for statins, associated with necrotising autoimmune myopathy (NAM).

> Anti-signal recognition particle (anti-SRP) – this is associated with NAM.

> Anti-transcriptional intermediary factor 1γ (anti-TIF-1γ; also known as anti-p155) – this is associated with cancer-associated dermatomyositis.

> Anti-cytosolic 5'-nucleotidase1A (anti-cN1A) – this is associated with inclusion-body myositis.

> Anti-PM-Scl – this is associated with overlap syndrome characterised by features of polymyositis and scleroderma.

Detection of autoantibodies is often helpful, although around one-third of patients with PM/DM do not have any recognised pattern of autoantibodies. The presence of high-titre antinuclear antibodies greatly increases the diagnostic likelihood of PM/DM or other CTDs. A variety of distinctive patterns of autoantibody production are seen in defined subtypes of myositis and overlap syndromes. These include anti-Jo-1, anti-SRP, anti-HMGCR, anti-TIF-1γ, anti-PM-Scl and anti-cN1A (see 'key point' box).

Differential diagnosis
See Section 1.1.11.

Hazard

Do not automatically assume that:

> a normal CK level excludes myositis

> a raised CK level is the result of myositis without additional investigation

> lymphocytic infiltrates in a muscle are always caused by myositis.

Treatment
Corticosteroids form the mainstay of treatment, initially at high doses. Most patients require a steroid-sparing drug as their dose of steroids is reduced. Methotrexate can be used if there is no evidence of inflammatory lung disease. Another alternative is azathioprine. Cyclosporin as monotherapy, or in combination with methotrexate other immunosuppressant drugs including intravenous cyclophosphamide and high-dose intravenous immunoglobulin – can be used where the response to treatment is poor. Assessing response to treatment is usually by serial measurement of CK and muscle strength. Lung function tests including transfer factor and high-resolution CT of the lungs are useful in patients with inflammatory lung disease. Physiotherapy is an important adjunct to pharmacological treatment.

Key point

Reassessment
Where response to treatment is poor, consider re-biopsy to reassess the following:

> Initial diagnosis: is this really PM/DM? Inherited myopathies can sometimes be confused. Inclusion body myositis is a variant of PM that is much less responsive to immunosuppression. Patients with inclusion body myositis often have distal muscle weakness as well as proximal weakness.

> Treatment or disease: could persistent weakness be corticosteroid induced?

Skin and lung involvement will usually respond in parallel with the muscle disease, but topical steroids and antimalarials may be useful in skin disease and more aggressive immunosuppression may be required for lung disease. Rapid, non-specific deterioration may reflect the progression of underlying malignancy rather than the muscle disease itself.

Prognosis
Morbidity
Although most patients will show some response to immunosuppression, the morbidity of those with PM and DM is high. Overall, more than 50% of patients will have some long-term muscle weakness. The response to treatment in DM and myositis associated with other CTDs is better than in PM. Onset over the age of 65 is a poor prognostic sign.

2.3.6 Crystal arthritis: gout
Aetiology/pathophysiology/pathology

Key point

Poorly soluble crystals
A variety of poorly soluble crystals can be found in joints, some of which can induce inflammation, including the following:

> monosodium urate – the cause of gout

> calcium pyrophosphate – the cause of pseudogout

> apatite – possibly associated with aggressive forms of osteoarthritis (OA) (rare and not discussed further here).

Formation of monosodium urate crystals is a consequence of hyperuricaemia, resulting from overproduction or inefficient renal excretion of uric acid (or a combination of the two). Poor excretion is probably the major factor in most cases of gout.

There are a number of factors associated with gout, including male sex, increasing age and ethnicity (Polynesian populations are at particular risk). Medical conditions associated with gout include chronic kidney disease, obesity, cardiovascular disease, type 2 diabetes, hypertriglyceridaemia and psoriasis. Drugs are an important contributory cause, particularly diuretics and ciclosporin.

Crystals, which induce inflammation by activating leukocytes and/or the complement cascade, tend to form:

> in joints

> subcutaneously – forming discrete masses or tophi

> in the kidney and renal tubules.

Epidemiology

Gout is common, affecting more than 1% of the population, and is the most common cause of an acute hot joint. Gout is predominantly a male disease, and only occurs in significant numbers of women among those over the age of 60, when it is almost invariably associated with diuretic usage.

Clinical presentation

A number of overlapping syndromes are associated with urate crystal deposition:

> acute gout

> tophaceous gout

> nephrolithiasis

> uric acid nephropathy.

Acute gout

This usually presents with an episodic, self-limiting, flitting monoarthritis or oligoarthritis. This is most commonly of the first metatarsophalangeal joint ('podagra') and knee, but can produce an asymmetrical polyarthritis. Extra-articular acute attacks can occur in bursae (especially the olecranon). The inflammation is usually severe and exquisitely painful, although polyarthritic gout tends to be less florid. The attacks may be associated with systemic ill-health and fever. Precipitants include the following:

> alcohol excess

> intercurrent illness (including surgery), particularly if dehydration is present

> starvation

> the introduction of any drug that interferes with the handling of uric acid (including allopurinol).

The joint generally returns to normal between attacks, but may accrue erosive damage if there are recurrent attacks over many years.

Tophaceous gout

Widespread tophus formation can occur on a background of recurrent long-standing acute gout, but it can also occur in older women on diuretics in the absence of acute attacks (Fig 26). Tophi are usually pea sized, but can be very large. They tend to occur on the pinnae and on pressure points, such as extensor surfaces.

Nephrolithiasis

Uric acid crystals account for around 8% of all renal/ureteric calculi. They are radiolucent.

Uric acid nephropathy

Hyperuricaemia is a common finding in renal impairment, usually as a consequence of impaired kidney function, hypertension or drug treatment rather than the cause. The important exception is acute uric acid nephropathy which occurs in high cell turnover states, particularly leukaemias and lymphomas during the early stages of chemotherapy. Systemic illness and poor renal perfusion increase the risk of renal failure.

Physical signs

For physical signs see Section 1.3.6. Gout and sepsis are the only common causes of a red-hot joint, and it is important to differentiate the two by joint aspiration if there is any doubt. Gout may also mimic infection by producing spreading cellulitic changes, which may desquamate as recovery occurs. The affected joint is usually red, hot, swollen and very tender and painful to palpation.

Investigations

> Aspiration of synovial fluid is the only definitive diagnostic manoeuvre (see Section 3.5). The crystals are negatively birefringent under a polarised light microscope and are needle-shaped. Uric acid crystals can be found in between acute attacks, and the diagnosis can be made by aspiration of a quiescent joint – only a tiny amount of fluid is required. Crystals can also be seen in material aspirated from bursae and tophi.

> Measurement of serum uric acid is of little value: hyperuricaemia is far more common than clinical gout and, furthermore, the level may be normal during an acute attack.

> Uric acid excretion can be used to define overproducers and underexcretors, but this is rarely of clinical value.

> Assess renal function and consider screening for common comorbid conditions: hypertension, diabetes mellitus and hypercholesterolaemia (metabolic syndrome X / insulin resistance syndrome).

> Radiographs may be useful in chronic disease: periarticular tophi produce a distinctive punched-out pattern, which can be distinguished from other erosive arthropathies.

Differential diagnosis

This includes the causes of the acute hot joint that is discussed in Section 1.4.4. Chronic tophaceous gout can be confused with:

> rheumatoid arthritis

> psoriatic arthritis

> nodal OA.

Treatment

Management of gout has three goals: treating acute flares, prevention of acute attacks, and prevention of chronic gout (with urate-lowering therapy). Treatment of an acute flare should be commenced as soon as possible, aiming to reduce pain and inflammation.

Short term

Non-steroidal anti-inflammatory drugs

These are the mainstay of acute treatment, but beware the use of non-steroidal anti-inflammatory drugs (NSAIDs) in cases of renal impairment, and of the marked deterioration that can occur in patients with congestive cardiac failure and ischaemic heart disease. Where indicated, fast-acting NSAIDs at full therapeutic doses should be used (such as naproxen 500 mg twice daily or indomethacin 50 mg three times daily). Cyclooxygenase (COX)-2 inhibitors such as etoricoxib 120 mg daily appear equally effective. Aspirin is avoided because it impairs urate excretion.

Colchicine

This may be poorly tolerated. In high doses it causes diarrhoea, so has little to recommend it as a first-line treatment. However, it is sometimes used in low doses (500 µg bd) in patients who are unable to tolerate NSAIDs with good effect. It should be used with caution in those with renal or liver disease.

Corticosteroids

These are invaluable, particularly in patients unable to tolerate NSAIDs. Intra-articular administration is preferred when one or a small number of joints are affected, once sepsis has been ruled out. Alternatively, consider a short 5–7 day oral burst (eg prednisolone 30 mg daily). Some advocate tailing off the dose over a week or two, but others do not feel that this is necessary.

Long term

Most of the predisposing causes of gout are reversible. Alongside medical management, attention should be paid to modifying lifestyle risk factors (especially alcohol intake) and, where possible, altering precipitating medications. Urate-lowering agents can

be divided into three groups: xanthine oxidase inhibitors, uricosuric agents and recombinant uricase. Therapy is tailored to match the individual, with the ideal aim of reducing serum urate levels to below 0.3 mmol/L.

Key point

Prophylaxis
Prophylactic treatment should be considered in the following circumstances:

> recurrent acute attacks

> chronic tophaceous gout

> renal impairment

> the presence of leukaemias / lymphomas / bulky solid tumours prior to aggressive chemotherapy

> inherited syndromes with uric acid overproduction, eg Lesch–Nyhan syndrome.

The xanthine oxidase inhibitor allopurinol is the mainstay of prophylaxis, at doses between 300 mg and 900 mg daily unless renal impairment is present. Initiation of treatment is usually delayed until around 2 weeks after an acute attack as this can precipitate further attacks. For this reason, an NSAID or low-dose colchicine is often co-prescribed for the first few weeks of allopurinol treatment. Allopurinol is usually well tolerated, but it can provoke severe mucocutaneous reactions, including Stevens–Johnson syndrome. Febuxostat, another xanthine oxidase inhibitor, is used in patients who fail to respond to or fail to tolerate allopurinol. It may be especially useful in those with renal impairment, when allopurinol dosing can be complex, but clinical experience of its use in the context of severe renal or hepatic disease is limited. Recurrent gout on allopurinol/febuxostat usually reflects poor compliance or persistent high alcohol use.

Uricosuric drugs – probenecid and sulfinpyrazone are useful when allopurinol is ineffective or not tolerated, and can be used as monotherapy or in combination with xanthine oxidase inhibitors. However, these drugs may be less effective in those with renal impairment, and are contraindicated in those with severe renal or liver disease. They also have the potential to promote urate stone formation and should therefore be avoided in those with a history of nephrolithiasis.

Recombinant uricase (eg rasburicase) – this leads to rapid and profound reductions of urate levels, but due to its short half-life, high cost and risk of hypersensitivity reactions, its use is essentially limited to the management of tumour lysis syndrome following chemotherapy.

Management of comorbidities, especially cardiovascular disease, is one of the great challenges in gout treatment. Thiazide diuretics should be avoided and replaced, where possible, with losartan and amlodipine which have modest urate-lowering effects. Likewise fenofibrate and atorvastatin may be particularly useful adjuncts in those with dyslipidaemia. Despite its mild urate-elevating effects, aspirin should not be withheld in those with cardiovascular disease.

Hazard

Beware the interaction between the xanthine oxidase inhibitors allopurinol or febuxostat and azathioprine in organ recipients and patients with systemic autoimmune disease. Azathioprine toxicity including pancytopaenia may result due to accumulation of 6-mercaptopurine, the active metabolite of azathioprine, which is partially inactivated by xanthine oxidase.

2.3.7 Calcium pyrophosphate deposition disease

Aetiology/pathophysiology/pathology

This disease is poorly understood. Pyrophosphate crystals form in articular cartilage and are shed into the synovial fluid where they can provoke an inflammatory response. Pyrophosphate crystal formation occurs increasingly with age, but is also associated with a number of metabolic disorders:

> hereditary haemochromatosis

> primary hyperparathyroidism

> previous joint trauma (including surgery)

> previous intra-articular bleeding

> hypophosphatasia (rare inherited alkaline phosphatase deficiency).

Epidemiology

Acute pseudogout is largely a disorder of older people, unless it is secondary to a metabolic disorder. Incidence is about half that of gout. Radiographic chondrocalcinosis is common.

Clinical presentation

Acute pseudogout

This disease presents like any other acute hot joint (see Section 1.4.4), often with striking fever and systemic illness. Intercurrent illness is the most common precipitant.

Chronic joint disease

The spectrum of disease ranges from a rheumatoid-like picture with synovitis to a variant of osteoarthritis. There is shoulder, elbow, wrist and metacarpophalangeal joint (especially second and third) involvement in the upper limb.

Investigations

For investigations, see Section 1.4.4. In an acute monoarthropathy, synovial fluid aspirate is the gold-standard investigation,

with identification of brick- or rod-shaped weakly positive birefringence on polarised light microscopy. The rheumatoid-like picture is not associated with rheumatoid factor or anti-CCP antibodies, and is only occasionally associated with an acute phase response. Diagnosis of the chronic joint diseases is largely radiological, looking for chondrocalcinosis (Fig 60) and the distinctive pattern of degenerative joint disease.

Key point

Investigate potential secondary causes, especially haemochromatosis. Ferritin, serum iron and iron binding, calcium and alkaline phosphatase should be measured in most cases, especially in younger patients.

Treatment

Acute pseudogout is best managed with NSAIDs, colchicine or intra-articular steroid injection once sepsis has been excluded. Low-dose colchicine has been used to prevent recurrent attacks, but there are no target-specific treatments for chronic pyrophosphate arthropathies.

2.3.8 Fibromyalgia

Aetiology/pathophysiology/pathology

Fibromyalgia is a syndrome characterised by chronic widespread pain, fatigue and low mood, in the absence of convincing evidence of musculoskeletal inflammation, although it may arise on a background of definite rheumatic disease (eg rheumatoid arthritis (RA) or spinal pain).

The pathogenesis of fibromyalgia remains unknown. Current understanding focuses on dysfunctional pain processing due to a combination of central sensitisation, reduction in inhibitory pain pathways, altered neurotransmitters and psychosocial factors. Various factors seem to perpetuate the syndrome, including the following:

> sleep disturbance

> a tendency to cope with pain and fatigue by withdrawal and rest

> consequent profound loss of physical fitness

> depression.

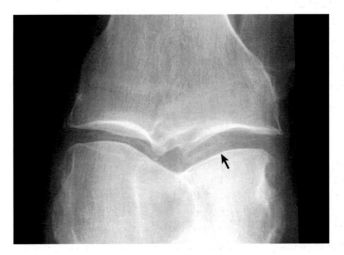

Fig 60 Chondrocalcinosis of the knee (arrowed).

Epidemiology

Fibromyalgia is common, affecting between 2% and 4% of the UK population. Its prevalence increases with age; women are more commonly affected than men, and it is associated with lower income, being disabled, divorced or separated, and having a lower educational status.

Clinical presentation

Patients with fibromyalgia present with widespread pain (ie affecting all four quadrants of the body), fatigue and consequent disability, which is often profound. Joint swelling or 'puffiness' and paraesthesiae may be reported, but synovitis or objective sensory change is not evident either clinically or following investigation unless there is a coexistent disorder such as RA or carpal tunnel syndrome. Fatigue is profound and out of keeping with low levels of activity; indeed there is considerable overlap with the chronic fatigue syndrome. In addition, patients may report headache, short-term memory loss and difficulty in concentrating.

Physical signs

In the absence of comorbidities, examination is normal, apart from pain on digital palpation of classic soft-tissue trigger points.

Investigations

Fibromyalgia is a clinical diagnosis. There is no investigation that will 'prove' that the patient has the condition. The purpose of investigation is to exclude other mimics or coexisting conditions. A reasonable set of tests to do in most cases would be the following:

> FBC

> renal, bone and liver biochemistry

> vitamin D

> blood glucose

> creatinine kinase

> thyroid function

> acute phase markers (C-reactive protein and erythrocyte sedimentation rate)

> myeloma screen in patients >50 years

> antinuclear antibodies, rheumatoid factor and anti-CCP antibodies

> chest radiograph, especially in smokers.

! Hazard

'Red flag' features in widespread pain

You should suspect that fibromyalgia is *not* the diagnosis if the patient has any of the following circumstances:

> onset age >50 years

> recent onset and a progressive history

> weight loss

> any previous history of malignancy or immunosuppression

> focal versus diffuse pain

> fever

> any abnormal physical signs other than tenderness

> abnormal blood tests.

Treatment

Patients with fibromyalgia have a high level of disability, often greater than that of those with RA. It is not acceptable simply to document the lack of severe physical disease in these patients and then discharge them: they deserve a constructive, multidisciplinary and positive approach to their diagnosis and management. Patient education is crucial, and reassuring them that they are believed and taken seriously is important. The condition is disabling but not destructive, and they have their own positive part to play in rehabilitation. Treatment should usefully be directed towards the factors that perpetuate an individual patient's disability. Cognitive behaviour therapy may be very effective for both depression and in correcting abnormal or unhelpful beliefs about pain.

Other standard approaches include:

> Improvement of sleep quality and pain levels with a low-dose tricyclic antidepressant, eg amitriptyline 10–50 mg nocte. Pregabalin or duloxetine are also useful options.

> The use of analgesics if they are helpful, but their withdrawal if they are not.

> Increase in physical fitness with a graded exercise programme, with emphasis on ultimately increasing aerobic capacity where possible.

> Treatment of any coexistent depression with full-dose antidepressant therapy.

Be realistic about the prognosis (see below); carefully assess any secondary gain and consider discussion with the family; and do not organise more and more investigations – try to limit further referrals.

Prognosis

Patients with a long history and a high degree of disability have a poor prognosis. Involvement of pain management services and liaison psychiatry may be useful. The issues of the sick role, secondary gain and involvement of the family and carers may also need to be addressed.

2.4 Autoimmune rheumatic disease

2.4.1 Systemic lupus erythematosus

Aetiology/immunopathogenesis

The cause of systemic lupus erythematosus (SLE) is unknown. It has a clear genetic element, as evidenced by the higher rate of concordance in monozygotic twins (25%) compared with dizygotic twins (3%). While genome-wide association studies (GWAS) and candidate gene studies have identified over 50 loci relating to B-cell activation, innate immune signalling (nuclear factor kappa B (NF-κB), type I interferon (IFN)), handling of apoptotic debris and clearance of immune complexes in patients with SLE, homozygous deficiency of early complement components (C1q) remains the strongest monogenic susceptibility risk factor for lupus. Several lines of evidence suggest that type I IFN is a primary pathogenic feature of SLE, with high circulating levels seen in patients of all ancestral backgrounds.

The onset of disease is triggered by ultraviolet (UV) light, drugs (eg minocycline, sulfasalazine, penicillamine, hydralazine and isoniazid) and possibly infection. There is a plethora of immunological abnormalities, characterised by marked polyclonal B-cell activation associated with hypergammaglobulinaemia, immune complex deposition and the production of autoantibodies.

Epidemiology

SLE is nine times more common in women than in men. Onset is commonly in the second and third decades. People of African-Caribbean and Asian origin are particularly susceptible. The prevalence of SLE in African-Caribbean women is one in 450, in Asian women it is one in 900 and in northern European women it is one in 2,000.

> **Key point**
>
> The factors responsible for exacerbations of SLE include:
>
> > exposure to sunlight (UV light)
> > psychological stress
> > infections
> > pregnancy and puerperium
> > drugs, eg minocycline, sulfasalazine, penicillamine, hydralazine and isoniazid.

Clinical presentation

Many patients present with fever, arthralgia, fatigue and a skin rash. The symptoms may sometimes be very non-specific and lead to a delay in diagnosis. Additional features and major organ involvement (eg kidneys and the central nervous system) may occur at disease onset or evolve. SLE has a long-term course characterised by exacerbations and remissions.

Musculoskeletal manifestations

The flitting arthralgia that is associated with early morning stiffness is common (90%). The arthritis rarely progresses to a deforming arthropathy. Hand deformities resulting from tendon disease may cause a rheumatoid-like but non-erosive arthropathy (Jaccoud's arthropathy) in a minority of patients (Fig 61). Only 4% of SLE patients develop erosions.

Skin and mucous membranes

UV light-induced skin photosensitivity is common. Malar rash (Fig 11) and recurrent mouth ulcers (Fig 12) occur in 50% of cases, non-scarring alopecia in 70% and Raynaud's phenomenon is a feature in 25%. Lupus confined to the skin is characterised by distinctive rashes: discoid lupus (Fig 10) or subacute cutaneous lupus.

Kidney disease

Almost all patients with SLE have histological abnormalities on renal biopsy, but only 50% of patients develop overt renal disease. Early disease should be screened for at each

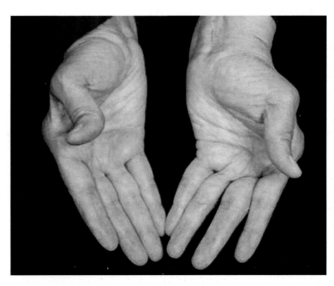

Fig 61 Jaccoud's arthropathy in a patient with SLE.

visit by performing urine analysis looking for blood and protein, and by checking the patient's blood pressure.

Nervous system
Neurological involvement affects up to two-thirds of patients at some point in their disease (see Section 1.4.3).

Key point

Neuropsychiatric manifestations of SLE

Neuropsychiatric manifestations of SLE are, in decreasing order of frequency:

> organic brain syndrome: cognitive impairment and psychosis (may be steroid induced)

> seizures

> cranial neuropathy

> peripheral neuropathy

> stroke

> movement disorder

> transverse myelitis

> headaches.

Pulmonary
Pleurisy with or without radiological evidence of effusion occurs in 40% of cases. Pulmonary emboli may occur in patients who are antiphospholipid-positive. Inflammatory lung disease, shrinking lung syndrome and pulmonary hypertension are rare manifestations in SLE.

Cardiovascular
Pericarditis (30%) is usually mild and very rarely progresses to tamponade. Non-infective thrombotic endocarditis (Libman–Sacks endocarditis) is rare and is associated with the antiphospholipid syndrome.

Haematological abnormalities
Normocytic normochromic anaemia, mild lymphopenia and mild thrombocytopenia occur in a substantial number of patients. Severe thrombocytopenia, severe leukopenia and haemolytic anaemia may sometimes occur. Reactive lymphadenopathy (in 40% of cases) and splenomegaly (in 10% of cases) occur, especially during disease activity. The antiphospholipid syndrome occurs in 20% of patients with SLE.

Overlap syndromes
This term describes patients who have coexisting features of two or more connective tissue diseases (Fig 62). The following are common examples:

> scleroderma/SLE overlap

> scleroderma/polymyositis (PM) overlap.

Mixed connective tissue disease
Patients are defined as having mixed connective tissue disease (MCTD) if they have features of:

> SLE

> scleroderma

> PM.

This is on the basis of high antibody titres to U1 ribonucleoprotein, arthritis/arthralgia (in 95% of cases), Raynaud's (in 85% of cases) and minimal renal disease. The existence of MCTD as a distinct diagnostic entity has since been questioned because none of the clinical or laboratory criteria used for the definition of the disease have proven specific.

Investigations for systemic lupus erythematosus
See Section 1.1.8.

Differential diagnosis
See Section 1.1.8.

Treatment
See Section 1.4.3.

Prognosis
The 5-year survival rate for patients with SLE is now over 90%. Patients with renal disease have a higher mortality rate than non-renal patients. Mortality is caused by severe disease activity, sepsis and cardiovascular complications due to atherosclerosis leading to premature coronary heart disease. Screening for disease activity, excluding infection and screening for risk factors for atherosclerosis are all important in the management of the lupus patient.

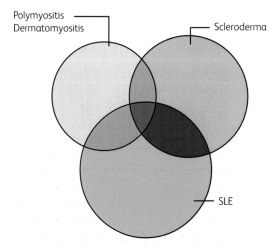

Fig 62 Venn diagram depicting overlap of SLE, scleroderma and myosis. SLE, systemic lupus erythematosus.

2.4.2 Sjögren's syndrome

Key point

Sjögren's syndrome is a chronic autoimmune exocrinopathy predominantly affecting the salivary and lacrimal glands. The clinical picture is dominated by keratoconjunctivitis sicca (KCS) and xerostomia. It may occur by itself (primary Sjögren's syndrome) or in association with one of the connective tissue diseases or rheumatoid arthritis (secondary Sjögren's syndrome, see Fig 63). Primary Sjögren's syndrome is classically associated with anti-Ro and anti-La antibodies.

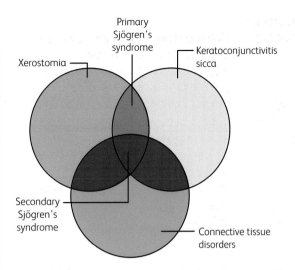

Fig 63 Relationship between KCS, xerostomia, and primary and secondary Sjögren's syndrome. (Adapted with permission from Manthorpe R, Jacobsson LT. Classification and assessment of rheumatic diseases. *Baillière's Clin Rheumatol* 1995;9:483–96.)

Epidemiology

> marked female preponderance

> male:female ratio is 1:10

> typically affects middle-aged women.

Aetiology/pathology

The cause of Sjögren's syndrome is unknown but believed to be multifactorial and due to a combination of genetic and environmental factors. Genetic markers include certain human leukocyte antigen (HLA) types, eg HLA-DR3 and HLA-DQ2. Possible viral factors include hepatitis C virus, cytomegalovirus and the Epstein–Barr virus. The cardinal pathological lesion is inflammatory destruction of salivary glands, mediated by focal periductular CD4$^+$ T-cell infiltrates.

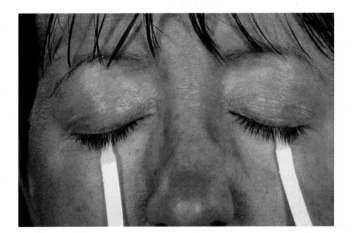

Fig 64 Dry eyes in Sjögren's syndrome demonstrated by Schirmer's test: wetting of <5 mm of filter paper in 5 minutes is considered abnormal.

Clinical presentation

KCS manifests as dry, gritty eyes (Fig 64) and can vary in severity from mild and episodic to constant, severe and disabling with visual disturbance. Photophobia is common and may be due to uveitis. Poor salivary secretion leads to dysphagia for dry foods, reduced taste perception, bad breath and increased rate of dental decay. Salivary gland enlargement (parotid and submandibular) occurs in 50% of cases. Other exocrine glands may be involved in Sjögren's syndrome, eg impaired glandular function in the nasal and sinus epithelium and the vagina, leading to recurrent sinusitis and dyspareunia, respectively. Fatigue is a major problem, similar to those affected by other rheumatic diseases; it is often exacerbated by poor sleep, anxiety and low mood.

Extraglandular features of Sjögren's syndrome

> an intermittent non-deforming non-erosive symmetrical polyarthritis

> Raynaud's phenomenon

> dry skin and cutaneous vasculitis

> mixed cryoglobulinaemia

> alveolitis

> interstitial nephritis

> renal tubular acidosis

> peripheral neuropathy

> mononeuritis multiplex

> risk of neonatal lupus rash or congenital heart block in babies of Ro/La-antibody-positive mothers.

Investigation

For laboratory findings, perform tests for KCS, the rose bengal test and tests for xerostomia – see Section 1.1.10.

Blood tests

The FBC usually reveals a mild normochromic anaemia, with leukopenia or thrombocytopenia, and an autoimmune haemolytic anaemia is occasionally seen. The acute-phase reactant erythrocyte sedimentation rate (ESR) is elevated as a consequence of hypergammaglobulinaemia, while the C-reactive protein (CRP) is often normal. Most patients are antinuclear antibody (ANA)- and rheumatoid factor (RhF)-positive. The best-described autoantibodies in Sjögren's syndrome are anti-Ro and anti-La antibodies, which are present in two-thirds and one-third of patients, respectively. Hypocomplementaemia in Sjögren's patients is associated with a higher frequency of vasculitis, lymphoma and cryoglobulinaemia.

Assessment of sicca symptoms

The Schirmer's test (see Fig 64) is the gold-standard screening test for dry eyes. A filter paper strip is inserted into the conjunctival sac over the lower lid margin, one-third in from the outer edge of the eye. The strips stimulate tear production and less than 5 mm wetting in 5 minutes is diagnostic of dry eye.

Salivary gland involvement can be measured by salivary flow rates and minor gland biopsy.

Treatment

Oral manifestations

Preventative measures – regular dental visits and scrupulous dental hygiene, minimise chronic use of alcohol and caffeine, and avoid drugs that can worsen sicca symptoms (eg antidepressants etc)

Salivary gland stimulation – sugar-free gum or lozenges, parasympathomimetic secretagogues such as pilocarpine or cevimeline

Saliva replacement – increase humidification, frequent sips of water, saliva substitutes.

Ocular manifestations

Preventative measures – avoidance of exacerbating factors and irritants, use of moisture glasses

Improved lubrication – tear substitutes such as eye drops and ointments, parasympathomimetic secretagogues (pilocarpine, cevimeline), tear retention measures (lacrimal punctum plugs), reduction of ocular surface inflammation (corticosteroid or ciclosporin eye drops)

Extra-glandular manifestations – arthralgia and skin disease usually respond to hydroxychloroquine or other disease-modifying antirheumatic drugs (DMARDs); pulmonary and neurological complications may require more powerful immunosuppression, depending on the severity of the disease. Vaginal dryness and dyspareunia respond to lubricants.

Poor sleep and fatigue are notoriously multifactorial and may be harder to treat. Identify and focus on any key features or exacerbating factors such as pain, irritable bladder, depression, nocturia from overhydration to counteract daytime sicca symptoms, and reduced physical capacity. Coaching, behavioural therapy and learning coping/pacing strategies may be useful in those with disabling fatigue.

See Section 1.1.10.

Complications

There is an increased risk of B-cell lymphoma (most commonly of mucosa-associated lymphoid tissue (MALT) type) and the risk is greatest in Ro/La-positive individuals. Other predictive features include neutropaenia, lymphadenopathy and low C4 levels. The usual presentation is of a discrete firm swelling within the parotid gland, which should prompt rapid evaluation with an open biopsy. The prognosis is good, with complete response to chemotherapy reported at greater than 90%.

Key point

Lymphoma in Sjögren's syndrome
Consider lymphoma if there is:

> persistent cervical lymph node enlargement

> persistent hard or nodular salivary or lacrimal gland enlargement

> lung shadowing

> monoclonal cryoglobulins

> a progressive fall in serum immunoglobulins.

2.4.3 Systemic sclerosis (scleroderma)

Scleroderma is an autoimmune disorder characterised by the excessive deposition of collagen. It leads to fibrosis and vascular obliteration within the skin, and frequently within other organs including the lung, heart, kidneys and gastrointestinal (GI) tract.

Aetiology/immunopathogenesis

Despite wide-ranging immunological activation, it has been difficult to propose a single unifying immunopathogenic model for scleroderma. Several environmental agents (silica and organic solvents) have been implicated in disease initiation, but conclusive epidemiological evidence is lacking. A genetic component is exemplified by human leukocyte antigen (HLA) associations (various HLA-DR alleles) with certain disease subsets. One recent hypothesis argues that microchimerism as a result of the persistence of fetal T-cells in the mother might cause scleroderma by initiating a graft-versus-host response; another describes the presence of stimulatory autoantibodies against the platelet-derived growth factor receptor that can activate collagen gene expression in fibroblasts.

Key point

The key immunological features in scleroderma are:

> skin and lung lesions infiltrated by activated CD4+ and CD8+ T-cells

> increased expression of adhesion molecules from selectin/integrin and the immunoglobulin gene superfamily

> increased production of T-helper (Th)-1 and Th-2 cytokines: interleukin (IL)-1, IL-2, IL-4, IL-6, IL-8, tumour necrosis factor and transforming growth factor β

> polyclonal B-cell activation leading to hypergammaglobulinaemia and autoantibody production.

Epidemiology

There is an annual incidence of 18 cases per 10 million in the UK. The prevalence is estimated to be one in 10,000. The female:male ratio is 3:1 and the incidence increases with age: it is most common in those aged between 30 and 50 years.

Clinical presentation

The classification of scleroderma is shown in Table 36.

Diffuse cutaneous scleroderma

The onset of diffuse cutaneous systemic sclerosis (DCSSc) may be abrupt and may present as swollen hands (Fig 25), face and feet, which is also associated with new or recent onset of Raynaud's phenomenon. Fatigue is common and overt weakness may be present due to coexisting myositis. Examination reveals an inability to pinch skin folds, and the loss of skin lines and creases in involved areas. An evaluation of swallowing, breathing, renal and cardiac functions may reveal abnormalities (Table 37).

Limited cutaneous systemic sclerosis

Limited cutaneous systemic sclerosis (LCSSc) was previously known as CREST (calcinosis, Raynaud's, oesophageal dysfunction, sclerodactyly, telangiectasia). Typically the patients are female, aged 30–50, have a long history of Raynaud's phenomenon and have recent skin involvement limited to the

hands, face and feet (Table 37). Other features include the following:

> calcium deposition in the skin (calcinosis) (Fig 65)

> dilated blood vessels (telangiectasia, Fig 66) in the palms and face

> oesophageal dysmotility with or without reflux (Fig 67).

Systemic sclerosis without scleroderma

Some patients have visceral disease without cutaneous involvement. The presence of anticentromere, antiscleroderma-70 or antinucleolar antibodies is helpful in making the diagnosis.

Visceral involvement

The clinical spectrum of visceral involvement in scleroderma includes the following:

> GI tract:

> small mouth aperture and oesophageal hypomotility (90% of cases)

> malabsorption, wide-mouthed colonic diverticulae and rarely pneumatosis cystoides intestinalis

> faecal incontinence

> gastric antral vascular ectasia (GAVE) (in DCSSc only), a form of vasculopathy, may present with chronic anaemia or an acute upper GI bleed. Diagnosis is made at endoscopy, with identification of

Table 36	Classification of scleroderma	
Disease extent	**Features**
Systemic	DCSSc LCSSc SS without scleroderma Overlap syndrome
Localised	Morphoea (localised and generalised) Linear scleroderma

DCSSc, diffuse cutaneous systemic sclerosis; LCSSc, limited cutaneous systemic sclerosis; SS, systemic sclerosis.

Table 37 Features helpful in differentiating DCSSc from LCSSc

	DCSSc	LCSSc
Extent of skin thickening	Truncal and acral	Acral
Timing of relationship between skin thickening and Raynaud's phenomenon	Simultaneous or skin first	Prolonged Raynaud's phenomenon before skin
Joints and tendon	Contractures and tendon friction rubs	Infrequent involvement
Calcinosis	Inflammatory lung disease	Prominent
Visceral involvement	Renal and myocardial disease	Pulmonary vasculopathy
Serum autoantibodies	Anti-Scl 70 (30%)	Anticentromere (70%)

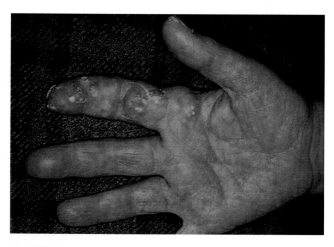

Fig 65 Calcinosis cutis in the index finger of a patient with LCSSc.

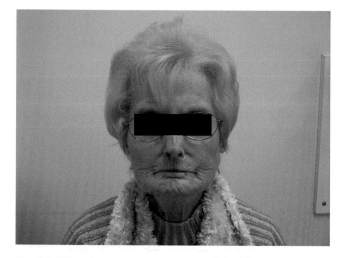

Fig 66 Telangiectasia in a patient with LCSSc.

the characteristic 'watermelon stomach'. Endoscopic laser therapy can be highly effective.

> lungs:

> > pulmonary arterial hypertension (PAH) may develop in both DCSSc and LCSSc but with differing underlying pathologies. PAH in diffuse disease tends to be driven by inflammatory parenchymal disease; in limited disease it is caused by vasculopathy

> > other patterns of respiratory involvement – these include aspiration pneumonia, recurrent chest infections, pleural thickening, effusion and calcification, spontaneous pneumothorax, pulmonary vasculitis and bronchoalveolar carcinoma

> cardiovascular system:

> > pericarditis with effusion

> > myocardial fibrosis causing dysrhythmias and congestive cardiac failure

> kidney:

> > hypertension

> > scleroderma renal crisis (accelerated hypertension)

> > progressive renal failure.

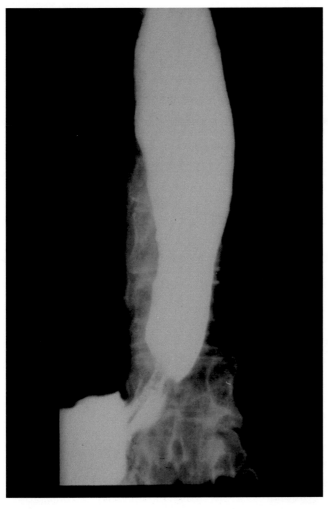

Fig 67 Oesophageal dysmotility in a patient with scleroderma.

Visceral involvement

Assess the extent of GI involvement (use manometry, endoscopy and contrast studies) and lung involvement (use pulmonary function tests including transfer factor to look for restrictive defect, as well as high-resolution CT scans). Regular monitoring of blood pressure, renal function and urinalysis is essential in a diffuse disease (owing to the risk of scleroderma renal crisis). Use Doppler echocardiography to detect pulmonary hypertension.

Treatment

Scleroderma is incurable. Treatment is aimed at the following:

> alleviating the symptoms of Raynaud's phenomenon by stopping smoking, wearing thermal gloves, avoiding cold temperatures and the prompt treatment of digital infections and ulcers. Oral vasodilators (calcium channel blockers) are useful for frequent attacks. Prostacyclin infusions are useful in treating severe digital ischaemia

> alleviating the symptoms of reflux oesophagitis and GI hypomotility

Investigations

Antinuclear antibodies

Antinuclear antibodies occur in 90% of patients. Three well-defined, mutually exclusive specificities have been defined for investigation (Fig 68), each associated with certain clinical features.

Hand radiograph

Look for loss of terminal phalangeal tufts and soft-tissue calcification (calcinosis).

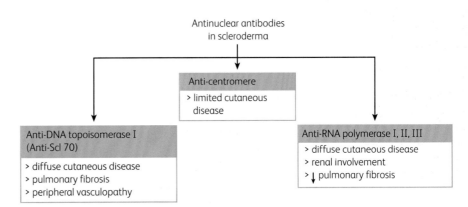

Fig 68 Antinuclear antibodies in scleroderma enable the definition of three mutually exclusive specificities.

- preventing the progression of lung fibrosis through the judicious use of immunosuppressive therapy; combined care with respiratory specialists is advised

- preventing the progression of pulmonary hypertension with prostaglandins (eg iloprost), endothelin blockers (eg bosentan) and PDE5 inhibitors (eg sildenafil); liaison with a specialist centre is recommended

- preventing renal crisis by using a prophylactic low dose of an angiotensin-converting enzyme (ACE) inhibitor and avoiding steroids where possible.

Prognosis

The 5-year survival rate ranges from 30% to 70%. Adverse prognostic features include male sex, extent of skin involvement, and heart, lung and renal disease.

2.4.4 IgG4-related disease

Aetiology/pathophysiology/pathology

IgG4-related disease (IgG4-RD) is a recently described fibro-inflammatory disorder with protean clinical manifestations. Its aetiology is unknown, but its characteristic histopathology in the form of lymphoplasmacytic inflammatory fibrosis and obliterative phlebitis, accompanied by prominent immunoglobulin G4 (IgG4)-expressing plasma cells, has enabled its delineation as a distinct clinical entity. The role of IgG4 in causation is a mystery given its inability to fix complement or activate Fc receptors, raising the possibility that its tissue deposition and elevation in serum are secondary events in response to an unspecified immunological stimulus. T-cells are likely to be involved in disease pathogenesis given the prominent presence of CD4$^+$ cells at sites of inflammation.

Epidemiology

The reported prevalence of 2.2 cases per 100,000 population for IgG4-related autoimmune pancreatitis is likely to be a substantial underestimate given its under recognition as a multisystem disease. In contrast to classic autoimmune disease, IgG4-RD is more common in men than in women.

Clinical presentation

Many patients will present with subacute salivary gland and or lymph node enlargement, or chronic pancreatitis, but IgG4-RD is truly protean in its ability to affect multiple organ systems (Fig 69). Typically, patients will have been symptomatic for months to years before diagnosis, but usually remain constitutionally well.

Salivary glands

Isolated enlargement of the submandibular glands, with or without xerostomia, is frequently seen. The historic diagnosis of Mikulicz's syndrome, which comprised chronic inflammatory enlargement of salivary and lacrimal glands, has now been recognised as IgG4-RD.

Pancreas

IgG4-RD was originally described in the pancreas as a form of steroid-responsive autoimmune pancreatitis with characteristic lymphoplasmacytic, sclerosing inflammation. Most affected patients would present with progressive obstructive jaundice because of concomitant sclerosing cholangitis.

Lymphadenopathy

Either localised or generalised painless lymph node enlargement mimicking lymphoproliferative disease is well recognised.

Aorta

IgG4-related aortitis resulting in aneurysmal dilatation or dissection may occur in the thoracic aorta.

Retroperitoneal fibrosis

Idiopathic retroperitoneal fibrosis has now been shown to be due to IgG4-RD in association with peri-aortitis. Common clinical presentations include backache, leg oedema and ureteric obstruction causing hydronephrosis.

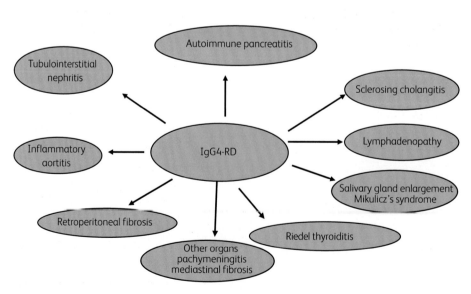

Fig 69 Multisystem manifestations of IgG4-RD. One or more features may be present in a single patient.

Investigation

Tissue biopsy, imaging and measurement of serum IgG4 are key investigations. Clinicopathological correlation of clinical features with tissue biopsy findings of lymphoplasmacytic infiltration with predominant IgG4-expressing plasma cells is critical in order to make a definitive diagnosis (Fig 70).

An elevated serum IgG4 is only seen in approximately 50% of cases, and in isolation does not provide diagnostic assurance given its elevation in a range of other disorders.

As important as tissue biopsy, imaging (CT or PET-CT) is essential to delineate organ involvement and the extent of systemic disease, including detection of asymptomatic pancreatic involvement.

Differential diagnosis

Its ability to mimic multisystem disease means that IgG4-RD should be considered as part of the differential diagnosis of patients thought to be presenting with a wide range of disorders, including suspected sarcoidosis, granulomatosis and polyangiitis, and Sjögren's syndrome. In patients presenting with obstructive jaundice due to pancreatic involvement, differentiation from pancreatic carcinoma is crucial to avoid unnecessary surgery. Presentations with lymphadenopathy and other organ involvement should be differentiated from lymphoma.

Treatment

IgG4-RD is highly sensitive to oral steroids to the extent that failure to respond to treatment should lead to a re-evaluation of the diagnosis. While no randomised controlled trials have been performed, there is sufficient experience with steroids to recommend them as first-line therapy. Most patients will require several months of therapy, with a few requiring additional steroid-sparing immunosuppressive therapy. B-cell depletion using rituximab has been shown to be effective in patients who are unresponsive to standard treatment.

2.5 Vasculitides

> **Key point**
> There is no single system of classification that would satisfy the heterogeneous group of vasculitides. In practical terms, it is best to classify the vasculitides using a combination of blood vessel size and underlying pathogenic mechanism(s), where these are known (Fig 71).

2.5.1 Giant cell arteritis and polymyalgia rheumatica

Aetiology/pathophysiology/pathology

> **Key point**
> Giant cell arteritis (GCA) and polymyalgia rheumatica (PMR) are related disorders with common epidemiological, clinical and serological features. Although GCA is a large-vessel vasculitis, PMR is a clinical syndrome characterised by prolonged proximal girdle pain and stiffness.

The aetiology of GCA and PMR is unknown. The clear preponderance of both disorders in older people remains unexplained. There is a genetic association with human leukocyte antigen (HLA)-DR4, similar to rheumatoid arthritis (RA), which indicates a role for T-cells. CD4 and CD8 T-cells are found in inflammatory lesions and both interferon-gamma- and interleukin-17-secreting T-cells may play an important role in pathogenesis, especially in activating CD68[+] macrophages.

GCA affects all layers of the vessel wall, but is marked in the internal elastic lamina, where intimal hyperplasia can lead to occlusion of the arterial lumen and consequent ischaemic complications.

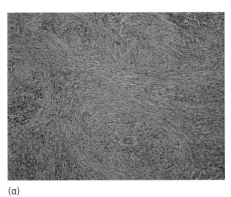

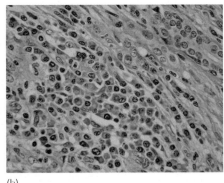

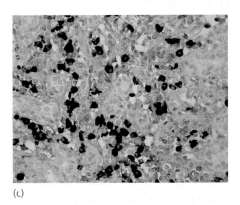

(a)   (b)   (c)

Fig 70 Biopsy of an inflammatory mass in a patient with IgG4-RD. **(a)** Low-power view showing storiform fibrosis. **(b)** High-power view showing plasma cells on a background of fibrosis. **(c)** High-power view showing predominant IgG4-positive plasma cells. (Courtesy of Dr Ketan Shah, Oxford University Hospitals.)

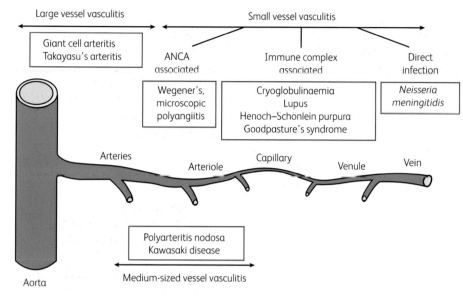

Fig 71 Classification of vasculitides according to vessel size and underlying mechanisms. (Modified with permission from Jennette JC, Falk RJ. Small vessel vasculitis. *N Engl J Med* 1997;337:1512–23.)

The thoracic aorta and its branches are commonly affected. Many of the characteristic clinical manifestations are the result of involvement of the branches of the external carotid artery.

Epidemiology

Ninety per cent of patients are over 60 years of age with a female preponderance. GCA is the most common of the primary systemic vasculitides and individuals of northern European descent have the highest incidence (the incidence is 178 per 10 million).

Clinical presentation

Symptoms in GCA are due to:

> ischaemia – mild or severe headache occurs in two-thirds of patients. Claudication of the jaw muscles, which produces pain on chewing, occurs in 40% of sufferers, whereas visual symptoms resulting from ophthalmic artery involvement occur in 20%.

> systemic inflammation with fatigue, fever and weight loss – PMR, with its characteristic proximal girdle pain and stiffness, occurs in 50% of patients with GCA and is the presenting feature in 25% of cases.

Occasionally, patients may present with a pyrexia of unknown origin or dissecting aneurysms of the aorta.

Physical signs

Scalp tenderness, frequently over the superficial temporal and occipital arteries, is highly suggestive of GCA and occurs in 40% of patients.

These include arterial bruits, asymmetrical blood pressure and absent pulses in extremities, and ophthalmoscopic evidence of ischaemic optic neuritis.

Investigations

There is no specific serological test. Elevated acute phase markers, in particular the erythrocyte sedimentation rate (ESR) (>40 mm/h) and C-reactive protein (CRP), occur in 80% of patients and are useful indices for monitoring treatment. Arterial biopsy is recommended for diagnostic confirmation of GCA (Fig 72). Arterial biopsy is not required in PMR, although it is positive in 10–20% of patients.

Alternative approaches using imaging have been used in patients with GCA to avoid the need for surgical biopsies and the associated morbidity. Colour Doppler ultrasonography can detect perivascular hypoechoic abnormalities

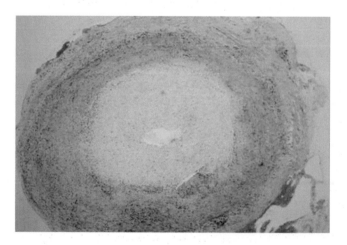

Fig 72 Occluded temporal artery in a patient with GCA showing thickening and lymphocytic infiltration throughout the vessel wall. (Courtesy of Dr L Bridges, Leeds General Infirmary.)

('halo sign') in the vessel wall as well as vascular stenosis and occlusion. 18F-fluorodeoxyglucose (FDG) positron emission tomography (PET) is indicated in poorly responding disease. FDG uptake can be demonstrated in the vessel walls of the aorta and its main branches, and interestingly can also be demonstrated in some individuals with PMR.

Differential diagnosis

A wide range of disorders may occasionally mimic PMR. Consider the alternative diagnoses listed in the 'key point' box below in cases of diagnostic doubt or the patient failing to respond promptly to steroid therapy.

Key point

Differential diagnosis of PMR:

> infection: tuberculosis and endocarditis

> autoimmune rheumatic disease: RA, inflammatory muscle disease and systemic lupus

> neoplasia

> Parkinsonism

> hypothyroidism

> chronic fatigue syndrome.

Treatment

Both GCA and PMR are exquisitely sensitive to steroids. Indeed, failure to respond to steroids is sufficient cause for the original diagnosis to be questioned. The dose of steroids required to suppress inflammation is higher in GCA (40–60 mg/day), whereas 10–20 mg is sufficient in PMR. The response to treatment is monitored using a combination of clinical and acute phase end points (ESR and CRP). As most patients require treatment for 1–2 years, it is essential to be alert to the problems of long-term corticosteroid therapy.

Complications

Permanent visual loss occurs in 15–20% of patients with GCA. A smaller percentage develop strokes and aortic aneurysms.

Prognosis

The overall prognosis for PMR is good, with 75% of patients stopping steroids by 2 years. The prognosis in GCA is determined by visual involvement (see above).

2.5.2 Granulomatosis with polyangiitis (previously known as Wegener's granulomatosis)

Aetiology/pathophysiology/pathology

Key point

Granulomatosis with polyangiitis (GPA) and microscopic polyangiitis (MPA) represent a spectrum of small-vessel vasculitides associated with antineutrophil cytoplasmic antibodies (ANCAs).

The aetiology is unknown. GPA is characterised by necrotising granulomatous vasculitis with little or no immune deposits. Kidney biopsies typically show a pauci-immune glomerulonephritis. Evidence from genome-wide association studies (GWAS) suggests that ANCA directed against proteinase 3 (PR3-ANCA) and myeloperoxidase (MPO-ANCA) define genetically distinct disorders. While the pathogenesis of ANCA-associated vasculitis is complex, a central role for polymorphonuclear leukocytes (PMN) and neutrophil extracellular traps (NETs) in ANCA induction in a genetically predisposed host is likely to be an important factor. The recent success of rituximab suggests an important role for B-cells in driving disease.

Epidemiology

Wegener's granulomatosis affects both sexes equally. The peak incidence is in the fourth decade. The incidence of ANCA-associated vasculitis in the UK is estimated to be 20 per 10 million members of the population per year.

Clinical presentation

Common

Most patients present with a pulmonary–renal syndrome (Fig 73) on a background of upper respiratory tract involvement (haemoptysis, sinusitis, destruction of the nasal septum and epistaxis); 50% of them have ocular involvement in the form of conjunctivitis, scleritis and uveitis.

Uncommon

An uncommon presentation is cutaneous vasculitis with nailfold infarcts and purpura.

Physical signs

Common

Despite the severity of systemic vasculitis, overt physical signs may be limited to a red eye in early disease. A collapsed nasal septum leading to a saddle nose is characteristic of established disease.

Uncommon/rare

> proptosis caused by retro-orbital granulomas (Fig 74)

> cranial nerve deficits resulting from the spread of inflammation from the sinuses.

Investigations

Antineutrophil cytoplasmic antibodies (ANCAs) directed against proteinase-3 (PR3-ANCA) in high titre that appear in this clinical setting are highly suggestive of GPA (see Section 3.2.6). MPO-ANCAs are predominantly associated with MPA or renal-limited vasculitis. Histological confirmation of vasculitis on tissue biopsy (of kidneys, nose or lungs) is essential.

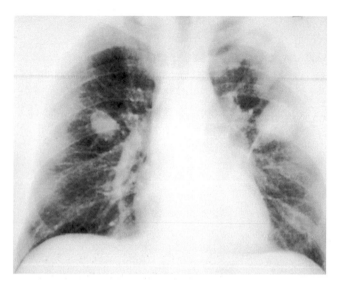

Fig 73 Chest X-ray depicting bilateral lung nodules caused by pulmonary vasculitis in a patient with Wegener's granulomatosis.

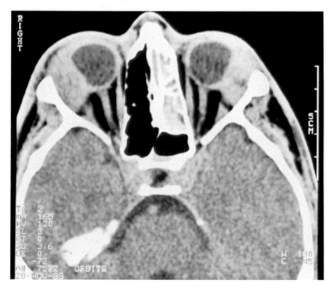

Fig 74 Bilateral orbital masses in a patient with Wegener's granulomatosis. (Courtesy of Dr R Melsom, Bradford Royal Infirmary.)

Approximately 10% of patients are ANCA-negative. The severity of an inflammation is established by measuring serum C-reactive protein.

Differential diagnosis
The diagnosis is clear cut in patients presenting with ANCA-positive granulomatous vasculitis on a background of sinus, lung and kidney disease. Other disorders that present with a pulmonary–renal syndrome (Table 38) may occasionally pose problems.

Treatment
Emergency / short term
Combined treatment with steroids and cyclophosphamide induces remission in 90% of patients. In keeping with the key role of B-cells in ANCA-associated vasculitis (AAV), rituximab has been shown to be as efficacious as cyclophosphamide in inducing and maintaining remission, even in patients with severe renal disease. In patients without critical organ involvement, low-dose methotrexate is a suitable alternative to cyclophosphamide for remission induction.

Long term
Recent evidence from randomised controlled trials shows that remission can be maintained by the early substitution of cyclophosphamide by azathioprine, thus limiting cyclophosphamide-induced toxicity. However, 50% of patients will relapse within 5 years. Note the increased risk of bladder malignancy and acute leukaemia with long-term cyclophosphamide therapy.

> **!** **Hazard**
> Be vigilant for infective problems (eg *Pneumocystis* pneumonia) that are associated with long-term immunosuppression.

The role of co-trimoxazole in preventing infection-induced relapse is controversial.

> **!** **Hazard**
> In patients treated with rituximab, relapses are rare during the period of B-cell ablation (up to 18 months), but some patients may go on to develop secondary hypogammaglobulinaemia.

Complications
Common

> chronic renal failure in 40% of cases

> collapsed nasal septum and subglottic stenosis in 30% of cases

> iatrogenic infertility in 50% of cases.

Table 38	Differential diagnosis of the pulmonary–renal syndrome
Disorder	Key investigations
Wegener's granulomatosis / MPA	ANCA and histology
Goodpasture's syndrome	Antiglomerular basement membrane antibody and renal histology
Lupus	Antinuclear antibody and serum complement
Mixed cryoglobulinaemia	Cryoglobulin, rheumatoid factor and serum complement

ANCA, antineutrophil cytoplasmic antibodies; MPA, microscopic polyangiitis.

Uncommon/rare

> nasolacrimal duct obstruction.

Prognosis

The 5-year survival rate is >80%. This is largely determined by the patient's renal function at presentation. Significant long-term morbidity is caused by complications of the disease and its treatment.

2.5.3 Polyarteritis nodosa

Aetiology/pathophysiology/pathology

Polyarteritis nodosa (PAN) is an immune complex-mediated vasculitis affecting medium-sized blood vessels.

The aetiology is unknown. The proportion of cases associated with hepatitis B virus infection has been reduced to less than 5% with the widespread adoption of vaccination. Vasculitic lesions are triggered by the deposition of immune complexes in endothelium with a marked granulocytic infiltration of media, which leads to aneurysmal dilatation.

Epidemiology

The peak incidence is in the fourth decade. The estimated annual incidence in Europe ranges from 0 to 1.6 in 1 million of the population.

Clinical presentation

Common

Some 40–70% of patients present with a purpuric or urticarial rash, myalgia, arthralgia and peripheral neuropathy, on a background of weight loss, hypertension and renal impairment.

Uncommon/rare

> bowel perforation

> orchitis

> congestive heart failure.

Physical signs

Common

> cutaneous signs

> 'glove and stocking' sensory loss

> mononeuritis multiplex

> areflexia.

Uncommon/rare

> testicular swelling

> papilloedema

> retinal detachment.

Investigations

In the absence of a single diagnostic test, the following are the key diagnostic investigations:

> visceral/renal angiography to demonstrate aneurysms (Fig 75) – the presence of multiple aneurysms in medium-sized arteries is a key finding

> tissue biopsy (muscle, sural nerve or kidney) for evidence of vasculitis.

Also assess renal function and hepatitis B status. Use C-reactive protein to assess the severity of the inflammation.

Differential diagnosis

The absence of glomerulonephritis and negative antineutrophil cytoplasmic antibody in PAN helps differentiate it from microscopic polyangiitis. Consider the possibility of drug-induced vasculitis in young males, eg amphetamine or cocaine abuse may cause aneurysms.

Treatment

Systemic disease requires combined therapy with steroids and cyclophosphamide for about a year. Steroids alone are adequate for PAN confined to the skin.

PAN associated with hepatitis B is best treated with a combination of antiviral agents, ie vidarabine/lamivudine combined with interferon-α.

Complications

Common

> chronic renal failure

> hypertension.

Uncommon/rare

> bowel infarction

> acute bowel perforation.

Prognosis

Adverse prognostic factors causing increased mortality are: proteinuria >1 g/day, raised serum creatinine and visceral involvement. The 5-year mortality rate in patients with all three factors is 46%.

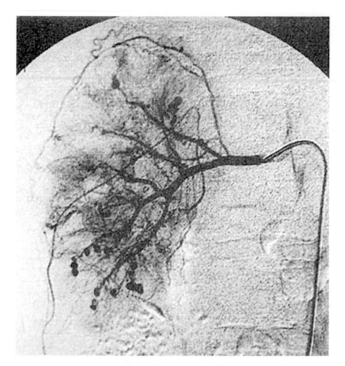

Fig 75 Multiple aneurysms affecting medium-sized vessels in the right kidney in a patient with hepatitis B-associated PAN. (Reproduced with permission from Chauveau D, Christophe JL. Renal aneurysms in hepatitis B-associated polyarteritis nodosa. *N Engl J Med* 1995;332:1070.)

2.5.4 Cryoglobulinaemic vasculitis

Aetiology/pathophysiology/pathology

This is an immune complex-mediated small-vessel vasculitis associated with mixed cryoglobulinaemia types II and III (see Table 7). The precise reasons why immunoglobulins cryoprecipitate is not known. Of cases of mixed cryoglobulinaemia, 60–80% are driven by an underlying hepatitis C virus (HCV) infection. Conversely, up to 50% of patients with HCV infections have a mixed cryoglobulinaemia, although only a small minority develop vasculitis. Clonal expansion of IgM-producing B-cells is a key feature of HCV-associated mixed cryoglobulinaemia.

Type I cryoglobulins are associated with lymphoproliferative disease and rarely cause vasculitis.

Epidemiology

> female preponderance

> estimated incidence one in 100,000

> higher incidence in southern Europe, reflecting the prevalence of hepatitis C.

Clinical presentation

Common

> triad of cutaneous vasculitis, glomerulonephritis and arthralgia (see Fig 8)

> skin involvement occurs in almost all cases.

Uncommon/rare

> mononeuritis multiplex

> abdominal pain.

Physical signs

Common

> purpuric skin rash

> Raynaud's phenomenon.

Uncommon/rare

> sensory deficits

> areflexia.

Investigations

Key point

Important serological clues to the presence of mixed cryoglobulinaemia are a markedly low C4 and a positive rheumatoid factor. Ensure that a blood sample for cryoglobulins is collected correctly at 37°C and transported immediately to the laboratory (Fig 76).

Check hepatitis C serology, including hepatitis C RNA in the cryoprecipitate. Routine investigation for other infective triggers (endocarditis, syphilis, Lyme disease, malaria and HIV) reportedly associated with mixed cryoglobulinaemia is not warranted in the absence of suggestive clinical clues. Perform a renal biopsy to assess renal damage.

Differential diagnosis

See Table 6.

Treatment

Mixed cryoglobulinaemia with hepatitis C infection

Depending on viral genotype, anti-HCV therapy comprising interferon-α, ribavirin and a protease inhibitor (boceprevir or telaprevir) achieves a sustained virological and clinical response. It is likely that recently licensed interferon-free oral regimens comprising direct protease inhibitors such as sofosbuvir will also be effective.

Idiopathic mixed cryoglobulinaemia with progressive renal or hepatic disease

Treat with immunosuppressive therapy using steroids and cyclophosphamide or azathioprine. Plasmapheresis is a useful adjunct for the treatment of acute exacerbations, irrespective of the underlying aetiology.

In keeping with the clonal expansion of B-cells in mixed cryoglobulinaemia, rituximab, an anti-CD20 monoclonal

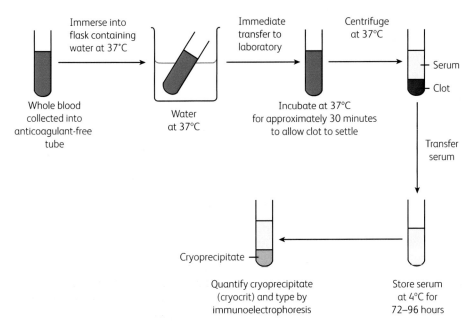

Fig 76 Steps in the detection of cryoglobulins in the laboratory.

antibody, is an effective alternative therapeutic option for severe disease in both hepatitis C-associated and idiopathic mixed cryoglobulinaemia.

Complications

Common

> chronic renal failure in 50% of patients

> hypertension

> leg ulcers.

Uncommon/rare

> liver failure

> B-cell lymphoma.

Prognosis

The long-term outcome is determined by the extent of the renal disease.

2.5.5 Behçet's disease

Aetiology/pathophysiology/pathology

Behçet's disease is a syndrome of unknown aetiology, with vasculitis of veins and arteries of all sizes, hypercoagulability and neutrophil hyperfunction. It is diagnosed on clinical grounds, after the exclusion of similar diseases.

Epidemiology

It is most common in populations living along the Silk Route. The incidence and severity of the disease are associated with human leukocyte antigen (HLA)-B51 in these populations, but not in Caucasians.

Clinical presentation

The disease typically presents with exacerbations and remissions.

Common

Skin

There will usually be:

> aphthous ulcers

> genital ulcers

> erythema nodosum

> vasculitic and acneiform lesions

> superficial thrombophlebitis at venepuncture sites

> pathergy: pustules at sites of skin puncture or minor trauma (such as bra straps, see Fig 77).

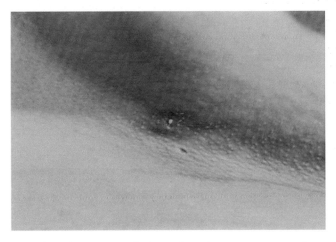

Fig 77 Pathergy: pustular/acneiform lesions occurring along the line of the bra strap in a woman with Behçet's disease.

Eye

Look for:

> anterior or posterior uveitis: red, painful eye; loss of visual acuity and hypopyon

> retinal vasculitis: loss of visual acuity.

Urgent ophthalmological opinion is necessary, even in patients who are asymptomatic, because uveitis and retinal vasculitis are common causes of blindness in Behçet's disease.

Joints

In 50–60% of cases joints are affected by arthralgia or arthritis, which usually affects large joints and which is non-erosive.

Uncommon

> nervous system (affected in 10–20% of cases): cerebral vasculitis (transient ischaemic attacks, stroke, fits, progressive dementia and meningoencephalitis) and venous sinus thrombosis

> respiratory system: pulmonary vasculitis (episodes of dyspnoea and haemoptysis) and pulmonary embolism

> gastrointestinal (GI) system: intestinal vasculitis (abdominal pain, constipation, mesenteric angina and occasionally infarction with bloody diarrhoea)

> cardiovascular: myocardial ischaemia or infarction, deep vein thrombosis.

Investigation

> Erythrocyte sedimentation rate and C-reactive protein are often elevated in cases of active disease.

> Biopsies show vasculitis, with neutrophil infiltration of small and medium-sized vessels.

> In cerebral disease CT is usually normal, but MRI may show multiple high-signal white matter lesions (Fig 78).

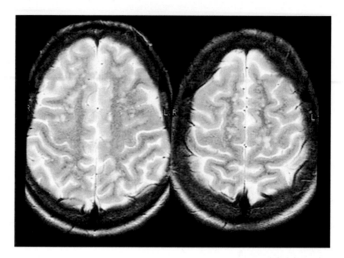

Fig 78 MRI of the brain of a woman with Behçet's disease, who was suffering from transient ischaemic attacks. Note multiple high-signal lesions.

> A lumbar puncture may show raised protein, cells (lymphocytes and neutrophils) or neither.

> There is no diagnostic test – most investigations are conducted to exclude other diseases. The presence of raised serum angiotensin-converting enzyme, strongly positive antinuclear antibodies, rheumatoid factor or antineutrophil cytoplasmic activity should prompt you to consider an alternative diagnosis.

Differential diagnosis

> herpes simplex (recurrent oral and genital lesions)

> inflammatory bowel disease (GI lesions)

> multiple sclerosis (central nervous system lesions)

> seronegative arthritis (arthritis and uveitis)

> sarcoidosis (erythema nodosum, arthritis and uveitis)

> Sweet's syndrome (pathergy).

Treatment

Key point

'There are some remedies worse than the disease.' (Publilius Syrus, 42 BC)

Mucocutaneous disease – this is usually controlled by topical corticosteroids, sometimes in combination with topical antibiotics and antifungals. Colchicine is used if topical agents are insufficient.

Acute sight problems or life-threatening disease – controlled by high-dose corticosteroids or tumour necrosis factor (TNF) inhibitors.

For long-term suppression of systemic disease the following have been used:

> azathioprine for eye, vascular or cerebral disease

> anti-TNF agents appear globally effective, although evidence is largely confined to observational studies

> cyclosporin for eye disease

> interferon-α for mucocutaneous disease, thrombophlebitis, arthritis and (sometimes) eye disease

> benzathine–penicillin for joint disease

> dapsone for mucocutaneous disease and arthritis.

Cyclophosphamide, chlorambucil, methotrexate and thalidomide are less commonly used.

Key point

Whatever the therapy chosen, you will need to monitor clinical and laboratory indices for side effects. Remember that Behçet's disease is a relapsing–remitting disease and the patient may be able to enjoy periods of little or no drug therapy.

Hazard

> Methotrexate and thalidomide cause severe teratogenicity and are contraindicated in pregnancy, which must be avoided for at least 6 months after stopping methotrexate.

> Cyclophosphamide and chlorambucil are teratogenic and may cause premature ovarian failure, particularly at high doses.

These drugs are best avoided in a young female patient but, if considered essential, it is important that she is willing to use reliable contraception and accept the risk of infertility.

Complications

Common

> venous (including sagittal sinus) thrombosis and pulmonary embolism

> pulmonary haemorrhage.

Venous thrombosis is common and presents a management dilemma because anticoagulation, the common treatment, may precipitate

life-threatening bleeding from the vasculitic lesions present from Behçet's disease. In practice most patients are anticoagulated without problems, although you would be wise to make a careful risk–benefit assessment and to distinguish pulmonary embolism from pulmonary vasculitis before commencing therapy.

Prognosis

This depends on the site and severity of the disease. HLA-B51 is associated with a worse prognosis.

Morbidity

Blindness occurs in 25% of those with ocular lesions.

Mortality

Death is from thrombosis, haemorrhage or organ failure as a result of the vasculitis.

2.5.6 Takayasu's arteritis

Aetiology/pathology

The cause of this arteritis is unknown; the pathology of the arterial lesion is similar to that of giant cell arteritis (GCA), with focal granulomatous panarteritis associated with infiltration of CD4$^+$ and CD8$^+$ T-cells. Fibrosis is a feature of advanced disease.

Epidemiology

It predominantly affects young females of Asian and South American origin. The precise incidence rates in these countries are unknown. The annual incidence in the USA is 2.6 per 10 million members of the population.

Clinical features

Early manifestations include:

> malaise

> arthralgia

> myalgia

> an elevated erythrocyte sedimentation rate (ESR).

Later in the course of the disease patients present with symptoms of vascular insufficiency, particularly in the upper limbs, with a range of feelings of numbness or coldness to claudication and Raynaud's phenomenon. Hypertension due to renal artery disease occurs in approximately 50% of patients.

Other features include:

> neurological manifestations due to carotid and/or vertebral artery disease

> ocular disease due to hypoperfusion or untreated hypertension

> cardiac disease, which may be multifactorial.

Bruits and an absence of peripheral pulses are noted on physical examination (hence the term 'pulseless disease').

Key point

Pattern of disease

The disease primarily affects the aorta and its major branches (subclavian and carotid). A triphasic pattern of disease progression is seen:

> stage I: pre-pulseless stage – fever, arthralgia and weight loss

> stage II: vessel inflammation – vessel pain, tenderness (carotidynia) and vascular insufficiency

> stage III: burnt-out stage – bruits and ischaemia predominate.

Differential diagnosis

Other disorders that may cause diagnostic confusion (Table 39) should be considered and distinguished on the basis of their distinctive features.

Investigation

Investigations should be aimed at documenting a patient's acute phase

Table 39 Differential diagnosis of fever and absent radial pulses

Disorder	Comments
Takayasu's arteritis	See text
GCA	May be difficult to differentiate in women >40 years old Far Eastern, Japanese and Asian sub-continent background, and subclavian and renal artery involvement favour Takayasu's arteritis
Polyarteritis nodosa	Multisystem involvement and aneurysms of visceral/renal circulation (see Sections 1.1.15 and 2.5.3)
Connective tissue disorders (systemic lupus erythematosus, rheumatoid arthritis and scleroderma)	Characteristic clinical picture accompanied by positive serology (see Sections 2.3.3, 2.4.1 and 2.4.3)
Tuberculous aortitis	Causes aneurysms rather than stenosis Look for evidence of tuberculosis elsewhere: chest radiograph, Mantoux test and sputum for acid-fast bacilli
Syphilitic aortitis	Very rare but worth considering Causes aneurysms rather than stenoses Check treponemal serology
Fibromuscular dysplasia	Proliferation of fibrous tissue in the media of large arteries Probably congenital in origin but produces progressive stenoses in young adulthood May be multifocal inflammatory: unresponsive to steroids
Atherosclerosis	Rare cause of absent pulses in young people Consider in the presence of hyperlipidaemia

GCA, giant cell arteritis.

response as an indirect measure of disease activity, excluding other possible diagnoses and performing the appropriate imaging to document the extent of vascular involvement. Most patients will have a normocytic anaemia and leucocytosis/thrombocytosis.

Serology
Both C-reactive protein (CRP) and ESR are elevated in 50–70% of cases. Hypergammaglobulinaemia is found in up to one-third of patients, but autoantibodies (eg antinuclear antibodies and antineutrophil cytoplasmic antibodies) are not a feature of Takayasu's arteritis.

Aortic arch angiography
The procedure of choice to detect arterial obstruction is magnetic resonance (MR) angiography (Fig 79). The majority of lesions are found in the branches of the aortic arch, but the renal arteries and abdominal aorta are involved in up to one-third of cases. Stenoses are the most common lesion, but occlusions, dilatations and aneurysms are also described. Angiography may also differentiate congenital aortic coarctation from Takayasu's arteritis.

Non-invasive imaging techniques
Ultrasonography, MRI, CT and 18F-fluorodeoxyglucose (FDG)-PET all provide useful information regarding aortic wall thickness and/or inflammatory cell infiltration and therefore delineate both disease activity and extent.

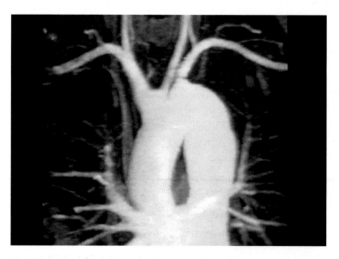

Fig 79 Magnetic resonance angiogram of aortic arch in a young woman with Takayasu's arteritis showing occlusion of the left subclavian artery at its origin. (Courtesy of Dr H Marzo-Orteza.)

Arterial biopsy

Such a biopsy is seldom required for the diagnosis.

Key point

The usual biopsy finding in Takayasu's arteritis is a granulomatous panarteritis, underlining the difficulty in differentiating this condition from GCA.

Treatment

The following are the important principles:

> medical suppression of inflammation

> control of hypertension

> intervention to correct stenotic lesions (in selected cases).

Inflammation

Corticosteroids (prednisolone 1 mg/kg/day) are the treatment of choice for active Takayasu's arteritis; additional immunosuppressive therapy (cyclophosphamide, mycophenolate mofetil, azathioprine or methotrexate) is required for patients who fail to respond, or those who relapse with tapering or discontinuation of steroids. Response to therapy is usually monitored using CRP/ESR.

Hypertension

Management is with aggressive antihypertensive therapy.

Surgery

Surgery may be required in up to 50% of patients. Indications include:

> critical renal artery stenosis causing hypertension

> severe carotid stenosis

> significant aortic regurgitation.

Timing surgery to disease remission considerably reduces restenosis rates.

Prognosis

For all patients, the 5-year survival rate is about 90–95% but mortality is increased in those with severe vascular complications. Major causes of disability and/or mortality are heart failure, strokes and blindness.

2.5.7 Systemic Still's disease

Aetiology/pathology

Adult onset Still's disease (AOSD) is an acute systemic inflammatory disorder of unknown aetiology that frequently poses a diagnostic challenge because of the lack of pathognomonic clinical or laboratory features exhibited by those suffering from it. A key role in disease pathogenesis has been demonstrated for pro-inflammatory cytokines such as tumour necrosis factor alpha (TNF-α), interleukin (IL)-1, IL-6 and IL-18, leading to the use of biologics targeting these mediators.

Epidemiology

The disorder affects males and females approximately equally, with a slight preponderance in females. Three-quarters of patients are aged between 16 and 35 years at disease onset.

Clinical presentation

Typically presents as a pyrexia of unknown origin with spiking fever, arthralgia, an evanescent rash and multiorgan involvement.

Common

A fleeting maculopapular rash is characteristic and frequently mistaken for drug allergy because penicillin is often given for the sore throat associated with the disease prodrome. The other features that are usually present are:

> sore throat

> generalised myalgia without objective evidence of myositis

> arthralgia

> polyarthralgia affecting the knees, wrists and fingers is common, with some patients developing frank arthritis with effusions

> weight loss – this is a non-specific reflection of a persistent acute-phase response

> lymphadenopathy and splenomegaly

> pleuritis and pericarditis is associated with effusions in some patients.

Uncommon

> renal failure

> disseminated intravascular coagulation.

Investigation

In the absence of a specific marker, the diagnosis of AOSD is entirely based on clinical grounds (see Table 40).

Detailed laboratory investigations and appropriate imaging are essential to exclude infections, autoimmune rheumatic disease (see Section 2.4) and haematological malignancy. Neutrophil counts and inflammatory markers are raised: marked hyperferritinaemia (1,500–10,000 µg/L) (normal range 15–300) is a feature in >90% of patients and correlates with disease activity. Although ferritin is a non-specific acute-phase protein, the magnitude of its rise in this clinical setting is a useful pointer to AOSD.

Key point

The 'classic triad' occurs in <50% of patients with AOSD:

> arthritis

> persistent spiking fever

> a fleeting maculopapular rash.
Virtually all patients with AOSD have markedly elevated erythrocyte sedimentation rate, C-reactive protein and neutrophil counts. Serum ferritin levels are usually very high.

Table 40 Classification criteria for adult onset Still's disease (AOSD). A definite diagnosis requires a patient to fit five or more criteria, including two or more major criteria

Major criteria	Fever of 39° C or higher, lasting for 1 week or longer Arthralgia lasting 2 weeks or longer Typical rash Leucocytosis (>10 × 10^9/L) including >80% granulocytes
Minor criteria	Sore throat Lymphadenopathy and/or splenomegaly Liver dysfunction Negative rheumatoid factor and antinuclear antibodies
Exclusions	Infections (especially sepsis and infectious mononucleosis) Malignancies (especially malignant lymphoma) Rheumatic diseases (especially polyarteritis nodosa and rheumatoid vasculitis with extra-articular features)

Differential diagnosis

Prolonged fever with joint pains has a wide differential diagnosis covering a range of disorders (Table 41). A thorough history is therefore crucial.

Key point

The crucial clue in AOSD is the long list of negative investigations, which in a systemically unwell patient presenting with high fever, rash, arthralgia and myalgia accompanied by a pronounced acute phase response raises the distinct possibility of this disorder.

Management

Aspirin and other NSAIDs have traditionally been considered as first-line therapy, but are successful in only 20% of cases. Over 50% of patients require long-term steroid treatment. Patients with persistent arthropathy require treatment with disease-modifying antirheumatic drugs. A minority of patients who are unresponsive to such conventional immunosuppressive treatment may benefit from cytokine blockade directed against IL-1 or TNF or IL-6.

2.5.8 Autoinflammatory syndromes

Autoinflammatory syndromes are characterised by inappropriate activation of the innate immune system, leading to intermittent fever, systemic inflammation and multiorgan involvement. If inflammation is uncontrolled, there is a risk of organ damage and amyloidosis.

Key point

Autoinflammatory syndromes caused by single gene mutations include:

1 familial Mediterranean fever (FMF)

> autosomal recessive pyrin (*MEFV*) gene mutation

2 cryopyrin-associated periodic syndromes (CAPS)

> autosomal dominant gain of function mutation in *NLRP3*

> resulting (in ascending order of severity) in:

a familial cold autoinflammatory syndrome (FCAS)

b Muckle–Wells syndrome (MWS)

c neonatal onset multisystem inflammatory disease (NOMID) / chronic

> infantile neurological, cutaneous and articular syndrome (CINCA)

3 tumour necrosis factor-associated periodic syndrome (TRAPS)

> autosomal dominant mutation in *TNFRSF1A*

4 mevalonate kinase deficiency (MKD) including:

> hyper-IgD syndrome (HIDS) and the more severe mevalonic aciduria (MA)

> autosomal recessive caused by mutations in *mevalonate kinase* gene.

Newer genetic technologies, such as whole exome sequencing are identifying novel autoinflammatory syndromes.

Table 41 Differential diagnosis of fever and arthritis

Infection	Direct invasion: bacterial (mycobacterial), fungal and Whipple's disease Indirect: bacterial (acute rheumatic fever) and reactive arthritis
Crystal arthropathy	Urate
Inflammatory disorders	Calcium pyrophosphate Lupus and lupus overlap disorders Necrotising vasculitis AOSD Rheumatoid arthritis Sarcoidosis
Haematological malignancies	Arthritis associated with inflammatory bowel disease

Modified from Van De Putte LBA, Wouters JM. Adult onset Still's disease. *Bailliére's Clin Rheumatol* 1991;2:263–75.

Clinical presentation

Intermittent fever (all), arthralgia (all), urticarial (CAPS), maculopapular (MKD) or erysipelas-like rash (FMF), abdominal pain (FMF, MKD, TRAPS), serositis (FMF), mouth ulcers and lymphadenopathy (MKD) (see Table 42).

Physical signs

Between attacks, complications may result in physical signs of amyloidosis (all), growth retardation (MKD, CAPS, NOMID/CINCA), neuronal hearing or visual loss (CAPS/MWS/NOMID), ataxia and cognitive impairment (MKD/MA) and bone overgrowth of the lower limbs (CAPS).

Investigations

During attacks: raised neutrophil count and inflammatory markers, such as C-reactive protein and serum amyloid A (SAA).

Between attacks: raised SAA between attacks indicates subclinical inflammation and risk of amyloidosis.

Screening for complications listed above.

Genetic sequencing confirms the diagnosis and should also be offered to family members at risk.

Differential diagnosis

Infection

Arthritis

Acute abdomen with peritonitis, pleurisy, pericarditis, orchitis (FMF)

Still's disease (MKD).

Other autoinflammatory syndromes

Periodic fever, aphthous ulcers, pharyngitis and adenitis (PFAPA) is a self-limiting syndrome of unknown aetiology mainly affecting children.

Schnitzler's syndrome is an autoinflammatory syndrome associated with a monoclonal immunoglobulin G gammopathy.

Treatment

> Interleukin (IL)-1 blockade, with agents such as anakinra

(short acting) or canakinumab (long acting), controls symptoms and underlying inflammation, even if subclinical (all).

> colchicine (FMF)

Adjunctive treatment may be considered with:

> NSAIDs or corticosteroids (symptom control)

> etanercept (TRAPS/mevalonate kinase ((MVK))

Avoid the following which are ineffective and may worsen disease:

> infliximab or adalimumab in TRAPS

> colchicine or statins in MVK.

Prognosis

This depends on the degree and duration of inflammation. The outlook for patients with autoinflammatory syndromes has been transformed by prompt diagnosis, monitoring for subclinical inflammation and use of IL-1 blockade.

Table 42 Clinical features of autoinflammatory syndromes

Autoinflammatory syndrome	Symptoms	Frequency of attacks	Duration of attacks
FMF	Fever, abdominal pain, pleuritic pain, arthritis, orchitis, erysipeloid rash	Variable	12–72 hours
FCAS	Fever, urticaria, arthralgia	1–3 hours after exposure to cold	12–24 hours
MWS	As for FCAS plus deafness, papilloedema and headache	Frequent, triggered by cold	2–3 days
NOMID/CINCA	As for MWS plus ocular inflammation, aseptic meningitis, raised intracranial pressure and pericarditis	Continuous	Continuous
TRAPS	Fever, abdominal pain, arthralgia, red patch / migratory rash	Every 3–6 months	Days to weeks
MVK/MA	Fever, adenitis, oral ulcer	Every 2–12 weeks	3–7 days

CINCA, chronic infantile neurological, cutaneous and articular syndrome; FCAS, familial cold autoinflammatory syndrome; FMF, familial Mediterranean fever; MA, mevalonic aciduria; MVK, mevalonate kinase; MWS, Muckle–Wells syndrome; NOMID, neonatal onset multisystem inflammatory disease; TRAPS, tumour necrosis factor-associated periodic syndrome. From ter Haar NM, Oswald M *et al.* Recommendations for the management of autoinflammatory diseases. *ARD* 2015;74:1636–44.

3 Investigations and practical procedures

3.1 Assessing acute phase response

3.1.1 Erythrocyte sedimentation rate

Principle

> **Key point**
>
> The erythrocyte sedimentation rate (ESR), plasma viscosity (PV) and C-reactive protein (CRP) are well-established markers of the acute phase response (APR) (Tables 43 and 44).

The ESR is a measure of the rate of fall of red blood cells in a calibrated vertical tube.

> **Key point**
>
> ESR measures the acute-phase response indirectly by reflecting changes in plasma proteins, particularly:
>
> > fibrinogen
> > α_2-macroglobulin
> > immunoglobulins.
>
> The ESR is also significantly influenced by changes in the number, shape and deformability of red blood cells, causing the ESR to rise with a fall in the haematocrit.

Indications

As it is influenced by plasma proteins of varying half-lives, the ESR represents, at best, a relatively crude way of assessing a persistent acute-phase response. The PV mirrors changes in the same plasma proteins that influence the ESR, but it is not altered by changes in haematocrit or red cell aggregability. For this reason and the ease of performing automated assays, there is an increasing tendency to substitute PV for ESR. However, the traditional role of both ESR and PV in monitoring chronic inflammatory disorders is being supplanted by CRP, a highly sensitive marker of the acute-phase response.

Table 43 Comparative utility of CRP, ESR and PV as markers of tissue damage: I

	CRP	ESR	PV
Change driven by	Cytokines: IL-1, IL-6 and TNF Not dependent on changes in plasma proteins or red cells	Changes in plasma proteins and red cells	Changes in plasma proteins; unaffected by changes in red cells
Rapidity of change	Within 6 hours of onset of tissue damage; and returns to normal within 48 hours of resolution of inflammation/infection	Within 24–48 hours of onset of tissue damage; returns to normal over 4–6 days	Kinetics of response similar to ESR
Clinical utility	Highly sensitive and reproducible marker of inflammation, bacterial infection and tissue necrosis	Marker of chronic inflammation/infection	Marker of chronic inflammation/infection
	Levels correlate with severity	Poor correlation with severity	

IL, interleukin; TNF, tumour necrosis factor.

Table 44 Comparative utility of CRP, ESR and PV as markers of tissue damage: II

	CRP	ESR	PV
Disorders characterised by major elevation	Inflammatory disease: rheumatoid arthritis and systemic vasculitis Infection: septicaemia and pyogenic abscesses	Systemic vasculitis Hyperglobulinaemic state: plasma cell dyscrasias, SLE and Sjögren's syndrome Systemic bacterial infection, eg infective endocarditis	As for ESR
Clinical situations associated with discordant responses	Raised ESR with normal CRP: consider hyperglobulinaemia as in SLE, Sjögren's syndrome (without infection), anaemia and hyperlipidaemia		

SLE, systemic lupus erythematosus.

3.1.2 C-reactive protein

Principle

C-reactive protein (CRP) is a member of the pentraxin family of proteins and is synthesised in the liver in response to pro-inflammatory cytokines, ie interleukin (IL)-1, IL-6 and tumour necrosis factor, during an acute-phase response. Circulating CRP is easily and accurately measured using nephelometry, a technique that measures the amount of light scattered by immune complexes of analyte (in this case CRP) and exogenous antibody. Given a constant antibody concentration, the amount of light scattered reflects the concentration of the analyte.

Indications

Its rapid rise within 6 hours of the onset of tissue damage (peak at 48–72 hours) makes CRP the most useful marker for monitoring inflammatory disease and systemic bacterial infection. Unlike the erythrocyte sedimentation rate (ESR) or plasma viscosity (PV), CRP is not influenced by changes in plasma proteins or erythrocytes. For most clinical indications, there is little to be gained by requesting both CRP and ESR, with the following exceptions: an isolated rise in ESR may rarely be observed in giant cell arteritis while patients with systemic lupus erythematosus (SLE) and Sjögren's syndrome (disorders associated with hypergammaglobulinaemia) may exhibit a discordant rise in ESR with a normal CRP.

3.2 Serological investigation of autoimmune rheumatic disease

3.2.1 Antibodies to nuclear antigens

Principle

Antibodies to nuclear antigens are detected by indirect immunofluorescence (IIF). Human epithelial cells (HEp-2) are used as a source of antigen. HEp-2 cells are incubated with the patient's sera which contains autoantibodies. Immunoglobulin G (IgG) antibodies reacting with antigens within the HEp-2 cells are recognised by adding a second anti-IgG antibody (conjugate) that contains a fluorochrome tagged to its Fc end (Fig 80). Fluorescent microscopy is used to visualise the pattern of immunofluorescence produced by the autoantibody. Recently some laboratories have moved over to using enzyme-linked immunosorbent assays to detect antinuclear antibodies (ANAs).

Indications

Looking for ANAs is the key initial investigation (Fig 81) in patients with suspected systemic lupus erythematosus (SLE), lupus overlap disorders, Sjögren's syndrome and scleroderma (see Table 45). Using HEp-2 cells as antigenic substrate, virtually all patients with untreated SLE are ANA positive.

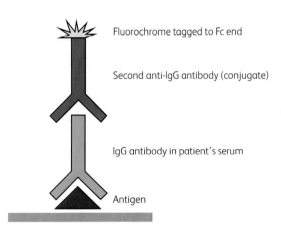

Fluorochrome tagged to Fc end

Second anti-IgG antibody (conjugate)

IgG antibody in patient's serum

Antigen

Fig 80 Diagrammatic representation of IIF for the detection of circulating antibodies.

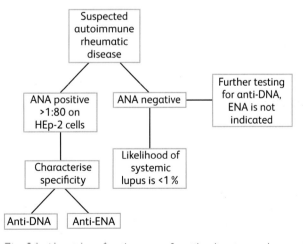

Fig 81 Algorithm for the use of antibodies to nuclear antigens. ANA, antibodies to nuclear antigens; ENA, extractable nuclear antigens. (Reproduced with permission from Kavanaugh A, Tomar R, Reveille J, Solomon DH, Homburger HA. Guidelines for clinical use of the antinuclear antibody test and tests for specific autoantibodies to nuclear antigens. *Arch Pathol Lab Med* 2000;124:71–81.)

Table 45 Prevalence of autoantibodies in autoimmune rheumatic disease

Disorder	ANA (%)	DNA (%)	Ro (%)	La (%)	Sm (%)	RNP (%)	ANCA (%)	Centromere (%)	Histones (%)	Jo-1 (%)	Scl-70 (%)
SLE	99–100	60–90	35–60	Accompanies anti-Ro; rare in isolation	30	30–40	25 (p-ANCA)	Rare	50–70 of idiopathic SLE; 90–100 of drug-induced SLE	0	0
Scleroderma	60–90	0–5	0	0	0	0	Not known	60	20	0	20–40
Primary Sjögren's syndrome	40–70	10	40–90	40–90	0	0	Not known	Rare	Not known	0	0
MCTD	100	0–5	0	0	0	100	Not known	Rare	Not known	Variable	Variable
Inflammatory myositis	40–70	0–5	0	0	0	0	Not known	0	Not known	30	0
Wegener's granulomatosis	?–5	0	0	0	0	0	80–95 (c-ANCA directed against PR3)	0	Not known	Not known	0
Microscopic polyangiitis	?–5	0	0	0	0	0	<80 (p-ANCA directed against MPO)	0	Not known	Not known	0

ANCA, antineutrophil cytoplasmic antibody; MCTD, mixed connective tissue disease; MPO, myeloperoxidase; PR3, proteinase-3; RNP, ribonucleoprotein.

> **Key point**
> Previous reports of rare patients with ANA-negative lupus were based on studies using rodent tissue.

ANAs are not specific for lupus and related disorders; they occur in normal people and in a wide range of inflammatory and infective disorders.

Variants of antinuclear antibodies

Anticentromere antibodies

Antibodies directed against centromere antigens are easily detected by their characteristic pattern on HEp-2 cells by IIF (Fig 82). Anticentromere antibodies are markers of the limited form of scleroderma, also known as the CREST syndrome (**c**alcinosis, **R**aynaud's, o**e**sophageal dysfunction, **s**clerodactyly, **t**elangiectasia). Diffuse disease in scleroderma is associated with antibodies to the enzyme DNA topoisomerase (anti-Scl 70). Anti-Scl 70 is associated with more severe diseases, especially pulmonary fibrosis.

Antihistone antibodies

Antibodies directed against histones, a group of highly conserved basic proteins in the nucleus, are associated with drug-induced lupus.

3.2.2 Antibodies to double-stranded DNA

Principle

These are detected by a variety of techniques:

> Farr radioisotope assay

> enzyme-linked immunosorbent assay (ELISA)

> indirect immunofluorescence using the haemoflagellate *Crithidia luciliae* (Fig 83).

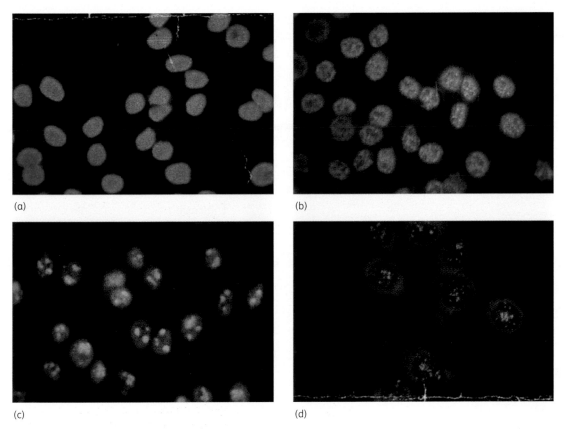

(a)

(b)

(c)

(d)

Fig 82 Staining patterns of ANAs on HEp-2 cells: **(a)** homogeneous; **(b)** speckled; **(c)** nucleolar; and **(d)** centromere (note the appearance of multiple fine dots representing staining of the kinetochores of 23 pairs of chromosomes). (Courtesy of Mr K Taylor, Leeds General Infirmary.)

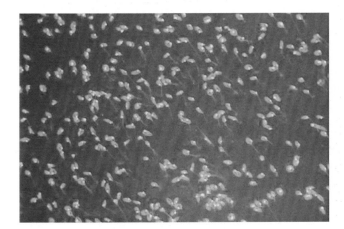

Fig 83 Fluorescence confined to the kinetoplast of *Crithidia luciliae* in a serum sample containing high concentrations of anti-DNA antibodies in a patient with active systemic lupus erythematosus (SLE).

In practice, ELISAs are increasingly used in view of their high sensitivity, ease of automation and ability to quantify results reliably (Table 46).

Indications

Antibodies to double-stranded-DNA are a specific marker of systemic lupus erythematosus (SLE) that is useful for the diagnosis and monitoring of disease activity in SLE. A steady rise in anti-DNA antibody levels heralds a lupus flare in many patients.

Table 46 Comparison of three commonly used anti-double-stranded DNA assays in SLE

	Farr	*Crithidia*	ELISA
Sensitivity	High	High	High
Specificity	High	High	Moderate
Detection of high-avidity antibodies	+++	++	++
Detection of low-avidity antibodies	+	++	+++
Ability to identify individual antibody isotypes (IgG, IgA and IgM)	No	Yes	Yes
Suitability for monitoring disease activity	Yes	No	Yes

ELISA, enzyme-linked immunosorbent assay; Ig, immunoglobulin.

3.2.3 Antibodies to extractable nuclear antigens

Principle

Key point
Extractable nuclear antigens refer to a group of saline-extractable antigens known individually as Ro, La, Sm and U1-RNP (uridine ribonuclear protein). Ro, La and Sm were named after the patients in whom they were first characterised: Robert, Lane and Smith. In conjunction with U1-RNP, these proteins are responsible for splicing and processing mRNA.

These antibodies are detected by a range of techniques including:

> immunoprecipitation assays such as countercurrent immunoelectrophoresis (CIE) or double diffusion

> immunoblotting.

These techniques are specific, but are not suitable for handling large numbers of samples. Enzyme immunoassay is increasingly the method of choice, but this may produce false-positive results in hypergammaglobulinaemic sera.

Indications

> investigation of systemic lupus erythematosus (SLE)

> lupus overlap disorders

> Sjögren's syndrome.

Anti-Ro antibodies

Anti-Ro antibodies correlate with cutaneous disease and vasculitis in SLE. In pregnant women with lupus, anti-Ro antibodies may cross the placenta to cause transient cutaneous lupus in the neonate (5–25% of babies) or permanent congenital heart block (1–3% of babies). Antinuclear antibody-negative, anti-Ro-positive lupus is extremely rare (<1% of lupus patients). Consider primary complement deficiency in such patients. Anti-La antibodies tend to accompany anti-Ro.

Anti-Sm and anti-U1-RNP antibodies

Anti-Sm antibodies are highly specific for SLE; their prevalence varies with the ethnic background of the patient. Anti-Sm and U1-RNP antibodies tend to occur together because of the shared peptide sequences between Sm and U1-RNP. The presence of anti-U1-RNP antibodies in isolation was thought to identify a group of patients with mixed connective tissue disease (MCTD) – a group of lupus overlap disorders with additional features of polymyositis and scleroderma. Long-term follow-up of the original cohort has raised questions about the existence of MCTD as a distinct entity.

3.2.4 Cyclic citrullinated peptide antibodies and rheumatoid factor

Indication

Measurement of cyclic citrullinated peptide (CCP) antibodies has replaced rheumatoid factor as a diagnostic test for rheumatoid arthritis (RA). CCP has comparable sensitivity (70–80%) and superior specificity (90–95%) in early RA and is detectable in the majority of patients with established RA. CCP is not usually used for disease activity monitoring.

Principle

In the presence of inflammation, arginine residues in synovial proteins may be converted to citrulline, 'citrullinated', and therefore visible to the immune system, initiating ongoing inflammation. CCP is detectable by ELISA or similar techniques.

3.2.5 Rheumatoid factor

Principle

Traditional sheep cell agglutination assays have been replaced by latex-enhanced turbidimetry or nephelometry (see Section 3.1.2).

Indications

> prognostic marker in rheumatoid arthritis (RA)

> immunoglobulin M rheumatoid factor (RhF) occurs in 50–90% of patients with RA and in a wide range of other inflammatory and infective disorders. The role of RhF as a marker of RA has largely been supplanted

by antibodies to cyclic citrullinated peptide

> RhF continues to be used in diagnosis of mixed cryoglobulinaemia and Sjögren's syndrome.

3.2.6 Antineutrophil cytoplasmic antibody

Principle

Indirect immunofluorescence using human neutrophil as substrate is used to define patterns of antineutrophil cytoplasmic antibodies (ANCAs). A cytoplasmic pattern of fluorescence (c-ANCA) is associated with antibodies directed against proteinase-3 (PR-3-ANCA), whereas a perinuclear pattern (p-ANCA) is associated predominantly with antibodies directed against myeloperoxidase (MPO-ANCA) (Fig 84). Antigenic specificity is confirmed by enzyme immunoassay.

Indications

PR-3-ANCA and MPO-ANCA are sensitive markers of Wegener's granulomatosis and microscopic polyangiitis, respectively. False positives may occur with infection, malignancy and other inflammatory disorders. In a routine clinical setting, the positive predictive value of ANCA is less than 50%, ie the majority of ANCA-positive patients do not have small vessel vasculitis.

3.2.7 Serum complement concentrations

Principle

C3 and C4 are assayed by nephelometry (see Section 3.1.2).

Indications

Indications are for the investigation of suspected systemic immune-complex disease. Hypocomplementaemia is a characteristic feature of systemic lupus erythematosus and mixed cryoglobulinaemia, but it may also occur as a transient feature with infection, eg bacterial endocarditis.

3.3 Suspected immune deficiency in adults

Principle

Key point

Immune deficiency
Suspect immune deficiency:

> when infections are severe, frequent, prolonged or disseminated

> when unusual (opportunistic) organisms are isolated

> in relatives of patients with known or suspected hereditary immunodeficiencies.

Antibody deficiency

Antibodies are most important for extracellular organisms and for secondary protection against some viruses. Ask about the following:

> bacterial infections

> *Giardia* spp

> enteroviruses.

Phagocyte defect

Phagocytes (neutrophils and macrophages) are scavengers, engulfing foreign material. They are important in the early response to infection (before the specific immune responses are under way) and, later, they are the effectors against organisms targeted by the

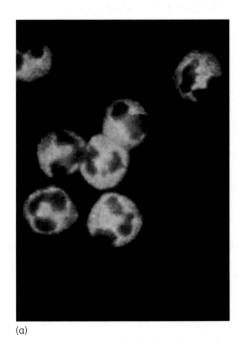

(a)

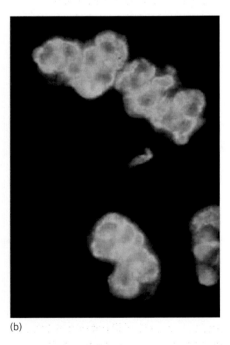

(b)

Fig 84 ANCA: **(a)** granular cytoplasmic fluorescence with interlobular accentuation characteristic of c-ANCA; **(b)** perinuclear immunofluorescence characteristic of p-ANCA.

specific immune response. Ask about the following:

> septicaemia, periodontitis or deep abscesses with Gram-negative bacteria or staphylococci, or invasive *Candida* or *Aspergillus* spp

> poor wound healing.

Key point

Screening for ciliary dysfunction

Ciliary dysfunction may masquerade as antibody deficiency. Test for this in non-smokers by placing a piece of saccharine tablet in the nose on the inferior turbinate. The patient should taste sweetness within 20 minutes if their ciliary function is normal.

T-lymphocyte defect

T-lymphocytes activate macrophages to kill organisms that they have phagocytosed, kill virus-infected cells and help B-cells produce antibodies. Severe cellular defects present in infancy but milder forms may be diagnosed only in adulthood. Ask about the following:

> viral infections: herpes simplex and zoster, cytomegalovirus (CMV), Kaposi's sarcoma and warts (including cervical intraepithelial neoplasia)

> intracellular bacterial infections: *Salmonella* infection and mycobacteria, including tuberculosis (TB)

> mucocutaneous candidiasis

Table 47 Common causes of secondary immunodeficiency	
Cause	**Deficiency**
Drugs:	
> Steroids and cytotoxics	Cellular or antibody deficiency, or neutropenia (quantitative/functional)
> Rituximab	Antibody deficiency
> Antiepileptics	Antibody deficiency
> Penicillamine, gold and sulfasalazine	Antibody deficiency
> Carbimazole	Idiopathic neutropenia
> Antibiotics	Disruption of normal bacterial flora
Smoking	Impaired mucociliary clearance
Viral respiratory tract infections	Impaired mucociliary clearance
HIV	Cellular deficiency
Haematological malignancy	Cellular, antibody or complement deficiency
Burns, wounds (skin) and severe eczema	Breach of protective barrier

> invasive cryptococci (meningitis)

> *Pneumocystis* spp (pneumonia).

Consider secondary immunodeficiencies (Table 47).

Complement defects

An intact complement pathway is essential for the opsonisation of micro-organisms and solubilisation of immune complexes. Patients with terminal complement component deficiencies are prone to neisserial infection (see Sections 1.1.2 and 2.1.5) whereas early component deficiencies predispose to systemic lupus erythematosus (SLE) and a broader range of bacterial infections.

Practical details

Key point

Detailed immunological investigations should be undertaken in conjunction with a clinical immunologist in order to ensure appropriate test selection.

Your investigations will depend on your clinical assessment. Your aim is to:

> define the immunodeficiency (if any)

> assess your patient's individual risk of opportunistic infection, with a view to avoidance, prophylaxis or early treatment.

Basic investigations

For most patients, a sensible starting point would be to check the following:

> FBC and a differential white cell count: lymphopenia is a feature of many cellular defects whereas a marked persistent neutrophilia (in the absence of sepsis or inflammation) would point to an adhesion molecule deficiency.

> Serum immunoglobulins as a basic screen of B-cell function. Exclude urinary loss of immunoglobulin G (IgG) by performing urine electrophoresis in patients with an isolated low IgG. Intestinal loss is unlikely when serum albumin is normal.

> Lymphocyte surface markers (eg CD3, CD4, CD8 for total, helper and cytotoxic T-cells; CD19 for B-cells; and CD16 / CD56 for natural killer cells) to quantify numbers of circulating lymphocytes. Close liaison with the clinical immunology laboratory is essential for selection of appropriate markers.

Antibody deficiency

Diagnosing antibody deficiency is relatively straightforward in patients with marked hypogammaglobulinaemia. If serum immunoglobulins are normal or moderately low, or if there is isolated IgA deficiency, check baseline antibody levels to common pathogens (*Streptococcus pneumoniae*) and routine immunisations (tetanus, diphtheria and *Haemophilus influenzae* type b).

Key point
A normal serum immunoglobulin profile does not exclude significant antibody deficiency.

If antibody levels are low, proceed to test immunisation with appropriate killed vaccines or toxoid (tetanus toxoid, Pneumovax (pneumococcal polysaccharide) and *H. influenzae* type b conjugate) and recheck antibody levels 3–4 weeks later. IgG subclass measurements may occasionally be helpful.

Key point
Live vaccines should be avoided in cases of suspected immunodeficiency because of the risk of vaccine-induced disease, eg paralytic poliomyelitis caused by oral polio vaccine.

Establishing the cause

Key point
Severe hypogammaglobulinaemia accompanied by lack of circulating B-cells is suggestive of a defect in B-cell differentiation.

If B-cells are absent consider checking for mutations in the following:

> Bruton's tyrosine kinase gene (X-linked)

> μ heavy chain gene (autosomal recessive)

> λ5 light chain gene (autosomal recessive)

> Igα (CD79a) gene, a component of the pre-B-cell receptor.

In male patients with hypogammaglobulinaemia and a normal or high serum IgM, exclude CD40 ligand deficiency.

Complement deficiency

Check the integrity of complement pathways by checking the haemolytic activity of the classic and alternate pathways (CH50 and AP50, see Section 2.1.5).

Also consider secondary causes: C3 nephritic factor, an IgG autoantibody that stabilises the alternate pathway C3 convertase causing consumption of C3 (associated with mesangiocapillary glomerulonephritis); and immune complex diseases, such as endocarditis or SLE.

T-lymphocyte defect

Total lymphocyte and individual lymphocyte subset numbers are usually low. Check additionally for human leukocyte antigen class I and II expression by flow cytometry. Check lymphocyte proliferation to mitogens, such as phytohaemagglutinin (stimulates all lymphocytes) and to antigens such as purified protein derivative (PPD) or tetanus toxoid (stimulates only lymphocytes with the appropriate T-cell receptor). Consider *in vivo* intradermal testing to a range of antigens (PPD, *Candida* spp and tetanus, streptokinase). Consider checking the T-cell repertoire by flow cytometry or a PCR-based method.

Establishing the underlying causes

Genetic analysis

Where a specific genetic defect is suspected this can be tested for in regional specialist laboratories.

Cytogenetics can be helpful for suspected syndromes such as Di-George (22qll deletion associated with combined immunodeficiency).

Next-generation sequencing holds great promise for the future diagnosis and management of rare and sometimes unique monogenetic disorders.

Enzyme assays can be used to diagnose adenosine deaminase and purine nucleoside phosphorylase (PNP) deficiency, which are associated with progressive combined deficiencies.

Key point
A useful clue to PNP deficiency is the presence of marked hypouricaemia, reflecting the key role of PNP in urate production.

Phagocyte defect

Check for cyclical neutropenia. Do neutrophil counts three times weekly for 1 month. Do a nitroblue tetrazolium or dihydrorhodamine test (see Fig 5).

Check for leukocyte adhesion defects: use flow cytometry to check for the presence of adhesion molecules, especially CD18. Assess neutrophil chemotaxis.

Determining risk of infection

Knowledge of the patient's individual immune defect, combined with their probable exposure to pathogens, will help determine the likelihood of infection (Table 48). Take a thorough history, including details of any travel or immunisation. Serological tests based on antibody detection are likely to be unreliable in the presence of immunodeficiency, but may give information about previous exposure (risk of reactivation) or immunity (risk of severe disease if non-immune). Cultures, biopsy and antigen-detection techniques (immunofluorescence or polymerase chain reaction) will usually be necessary to diagnose active infections because clinical features may be atypical in immunodeficient individuals. Invasive investigations may be required.

3.4 Imaging in rheumatological disease

3.4.1 Plain radiology

Principle

The primary use of radiography is to detect changes in bony structure. It is much less useful in soft-tissue pathology.

Table 48 Patterns of infection in immunodeficiency

	Antibody/complement	Cell-mediated	Phagocyte
Bacterial	*Streptococcus pneumoniae*	*Salmonella* spp	*Staphylococcus aureus* and *Staphylococcus epidermidis*
	Haemophilus influenzae	*Listeria* spp	*Escherichia coli*
	Neisseria meningitidis	*Nocardia* spp	*Klebsiella* spp
	Mycoplasma spp	Mycobacteria (TB and atypical)	*Pseudomonas* spp
	Staphylococcus aureus[1]		
	Pseudomonas spp[1]		
Viral[2]	Enteroviruses; including invasive echovirus, polio and persistent norovirus	Herpesviruses including HSV-1 and HSV-2, invasive CMV, lymphomas (EBV) and Kaposi's sarcoma (human herpes virus 8)	
	Persistent respiratory viruses	Papillomavirus (warts, cervical and anal neoplasia)	
	Recurrent HSV or VZV	JC virus (progressive multifocal leucoencephalopathy)	
Fungal		*Candida* spp (mucocutaneous)	*Candida* spp (invasive) and *Aspergillus* spp
		Pneumocystis spp	
		Cryptococci	
Protozoal	*Giardia* spp[2]	*Toxoplasma* spp	
		Cryptosporidium spp	
		Microsporidium spp	

1 More common in the presence of bronchiectasis.
2 *Giardia* and viral infections are not a feature of complement deficiency.
CMV, cytomegalovirus; EBV, Epstein–Barr virus; HSV, herpes simplex virus; JC, John Cunningham; TB, tuberculosis; VZV, varicella zoster virus.

Indications

Diagnostic

> Differential diagnosis of chronic arthritis: inflammatory and erosive arthritis can be distinguished from osteoarthritis (OA). Distinct forms of inflammatory arthritis can be further differentiated (Fig 85).

> Back pain: plain radiographs are greatly overused in the assessment of back pain. However, in 'red flag' back pain (see Section 1.1.13) plain radiographs may provide definitive diagnostic information (eg of osteoporotic fracture or ankylosing spondylitis) or might provide pointers to appropriate further investigation (eg in cases of suspected malignancy or septic discitis). Plain radiographs hardly ever help in the assessment of neurological problems.

> Metabolic bone disease: diagnostic in Paget's disease (increased trabecular markings; see Fig 86), supportive in osteomalacia and unhelpful in osteoporosis (unless a fracture is present).

> Malignancy: gives few definitive diagnostic findings, but often provides strong supportive evidence for both primary and metastatic bone tumours.

Prognosis / disease outcome

Plain radiographs play a major role in assessing the progress of inflammatory arthritis. The development of bony erosions, the progression of erosive changes and the development of secondary osteoarthritic changes are the most robust methods for assessing articular damage, prognosis and response to treatment (see Sections 1.1.14, 1.1.16 and 2.3.3).

In rheumatoid arthritis (RA), annual or biannual serial radiographs of the hands (Fig 87) and wrists are the most useful means of monitoring the rate of joint damage and assessing the effects of treatment. The early development of erosions is one of the best predictors of aggressive disease. Radiographs of larger joints in RA are only useful in documenting the development of secondary OA. Neck pain or neurological signs in the limbs should provoke a radiograph of the cervical spine, particularly to look for atlantoaxial subluxation. Views in cervical flexion and extension are required.

> **!** **Hazard**

> **Limitations of plain radiographs**
> > radiation exposure
>
> > failure to detect soft-tissue pathology
>
> > changes only appear late in the disease process; neoplastic and inflammatory bone destruction is usually well advanced before it is evident on a plain film.

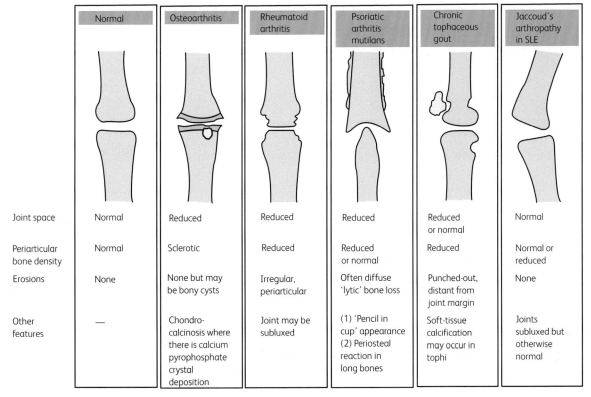

	Normal	Osteoarthritis	Rheumatoid arthritis	Psoriatic arthritis mutilans	Chronic tophaceous gout	Jaccoud's arthropathy in SLE
Joint space	Normal	Reduced	Reduced	Reduced	Reduced or normal	Normal
Periarticular bone density	Normal	Sclerotic	Reduced	Reduced or normal	Reduced	Normal or reduced
Erosions	None	None but may be bony cysts	Irregular, periarticular	Often diffuse 'lytic' bone loss	Punched-out, distant from joint margin	None
Other features	—	Chondrocalcinosis where there is calcium pyrophosphate crystal deposition	Joint may be subluxed	(1) 'Pencil in cup' appearance (2) Periosteal reaction in long bones	Soft-tissue calcification may occur in tophi	Joints subluxed but otherwise normal

Fig 85 Schematic representation of radiological changes in major arthritides. These changes are found in advanced, long-standing disease. Radiographs may be normal in early disease. SLE, systemic lupus erythematosus.

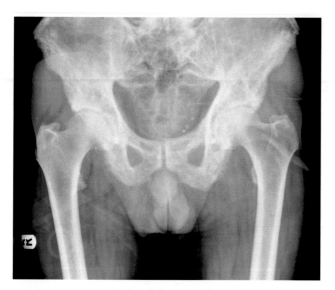

Fig 86 Pelvic radiograph showing characteristic trabeculation in a patient with Paget's disease.

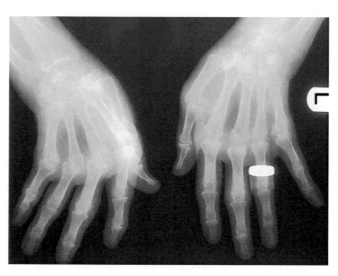

Fig 87 Radiograph of the hands in a patient with advanced RA showing deforming, erosive arthropathy.

3.4.2 Bone densitometry

Principle

Plain radiographs cannot provide a reliable assessment of bone mineral density (BMD). Several techniques exist for quantitating the absorption of radiation by bone while simultaneously compensating for any absorption by soft tissues. Dual-energy X-ray absorptiometry (DEXA) scanning is the most widely used technique, because it is highly accurate and involves low radiation exposure. BMD is usually measured at the hip and lumbar spine and results are expressed as the following:

> standard deviations above (+) or below (-) the mean for the patient's sex and age (*Z* score)

> standard deviation from the mean BMD for a young adult (*T* score)

> fracture risk varies continuously with a reduction in BMD, and approximately doubles with each standard deviation below the mean. However, osteoporosis is usually defined as BMD *T* score < -2.5.

Indications

Key point

BMD measurement should be used primarily when the result will influence treatment and it contributes to the overall fracture risk assessment. If a decision has been made to treat on clinical grounds (eg commencing prolonged steroid treatment), then DEXA scanning is unlikely to add anything useful. BMD measurement can also be used to assess response to therapy, and/or before commencing some types of antiresorptive medication (eg denosumab).

Key point

When to use DEXA
DEXA scanning should be considered in the following circumstances:

> plain radiographs suggest osteopenia or vertebral deformity

> previous fragility fractures have occurred

> patient has been on prednisolone therapy (or equivalent other corticosteroids) for >6 months at doses >7.5 mg

> gonadal failure (early menopause, prolonged amenorrhoea and hypogonadism in men)

> chronic systemic ill-health; especially if it involves weight loss, malabsorption or metabolic bone disease

> serial monitoring of BMD in response to treatment or risk factors such as corticosteroid treatment.

3.4.3 Magnetic resonance imaging

Principle

Magnetic resonance imaging (MRI) utilises the changes in magnetic field induced by excitation of hydrogen protons to produce cross-sectional imaging; these images can powerfully differentiate types of soft tissue, largely on the basis of water content. Cross-sectional images can be constructed in any plane. Scans are usually performed to detect two different patterns of change in magnetic field, known as T1-weighted (T1w) and T2-weighted (T2w) scans. T1w scans show high signal from fat, but not fluid, whereas T2w scans show both fat and fluid as high signal. The signal from fat can be suppressed from a T2w scan to give selective imaging of the fluid content.

Tissues with a low fluid and fat content (eg bone, ligament and tendon) appear dark on MRI, whereas pathological processes such as inflammation or neoplasia appear bright on T2w scans because of their rich blood supply.

Indications

> **Hazard**
> MRI is an extremely sensitive technique. Minor pathologies of doubtful significance are frequently demonstrated, eg scans of the lumbar spine are rarely 'normal' in patients over the age of 40. Great care needs to be exercised when requesting and interpreting MRI scans. Scans performed as a 'screening' exercise, without a sound diagnostic hypothesis, are more likely to confuse than to inform.

Key point

When to use MRI

MRI may provide diagnostic information in the following:

> 'red flag' pattern back pain – suspected malignancy, discitis or serious neurological involvement (see Section 1.1.13)

> cervical and lumbar pain with neurological involvement, particularly spinal cord pathology

> central nervous system disease in systemic lupus or systemic vasculitis

> suspected avascular necrosis of bone – changes may predate plain radiographs by several weeks, and surgical intervention is unlikely to be helpful once changes are seen on a plain radiograph

> polymyositis – useful in patchy disease, both diagnostically and to identify sites for biopsy

> mechanical knee pain – as useful as arthroscopy in demonstrating meniscal or ligament pathology

> shoulder pain – assessment of the rotator cuff

> suspected soft-tissue tumours – malignant and benign tumours can usually be distinguished, and pointers to histology can be found (eg haemangioma, neurofibroma, lipoma or synovial cyst)

> an MRI of inflammatory arthritis can be used to detect synovitis and early erosive changes, but currently it is largely a research tool.

Contraindications

> **Hazard**
> MRI is free from radiation hazards, although scanning anatomically fragile sites where mobile pieces of metal are present can have disastrous consequences: intracranial aneurysm clips, foreign bodies in the eye and permanent pacemakers all rule out the use of MRI. Imaging can be performed with fixed non-mobile metal such as joint prostheses, although the quality of imaging may be poor near the metal object.

3.4.4 Nuclear medicine

Principle

A short-lived radioisotope that emits gamma radiation is tagged on to either a pharmacologically active molecule or whole cells. After injection, the localisation of the isotope is visualised with a gamma camera. In general, scintigraphic techniques are strong in providing information on function, but relatively weak on anatomical definition. Radioisotope bone scanning is the most commonly used technique in rheumatology: this utilises technetium-99m-labelled bisphosphonates, which are taken up at sites of bone turnover.

Indications

Bone scintigraphy

> Suspected stress fracture: scintigraphic changes may predate changes visible on a plain radiograph by two or more weeks.

> Suspected osteomyelitis: again, scintigraphy precedes changes on a plain radiograph.

> Metabolic bone disease: scintigraphy may strongly support a diagnosis of Paget's disease (Fig 88) or of osteomalacia.

> Peripheral joint disease: scintigraphy has limited utility in defining the distribution of an arthritic process.

> Suspected bony malignancy: scintigraphy is sensitive but has low specificity.

Key point

Bone scintigraphy is usually normal in multiple myeloma.

Inflammation or infection

This is most commonly performed using radiolabelled autologous leukocytes. This is of particular use in locating occult sepsis (eg in pyrexia of unknown origin).

Amyloid

The diagnosis and response to treatment of all forms of amyloidosis is facilitated by scintigraphy, using radiolabelled serum amyloid P protein. Unfortunately this technique is restricted to a small number of centres.

3.4.5 Ultrasound

Principle

Modern high-frequency ultrasound machines can be used to provide high-definition dynamic imaging of the soft tissues. Although heavily dependent upon the skill of the operator, ultrasound can be used in the clinic to supplement information derived from conventional clinical assessment.

Indications

Ultrasound can be used to make accurate anatomical diagnoses of regional pathology involving tendons, entheses and joints (for example to differentiate causes of shoulder pain); to guide accurate aspiration and injection of joints; and to identify damage (such as erosions in early rheumatoid arthritis) with greater sensitivity than conventional radiology.

3.5 Arthrocentesis

Principle

Aspiration of synovial fluid is a useful diagnostic manoeuvre in the differential diagnosis of joint disease (see Section 1.4.4). Macroscopic examination of synovial fluid may demonstrate the clear, viscous synovial fluid found in osteoarthritis and other non-inflammatory disorders, and also the turbid fluid of inflammatory arthritis or haemarthrosis. The use of Gram stain, culture and polarised light microscopy will differentiate between septic arthritis, crystal arthritis and other inflammatory arthritides.

Indications

> any inflammatory arthritis or joint effusion of uncertain cause

> any established inflammatory arthritis that behaves in an unexpected fashion (eg a severe monoarticular flare in otherwise stable rheumatoid disease – this may be the result of septic arthritis).

Lack of experience in the technique is not an excuse – if you can't do it, find someone who can! Small joints may require ultrasound guidance to increase success rate / diagnostic yield.

Contraindications

There are very few contraindications:

> Probable periarticular sepsis (eg cellulitis overlying an inflamed joint) may lead to the introduction of sepsis into the joint.

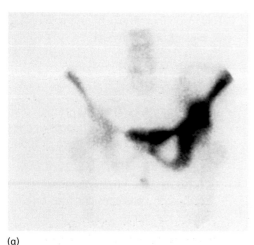

(a)

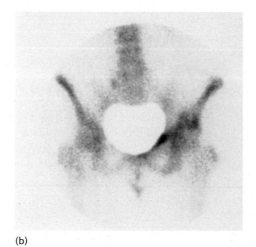

(b)

Fig 88 Isotope bone scan showing Paget's disease of the pelvis **(a)** before and **(b)** after treatment with pamidronate infusions.

> Prosthetic joints should usually be left to the orthopaedic surgeons.

> Warfarin treatment with international normalised ratio (INR) in the therapeutic range is not a complete contraindication, but severe bleeding tendencies (eg severe haemophilia or thrombocytopenia severe enough to cause spontaneous bleeding) should usually be corrected before aspiration. Be especially careful with shoulder injections as bleeds here can be very significant indeed.

Hazard

Prosthetic joint problems should be referred to the orthopaedic surgeons. Never aspirate a prosthetic joint without at least discussing this with your orthopaedic colleagues.

Practical details

Before the procedure

Arthrocentesis can be performed in the outpatient clinic or at the bedside. For medium to large joints (ie wrist and larger) no equipment is needed other than something to clean the skin and a needle and syringe. In general, use a green 21G needle for large joints such as the knee or shoulder, and a blue or orange needle for smaller joints. Use of too small a needle may prevent aspiration of viscous fluid. Choose a size of syringe appropriate to the size of the effusion – you are unlikely to aspirate more than 1–2 mL from the wrist, but an acutely swollen knee may contain >200 mL of fluid.

Most rheumatologists use a 'no-touch' technique, whereby the site of aspiration is identified and marked before skin preparation and aspiration is performed.

Most experienced aspirators do not use local anaesthetic because its infiltration can be as uncomfortable as the procedure itself, but it may be useful when aspirating the knee. Alternatively

cryogesic spray can transiently numb the skin and make the procedure more comfortable for the patient.

Key point

Virtually all extraspinal joints can be aspirated at the bedside, guided by surface anatomy. The exception is the hip, which is so deep-seated that aspiration under radiological or ultrasonic control is recommended. Radiological help can also be invaluable with effusions that are difficult to aspirate but clinically important.

The procedure

Detailed instructions for individual joints cannot be given here. However, some general points apply:

1 Palpate the inflamed joint.

2 Decide whether a fluctuant effusion is present.

3 Mark the point of entry and clean the skin with alcohol or iodine.

4 Insert the needle at the point of maximum fluctuation, taking care to avoid major neurovascular structures (eg the ulnar nerve at the elbow).

5 Entry to the joint cavity will usually be with a palpable 'give'.

6 Draw back on the syringe at intervals during the advance of the needle until fluid is obtained.

7 Aspirate as much fluid as possible without causing undue discomfort.

8 If no obvious effusion is present, fluid is less likely to be obtained. However, in some deep-seated joints such as the hip, shoulder and elbow, significant effusions may be present even when not palpable at the surface.

After the procedure

Samples for microbiological examination should be placed in a clean sterile container. Some laboratories prefer an anticoagulant sample for polarised light microscopy and cytology – check with your local laboratory first. Samples should arrive at the laboratory within the same working day, although samples stored overnight may be suitable for culture and detection of crystals (see Sections 1.4.4, 2.3.6 and 2.3.7).

Diagnostic microscopy and culture can be performed on samples of <0.5 mL. Also, crystals can sometimes be seen in the flushings from the needle of an apparently dry tap, so it may be worth taking the needle and syringe to the laboratory.

Complications

Complications are rare:

> Major – infection may be introduced into the joint on rare occasions, but the risk is less than one in 30,000.

> Minor – some discomfort is inevitable, but this is usually minor.

3.6 Corticosteroid injection techniques

Principle

A suspension of poorly soluble corticosteroid crystals is injected into an inflamed joint or soft-tissue lesion. This produces a prolonged, potent, local anti-inflammatory effect with minimal systemic corticosteroid action.

Indications

This technique is one of the most useful therapeutic manoeuvres in rheumatology and is useful in the following:

> non-septic inflammatory arthritis in any joint

> selected cases of non-inflammatory arthritis

> soft-tissue rheumatic disorders: tennis elbow, plantar fasciitis and trochanteric bursitis

> carpal tunnel syndrome, especially when resulting from an inflammatory cause.

Contraindications

Absolute

> septic or suspected septic arthritis

> septicaemia

> allergy to any component of the corticosteroid preparation

> prosthetic joints

> infected skin overlying the joint.

Relative

> a peritendinous injection may predispose the patient to subsequent rupture of the tendon, especially the Achilles tendon and the long head of the biceps. Injection at these sites should be at the discretion of a senior colleague

> bleeding tendency.

Practical details

The preparation and techniques for the introduction of a needle into a joint are described in Section 3.5. Aspiration of the joint before injection is not always required (if you don't know the diagnosis, you shouldn't be injecting) and may not be possible if no effusion is present. However, large or tense effusions should be aspirated because this will make the joint less uncomfortable. Some rheumatologists recommend that any fluid that can be aspirated should be sent for culture to exclude unrecognised infection. Figures 89 and 90 show the landmarks for injection of the knee and shoulder.

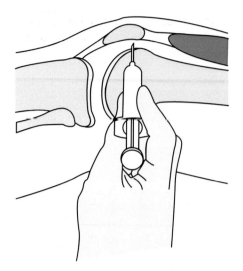

Fig 89 Injection of the medial aspect of the knee joint in extension. (Reproduced with permission from the Arthritis and Rheumatism Council.)

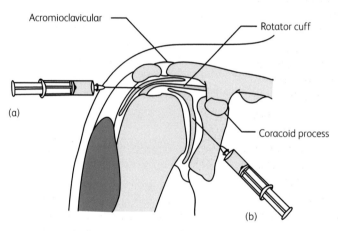

Fig 90 Injection of **(a)** the subdeltoid and **(b)** glenohumeral joint. (Reproduced with permission from the Arthritis and Rheumatism Council.)

If aspiration is being performed before injection, the syringe for aspiration should be removed leaving the needle *in situ*. Then the syringe containing the corticosteroid preparation should be carefully placed in the hub of the needle, taking care not to touch any sterile area. Even if aspiration is not performed before injection, gentle suction should be placed on the syringe containing the preparation as it aspirates the joint upon entry; reflux of synovial fluid confirms that you are in the joint space.

Key point

> Injection into the joint space should meet almost no resistance and be almost pain free.

> Accurate intra-articular placement gives a better response than periarticular injection.

Individual soft-tissue injection techniques cannot be described here. In general, the corticosteroid is injected directly at the site of pathology, into the most tender area. Soft-tissue injections are therefore usually more painful than intra-articular injections.

The steroid preparations used most commonly are poorly soluble salts of methylprednisolone, triamcinolone and hydrocortisone. Hydrocortisone preparations are the least potent and shortest acting, and are often preferred for use in superficial soft-tissue or peritendinous injections to reduce the risk of skin atrophy and tendon rupture. The differences between the other preparations are not great. The amount of steroid injected depends on the size of the joint, eg 40–80 mg (1–2 mL) methylprednisolone is appropriate for a large joint such as a knee, but only 5–10 mg (0.25–0.5 mL) is required for a small finger joint. Many rheumatologists use a mixture of steroids and local anaesthetic for injection. The evidence for any beneficial effect of any mixtures of local anaesthetic and steroid is small, but they may reduce discomfort after injection, particularly for soft-tissue injections. Only methylprednisolone and lidocaine (lignocaine) are available in a premixed form.

In theory, any number of joints may be injected in a single session, but in practice this is limited by discomfort and the cumulative dose of steroids. In practice, it is recommended that no more than three or four joints are injected in one session. Sometimes intramuscular steroid injections are considered in patients with multiple swollen joints, eg methylprednisolone 8–120 mg or triamcinolone 40–80 mg.

Outcome

Improvement usually occurs within 24–48 hours. Historically, most rheumatologists recommended 24–48 hours bed rest after receiving an injection in a weight-bearing joint, but this is no longer practical or necessary. However, advice to minimise the weight

borne by the affected joint does seem to be associated with a modest increase in efficacy.

Key point
The duration of the response after injection depends on the severity of synovitis with improvement usually occurring over a period of weeks to months. A rapid relapse of inflammation in a patient with a chronic arthritis should lead you, first, to question the diagnosis (Could this be sepsis? Is there an atypical infection?) and, second, to question whether the patient's systemic medication needs modification. The need for repeated injections should also lead to a review of the patient's disease-modifying therapy.

Complications

> Intra-articular infection is rare, occurring in around one in 30,000 procedures.

> Short-term increases in pain and inflammation after an injection are common, particularly with soft-tissue injections. Patients should be warned about this, although it usually settles within 48 hours and can be managed with analgesics. Rarely, a very florid flare in arthritis is seen, which must be differentiated from sepsis by re-aspiration.

> Tendon rupture may occur.

> Skin atrophy and depigmentation is more common after a superficial injection, particularly with the use of potent steroids and with repeat injections.

> Facial flushing may be experienced in the hour after the injection.

> Exacerbation of diabetes mellitus: changes in diabetic medication are not usually required because the

effect is generally mild and transient, but patients should be warned that their glucose readings may temporarily increase.

> Systemic side effects of corticosteroids: adrenal suppression and iatrogenic Cushing's syndrome may occur if frequent injections are used, or if there is concurrent use of oral steroids.

Key point
Local corticosteroid injections are generally used to minimise the systemic side effects associated with this class of drugs. However, some systemic absorption does occur and this can sometimes be therapeutically useful in the patient with a florid polyarthritis. Injection of the two to four worst affected joints will often enable sufficient systemic anti-inflammatory action to reduce more widespread joint inflammation and improve well-being, without resorting to oral steroids (which are often difficult to stop once started).

3.7 Immunoglobulin therapy

Principle

Intravenous immunoglobulin (Ig) therapy refers to the role that the replacement of immunoglobulin G (IgG) antibodies has in patients with defective B-cell function or its immunomodulatory role in autoimmune disease.

Immunoglobulin replacement may also be given subcutaneously.

Indications

Antibody deficiency

Intravenous Ig or subcutaneous Ig is the treatment of choice for severe antibody deficiencies (Fig 91). For milder antibody

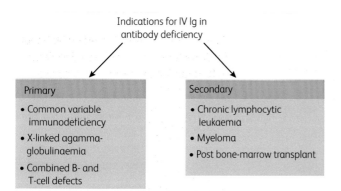

Indications for IV Ig in antibody deficiency

Primary
- Common variable immunodeficiency
- X-linked agamma-globulinaemia
- Combined B- and T-cell defects

Secondary
- Chronic lymphocytic leukaemia
- Myeloma
- Post bone-marrow transplant

Fig 91 Indications for intravenous Ig in antibody deficiency.

deficiencies, such as IgG subclass deficiency, antibiotic prophylaxis is usually sufficient. Immunoglobulin replacement should be reserved for cases with objective evidence of specific antibody deficiency or failure to respond to proven infection or test vaccination, or where antibiotic prophylaxis has failed.

Immunomodulation

Intravenous Ig therapy has been enthusiastically tried in a wide range of diseases, but proof of its efficacy has been demonstrated in relatively few.

Key point

Intravenous Ig as an immunomodulatory agent

Efficacy proven in randomised controlled trials (RCT):
- immune thrombocytopenia
- Guillain–Barré syndrome
- chronic inflammatory demyelinating polyneuropathy
- Kawasaki's disease
- dermatomyositis
- Lambert–Eaton syndrome
- multifocal motor neuropathy.

Ineffective in RCT:
- postviral fatigue (chronic fatigue syndrome)
- rheumatoid arthritis (RA)
- juvenile RA.

Contraindications

There are no absolute contraindications, but caution should be exercised in the following cases:

> Patients with total immunoglobulin A (IgA) deficiency and high titre anti-IgA antibodies, in view of the risk of anaphylaxis, though the strength of this association is debatable. Use an intravenous Ig product containing low levels of IgA for such patients or use subcutaneous Ig which is well tolerated by patients with a history of intravenous Ig-associated anaphylaxis.

> Patients with pre-existing renal impairment – infusion of high-dose intravenous Ig may precipitate reversible renal failure in this situation.

> Untreated bacterial infection: defer immunoglobulin for 24–48 hours and initiate antibiotic treatment.

> **! Hazard**

Infusion of intravenous Ig in the presence of bacterial sepsis may result in exogenous IgG complexing with bacterial antigen to cause an immune complex reaction.

Practical details
Before procedure
It is important to counsel patients on the risks and benefits of treatment with a blood product derivative. Measure

hepatitis B surface antigen, hepatitis C RNA and save serum before the first infusion and annually. Measure liver function and trough IgG every 3 months. Ensure the availability of a trained assistant and telephone if the patient is self infusing at home.

The procedure
Intravenous Ig: the usual dose is 0.4 g/kg every 2–3 weeks, and this should be sufficient to keep trough IgG well within the normal range. Higher levels may be required in established bronchiectasis or if granulomatous disease is present. Infuse at 0.01–0.07 mL/kg per minute. Slower rates are used when initiating treatment.

Key point

The dose of intravenous Ig used for immunomodulation is significantly higher than that used for antibody replacement. Empirically, high doses of the order of 1–2 g/kg are used.

Subcutaneous Ig: the usual dose is 0.1–0.2 g/kg every 1–2 weeks. Concentrated solutions formulated for subcutaneous use are used. Infusions are given via infusion pumps in the abdomen or thighs, giving 15–20 mL at each site. Local reactions are common but improve with time. Systemic and delayed reactions are much less common via this route.

Observe for adverse effects. Reduce the infusion rate if mild side effects occur. Discontinue if moderate or severe side effects occur. Flu-like symptoms occurring after 24–48 hours will respond to paracetamol.

After the procedure
Note batch number of intravenous Ig and any adverse events.

Complications

Complications may be divided into immediate infusion-related events, those related to infusing high doses of IgG, and transmission of infections as a result of infusing a blood product.

Infusion-related events
Serious anaphylactoid or immune complex-mediated reactions are rare. Milder infusion-related reactions, eg headache, flushing, low backache, nausea, chills and abdominal pain, occur in 2–6% of cases and respond rapidly to a reduction in the rate of infusion.

Sudden rise in serum IgG
These complications are seen predominantly with high-dose intravenous Ig:

> aseptic meningitis – aetiology unknown, occurs in approximately 10% of patients

> haemolysis caused by anti-blood group antibodies – this is exceptional but may occur if intravenous Ig contains high titres of blood group antibodies

> reversible renal failure as a result of osmotic tubular injury caused by the carbohydrate component of intravenous Ig

> arterial or venous thrombosis – occurs in patients with pre-existing hyperviscosity, cardiovascular disease or thrombophilia.

Blood-borne viral transmission
Stringent precautions in donor selection, plasma screening and the inclusion of antiviral steps in immunoglobulin preparation has minimised the risk of infection. Extrapolating from data on risks of viral transmission with blood transfusion, the current risk of hepatitis C viral transmission with intravenous Ig is estimated at one in 2–3 million. Emerging pathogens such as prions remain a theoretical concern. Minimise risk by monitoring batch numbers, thus enabling a swift recall in case of an infected batch. Do not change the intravenous Ig preparation except for strong clinical reasons.

Key point

HIV and hepatitis B virus have not been transmitted by intravenous Ig, presumably because these viruses do not survive Cohn ethanol fractionation, the manufacturing process for intravenous Ig.

3.8 Biologic therapy

Principle
Greater understanding of the pathogenesis of inflammatory conditions has allowed the specific targeting of key cells or cytokines that drive disease. Therapeutic use of monoclonal antibodies or fusion proteins has been exemplified best in the treatment of rheumatoid arthritis (RA), for which there are now four licensed targets: tumour necrosis factor alpha (TNF-α), interleukin (IL)-6, B-cells and T-cells (see Table 49).

Being antibodies, biologic treatments are complex and costly to manufacture, which has hampered their more widespread use. However, as originator biologic agents start to come off patent, biotechnology companies are increasingly able to produce so-called biosimilars; such competition may drive down price and allow greater access, but some concerns remain around their potential immunogenicity.

Indications
Biologic therapy is restricted by National Institute for Health and Care Excellence (NICE) guidance to those with severe disease who have failed standard treatment. In those whose disease activity is hard to assess, due to either concomitant fibromyalgia or biomechanical disease, the decision can be guided by more objective measures such as radiology (eg ultrasound in peripheral arthritis or MRI in spondyloarthropathy) or the acute-phase response. The most common conditions for which biologics are in routine use include rheumatoid arthritis (RA), psoriatic arthritis, ankylosing spondylitis and enteropathic arthritis. One of the great challenges of the biologic era is stratifying the use of these medicines for greatest clinical benefit – using the right drug in the right patient at the right time.

Contraindications
The most significant contraindications exist for TNF-α inhibition. Absolute contraindications include recent malignancy, severe heart failure and demyelinating disease. Septic arthritis is a relative contraindication (unless it involved a prosthetic joint and the metalwork has not been removed, in which case anti-TNF-α should be avoided indefinitely). The ongoing clinical concern is re-activation of latent tuberculosis (TB) following TNF-α inhibition: all patients are screened before treatment and if either latent or

Table 49	Mechanism of action of the four licensed biologics for treatment of RA	
Target	**Mechanism of action**	**Example**
TNF-α	Monoclonal antibody against TNF-α molecule	Adalimumab
	Fusion protein with TNF-α receptor (acts as decoy)	Etanercept
B-cell	Monoclonal antibody against CD20-positive B-cells	Rituximab
T-cell	Fusion protein with CTLA-4 (interrupts second T-cell signal)	Abatacept
IL-6	Monoclonal antibody against IL-6 receptor	Tocilizumab

IL, interleukin; RA, rheumatoid arthritis; TNF-α, tumour necrosis factor alpha.

active TB are identified, TNF-α inhibition is postponed until after adequate antimicrobial treatment. There are few contraindications for B-cell depletion, T-cell modulation or IL-6R inhibition.

Practical details

All patients should be screened for TB, hepatitis virus and HIV before commencing biologic therapy, and guidance sought if any of the above are identified. Conventional synthetic disease-modifying antirheumatic drugs (DMARDs) should be continued alongside biologic treatment, as there is increasing evidence that their use reduces the development of anti-drug antibodies and prolongs the life of the biologic agent. Patients need counselling and support from specialist nurses on the use of biologics, their storage (they must be refrigerated) and self-administration.

Complications

Biologic therapies are in general very well tolerated, but patients should remain aware of possible side effects. The most common problem is local skin reactions, but the severity of this can be reduced by rotating injection sites. The development of TB (especially extra-pulmonary disease) should always be borne in mind in patients on anti-TNF-α. Recurrent use of rituximab may cause persistent hypogammaglobulinaemia, and tocilizumab often causes hypercholesterolaemia, which may require treatment.

Rheumatology and clinical immunology: Section 4

4 Self-assessment

4.1 Self-assessment questions

MRCP(UK) Part 1 examination questions

Question 1

Clinical scenario

A 42-year-old man presented to the rheumatology outpatient clinic with inflammatory joint pain and swelling. On examination he had demarcated areas of a scaly rash over his forearms, synovitis affecting his proximal and distal interphalangeal joints bilaterally, and a sausage toe in his left foot.

Question

What is the most likely diagnosis?

Answer

A post-infectious arthritis

B psoriatic arthritis

C rheumatoid arthritis

D systemic lupus erythematosus

E vasculitis

Question 2

Clinical scenario

A 24-year-old woman with a history of Raynaud's phenomenon presented to the rheumatology outpatient clinic with hair thinning and oral ulcers. She complained of joint pains, but there was relatively little synovitis to detect. There was a circular patch of alopecia behind her right ear.

Question

Which investigation is most likely to establish the diagnosis?

Answer

A anticitrullinated peptide antibody (ACPA)

B antineutrophil cytoplasmic antibody (ANCA)

C antinuclear antibody (ANA)

D complement levels

E rheumatoid factor

Question 3

Clinical scenario

A 55-year-old woman was referred to the rheumatology outpatient clinic with a possible connective tissue disease. She suffered from disabling fatigue and joint pains, although she did not think that her joints had ever been swollen. She also complained of gritty eyes and a dry mouth. Examination revealed mild lymphadenopathy, injected sclera with reduced tear production and some mild synovitis.

Question

What would you expect her extractable nuclear antigen profile to show?

Answer

A centromere positive

B double-stranded DNA positive

C histone positive

D ribonucleoprotein (RNP) positive

E Ro/La positive

Question 4

Clinical scenario

A 62-year-old woman with rheumatoid arthritis, normally well controlled on methotrexate, was admitted to hospital with a community-acquired pneumonia, from which she appeared to be recovering. Her right wrist became painful over a period of 48 hours, and she felt tired and unwell, which she attributed to coughing all night. On examination she was afebrile but had a marked wrist monoarthritis.

Question

What is the investigation of choice?

Answer

A blood cultures

B C-reactive protein (CRP)

C serum urate

D synovial fluid culture

E ultrasound

Question 5

Clinical scenario

A 32-year-old man presented to the emergency department with an acutely painful swollen right knee. He was normally well and had returned from a holiday in America 3 weeks previously. While abroad he had experienced an episode of bloody diarrhoea, which lasted a few days and then resolved completely. On examination, apart from knee swelling, he had a palmar-plantar pustular rash.

Question

What is the most likely diagnosis?

Answer

A Behçet's disease

B enteropathic arthritis

C Lyme disease

D reactive arthritis

E septic arthritis

Question 6

Clinical scenario

A 65-year-old man with infective endocarditis due to *Streptococcus viridans* had a history of a penicillin-induced rash in childhood. His physicians wished to treat him with parenteral penicillin, but were concerned about the risk of anaphylaxis.

Question

Which would provide the highest level of reassurance regarding the safety of penicillin-based antibiotics in this patient?

Answer

A negative serum specific IgE to penicillin

B negative serum specific IgE to penicillin and normal serum tryptase

C negative skin-prick and intra-dermal tests to determinants of penicillin

D normal serum tryptase

E normal total serum IgE

Question 7

Clinical scenario

A 70-year-old man sustained a cardiac arrest after he presented to the emergency department with acute anaphylaxis following a wasp sting. He had a past history of ischaemic heart disease and hypertension, and took aspirin, bisoprolol, isosorbide mononitrate and ramipril as regular medications. After two cycles of cardiopulmonary resuscitation (CPR), including two adrenaline (epinephrine) injections, he had no cardiac output.

Question

Which drug would you use immediately to try and restore his circulation?

Answer

A diclofenac

B dobutamine

C glucagon

D isoprenaline

E prazosin

Question 8

Clinical scenario

A 78-year-old woman attended the emergency department with isolated orofacial angio-oedema and tongue swelling that had woken her from sleep. She had a history of cardiovascular disease and was unable to talk because of severe tongue swelling.

Question

What is the most likely cause?

Answer

A anaphylaxis

B aspirin

C C1 inhibitor deficiency

D hereditary angio-oedema

E lisinopril

Question 9

Clinical scenario

A 65-year-old Caucasian woman presented with a constant right-sided temporal headache. She had suffered from neck pain intermittently over the previous year and had been feeling generally tired and unwell for several weeks, during which time she had lost 4 kg in weight. On examination she had a temperature of 37.4°C, her neck was not stiff, and her right temporal artery was palpable and slightly tender.

Question

What is the most likely diagnosis?

Answer

A cervicogenic headache

B temporal arteritis

C tension headache

D trigeminal neuralgia

E tuberculous meningitis

Question 10

Clinical scenario

A 41-year-old woman presented with weakness and tingling in her right hand.

Question

Which feature would support a diagnosis of carpal tunnel syndrome?

Answer

A loss of sensation in the fifth finger

B wasting of the thenar eminence

C weakness of the first dorsal interosseous

D weakness of the third lumbrical

E weakness of wrist extension

Question 11

Clinical scenario

An 85-year-old man presented to the rheumatology outpatient clinic with a constant pain below his right knee. His right leg had been deformed for a number of years, and he had previously been diagnosed with osteoarthritis in his right knee, which caused knee pain after walking. On examination he had crepitus in his right knee, and the right tibia was bowed with a focal area of warmth. A diagnosis of Paget's disease was made.

Question

Which investigation is most appropriate to determine the extent of his Paget's disease?

Answer

A PET scan

B radionuclide bone scan

C serum alkaline phosphatase

D skeletal survey (MRI)

E skeletal survey (plain radiograph)

Question 12

Clinical scenario

A 23-year-old man with a history of joint hypermobility presented to the emergency department with a spontaneous pneumothorax. The chest X-ray that confirmed the presence of the pneumothorax showed an abnormal cardiac silhouette, and echocardiography subsequently revealed an aortic root aneurysm.

Question

Which additional feature would confirm a diagnosis of Marfan syndrome?

Answer

A ectopia lentis

B high arched palate

C pectus carinatum deformity

D scoliosis

E skin striae

Question 13

Clinical scenario

A 65-year-old man complained of intense pruritus just before developing marked hypotension (BP 30/? mmHg) followed by cardiac arrest soon after he received an injection of contrast during coronary angiography. Attempts to resuscitate him were unsuccessful. At post-mortem examination, atheromatous changes were noted in the coronary circulation, but this was felt to provide an insufficient explanation for the patient's collapse. The histopathologist was concerned about the possibility of contrast-agent-associated anaphylaxis.

Question

Which test is recommended for the post-mortem investigation of suspected anaphylaxis?

Answer

A carboxypeptidase

B interleukin-4

C platelet-activating factor

D total IgE

E tryptase

Question 14

Clinical scenario

A 50-year-old woman presented with a 6-month history of a purpuric rash on her lower limbs and intermittent arthralgia. Investigations by her general practitioner revealed a positive rheumatoid factor and elevated CRP, prompting a provisional diagnosis of rheumatoid arthritis. On assessment in the rheumatology outpatient clinic there was no evidence of synovitis, and the results of further investigations were as follows.

Anti-cyclic citrullinated peptide (CCP): antibody negative

Serum complement C3: 84 mg/dL (normal range 65–190)

Serum complement C4: 0.02 mg/dL (normal range 15–50)

Urine dipstick: non-visible haematuria 2+, proteinuria 2+

Question

Which is the most likely diagnosis?

Answer

A granulomatosis with polyangiitis

B Henoch–Schönlein purpura

C mixed cryoglobulinaemia

D rheumatoid vasculitis

E scleroderma

Question 15

Clinical scenario

A previously well 40-year-old motor mechanic was hospitalised in intensive care with acute respiratory failure. His chest CT showed diffuse inflammatory shadowing consistent with interstitial lung disease. The results of initial blood tests were normal, with the exception of CRP 70 mg/dL (normal threshold <10), a normochromic normocytic anaemia (Hb 104 g/L, normal range 130–180) and creatine kinase (CK) 2,204 U/L (normal range 24–195). An autoantibody screen revealed a positive antinuclear antibody accompanied by cytoplasmic staining on the HEp-2 cell testing substrate. Further investigation revealed a positive antibody to Jo-1.

Question

What is the most likely diagnosis?

Answer

A acute rhabdomyolysis

B granulomatosis with polyangiitis

C inflammatory myositis

D sarcoidosis

E systemic lupus erythematosus

MRCP(UK) Part 2 examination questions

Question 16

Clinical scenario

A 20-year-old student was hospitalised with acute meningococcal meningitis. He made a rapid recovery following prompt treatment, but review of his history revealed a previous episode of meningococcal meningitis at the age of 10 years (strain unknown), which raised concern about underlying immune deficiency.

Question

Which investigation is most likely to lead to a definitive diagnosis?

Answer

A antinuclear antibody

B CD4 count

C neutrophil respiratory burst

D serum immunoglobulins

E total haemolytic complement activity

Question 17

Clinical scenario

A 72-year-old retired publican presented to the emergency department with an acutely swollen left knee, which had developed over the preceding 2 days such that he now had difficulty weight-bearing. There was no history of trauma and he felt generally well. His past medical history includes chronic kidney disease stage 3. He was afebrile with a warm knee effusion. An X-ray of the knee confirmed the effusion, but was otherwise normal. A sample of synovial fluid was aspirated.

Question

What is the most likely finding from the synovial fluid?

Answer

A acellular aspirate

B Gram-negative rods

C Gram-positive cocci

D negatively birefringent needle-shaped crystals

E positively birefringent brick-shaped crystals

Question 18

Clinical scenario

A 24-year-old man presented to the rheumatology outpatient clinic with back and buttock pain. This was particularly severe in the early hours of the morning, waking him from sleep, and he was stiff for much of the morning. He had a history of iritis and Achilles tendinopathy, but systems review was otherwise unremarkable. An MRI confirmed bilateral sacroiliitis.

Question

What is the treatment of choice?

Answer

A anti-tumour necrosis factor (TNF)

B hydroxychloroquine

C methotrexate

D NSAIDs

E prednisolone

Question 19

Clinical scenario

A 45-year-old woman with Scl70-positive scleroderma and established pulmonary hypertension was reviewed in clinic after an interval of 2 years due to a number of failed attendances. She complained of gradually diminishing exercise tolerance and a dry cough. On examination she had features of diffuse cutaneous disease. Cardiovascular examination revealed that her jugular venous pressure (JVP) was elevated, and there was a parasternal heave, a loud S2, and peripheral oedema to mid-calf. Chest examination revealed fine bibasal crepitations.

Question

What complication is most likely to have arisen?

Answer

A chronic pulmonary thromboembolism

B interstitial lung disease

C left ventricular failure

D pulmonary vasculopathy

E renal failure

Question 20

Clinical scenario

A 65-year-old woman with systemic lupus erythematosus attended the rheumatology outpatient clinic for routine review. She complained of breathlessness and fatigue, with swelling of her ankles and periorbital puffiness each morning. Examination revealed pulse 78 beats per minute (sinus rhythm), BP 162/92 mmHg, JVP elevated +5 cm, normal heart sounds and peripheral oedema to mid-calf. In the chest there were some bibasal crepitations. Urine dipstick analysis was positive for blood (1+) and protein (3+).

Question

What is the most important investigation to determine management?

Answer

A chest X-ray

B CT chest

C echocardiography

D renal biopsy

E spirometry

Question 21

Clinical scenario

A 72-year-old woman with seronegative rheumatoid arthritis attended the rheumatology outpatient clinic for routine review. Despite several years of treatment with disease-modifying antirheumatic drugs (DMARDs), including methotrexate, her disease was severe, with a persistently high disease activity score (DAS). Her past medical history included an anterior resection for colorectal carcinoma 2 years previously, and longstanding chronic obstructive pulmonary disease (COPD), which was well controlled with Seretide.

Question

What is the best next therapeutic option?

Answer

A adalimumab

B cyclophosphamide

C rituximab

D tocilizumab

E ustekinumab

Question 22

Clinical scenario

A 39-year-old man attended the emergency department with acute orofacial angio-oedema and difficulty in breathing.

Question

Which feature most suggests the possibility of anaphylaxis?

Answer

A patient ate peanuts 4 hours before symptom onset

B patient is taking an angiotensin-converting enzyme (ACE) inhibitor as regular medication

C patient took amoxicillin 3 hours before symptom onset

D rapid progression of symptoms

E urticaria associated with the angio-oedema

Question 23

Clinical scenario

A 34-year-old woman presented to the emergency department with fever and a cough productive of green sputum, which had started 2 days previously. She was known to have common variable immunodeficiency and bronchiectasis, and was receiving weekly subcutaneous immunoglobulin. She had no known drug allergies. She appeared comfortable at rest, and vital signs included temperature 38°C, respiratory rate 20/min and oxygen saturation 97% (on room air). She had coarse crackles at both bases. Review of recent results showed trough IgG level of 8.4 g/L (normal range 6.0–13.0).

Question

What is the most appropriate treatment?

Answer

A co-amoxiclav

B co-trimoxazole

C fluconazole

D ganciclovir

E immunoglobulin

Question 24

Clinical scenario

A 72-year-old man who had previously been well presented to the emergency department with lobar pneumonia. He had had several episodes of sinusitis, requiring antibiotics, in the previous year. Blood test results included haemoglobin 112 g/L (normal range 130–180), white cell count $21,400 \times 10^9$/L (79% lymphocytes, 21% neutrophils) (normal range 4.0–11.0×10^9/L), platelets 142×10^9/L (normal range 150–400). Serum immunoglobulins were IgG 3.2 g/L (normal range 6.0–13.0), IgA 0.3 g/L (normal range 0.8–3.0), IgM 0.1 g/L (normal range 0.4–2.5) (ie all low).

Question

What is the most likely diagnosis?

Answer

A chronic lymphocytic leukaemia

B common variable immunodeficiency

C drug-induced antibody deficiency

D light chain myeloma

E protein losing enteropathy

Question 25

Clinical scenario

A 25-year-old Iraqi man was referred to the rheumatology outpatient clinic with joint pains. His past medical history included recurrent oral ulcers and treatment for uveitis. On examination he had no clear evidence of arthritis, but he did have extensive herpetiform aphthous ulcers on the buccal mucosa. His eyes and skin were normal.

Question

What is the most likely diagnosis?

Answer

A ANCA-associated vasculitis

B Behçet's disease

C sarcoidosis

D syphilis

E systemic lupus erythematosus

Question 26

Clinical scenario

A 60-year-old man presented with a history of low backache and recurrent urinary infections over the past 2 years. MRI of his abdomen demonstrated widespread retroperitoneal fibrosis associated with hydronephrosis. An ultrasound (U/S)-guided biopsy of fibrotic tissue revealed prominent lymphoplasmacytic inflammation with no evidence of lymphoma.

Question

Which investigation would be crucial in establishing the diagnosis?

Answer

A ANCA

B rheumatoid factor

C serum angiotensin-converting enzyme (ACE)

D serum immunoglobulins

E specific staining of biopsy tissue

Question 27

Clinical scenario

A 50-year-old woman with severe rheumatoid arthritis attended the rheumatology outpatient clinic for routine review. She had suffered from recurrent sinopulmonary infections over the past 12 months. Results of immunological investigations were as follows: serum IgG 2.1 g/L (normal range 6.0–13.0), IgA 0.1 g/L (normal range 0.8–3.0), IgM 0.2 g/L (normal range 0.4–2.5). Circulating lymphocyte surface marker profile revealed absent B-cells with moderate T-cell lymphopenia.

Question

Which treatment would account for these immunology results?

Answer

A adalimumab

B etanercept

C infliximab

D rituximab

E tocilizumab

Question 28

Clinical scenario

A 40-year-old man presented with a 2-year history of recurrent infections. Routine haematological and biochemical tests were performed. His full blood count and renal function were normal. The total serum protein level was 54 g/L (normal range 61–76) and serum albumin 41 g/L (normal range 37–49).

Question

Which is the key investigation to do next?

Answer

A CD4 lymphocyte count

B HIV serology

C high-resolution computed tomography (HRCT) chest scan

D neutrophil oxidative burst

E serum immunoglobulins

Question 29

Clinical scenario

An 18-year-old man presented with weight loss and haemoptysis. His chest X-ray showed bilateral cavitating pulmonary nodules. Further investigation results included a negative HIV test and a negative serum ANCA test. Biopsy of a nodule showed granulomatous disease with acid-fast bacilli, which were subsequently shown to be *Mycobacterium avium-intracellulare* (MAI).

Question

Which investigation is critical to establishing a definitive diagnosis?

Answer

A assessment of interferon-γ production by activated lymphocytes

B CD4 lymphocyte count

C lymphocyte transformation to mycobacterial purified protein derivative (PPD)

D sequencing of the mycobacterial genome

E total haemolytic complement

Question 30

Clinical scenario

A 28-year-old gas fitter presented with a 6-month history of lumbo-sacral back pain that frequently involved his buttocks. These symptoms were worse in the morning and sometimes woke him in the latter half of the night. Running tended to improve his back pain, as did ibuprofen. On examination he had a full range of movement in his spine and there was no peripheral synovitis.

Question

What is the most likely diagnosis?

Answer

A lumbar discitis

B mechanical back pain

C rheumatoid arthritis

D spondyloarthritis

E vertebral fracture

4.2 Self-assessment answers

Answer to Question 1

B: psoriatic arthritis

This patient has a polyarthritis and a rash. Although the differential could encompass all the above, the combination of scaly plaques and nail changes, in association with dactylitis and distal interphalangeal joint involvement makes psoriatic arthritis the most likely. Uncomplicated rheumatoid arthritis is not associated with a skin rash, while a vasculitic rash is usually non-blanching and displays discrete petechiae or purpura. Post-infectious rashes tend to be maculopapular, but can also appear vasculitic.

Answer to Question 2

C: antinuclear antibody (ANA)

The clinical scenario suggests systemic lupus erythematosus and a positive ANA (plus extractable nuclear antigens such as double-stranded DNA and Sm) would confirm the diagnosis. Complement levels are reduced in active disease but would not help with initial diagnosis if they were normal.

Answer to Question 3

E: Ro/La positive

This woman demonstrates features consistent with a diagnosis of Sjögren's syndrome, which is associated with anti-Ro and/or anti-La antibodies. Treatment is aimed at alleviating sicca symptoms and arthritis. Patients with Sjögren's are at a higher risk of developing lymphoma than the background population, hence regular review and monitoring of immunoglobulins is advised.

Answer to Question 4

D: synovial fluid culture

This patient is at high risk of septic arthritis as she has abnormal joints, is on DMARDs, and has a coexistent bacterial infection. Although synovial fluid microscopy may be helpful, it can be negative in patients exposed to antibiotics, so cultures are crucial. The diagnostic yield from blood cultures in septic arthritis is lower than that of synovial fluid aspirate. Although gout is a possible diagnosis, serum urate may be normal even during an acute attack.

Answer to Question 5

D: reactive arthritis

The combination of monoarthritis and a rash after a diarrhoeal illness makes reactive arthritis the most likely diagnosis. Enteropathic arthritis would be more likely if the history of bowel disturbance were more protracted, the bowel and peripheral joint disease coincided, and the rash was over the shins (erythema nodosum or pyoderma gangrenosum). Although Behçet's and Lyme disease can both cause a rash and arthritis, the clinical picture is not correct for either.

Answer to Question 6

C: negative skin-prick and intra-dermal tests to determinants of penicillin

The vast majority of patients who claim to be penicillin-allergic on the basis of an isolated skin rash many decades ago are not allergic to penicillin. This history suggests the risk of penicillin-induced anaphylaxis is very low, but the demonstration of negative skin-prick and negative intradermal tests provides added reassurance. Negative specific IgE antibodies to penicillin determinants cannot reliably exclude allergy because of their limited sensitivity, and total IgE and tryptase levels are of little value in excluding IgE-mediated allergy.

Answer to Question 7

C: glucagon

Adrenaline is frequently ineffective in patients on long-term beta-blockers because of chronic β-adrenergic receptor occupancy by these drugs, thus precluding the ability of adrenaline to exert inotropic effects. A drug that has cardiac inotropic effects and bypasses β-adrenergic receptors is required immediately. Glucagon fulfils both of these criteria.

Answer to Question 8

E: lisinopril

ACE inhibitors are associated with non-allergic slow-onset angio-oedema, which can cause life-threatening airway obstruction that is resistant to conventional treatments. Angio-oedema affects 0.1–0.7% of those treated with these agents and may occur even after many years of exposure. Hereditary or acquired angio-oedema due to C1 inhibitor deficiency may also present in this way, but are much less common. Salicylate hypersensitivity typically presents with urticaria and wheeze, would have more acute onset, and would be temporally associated with salicylate ingestion.

Answer to Question 9

B: temporal arteritis

The presence of constitutional symptoms, low-grade fever and tenderness of the temporal artery makes temporal arteritis the most likely diagnosis. Key investigations would be serum CRP and a temporal artery biopsy, but administration of steroids should not be delayed if the patient had any visual symptoms.

Answer to Question 10

B: wasting of the thenar eminence

Sensory loss with carpal tunnel syndrome typically involves the second and third fingers and weakness is associated with the thenar muscles. Ulnar nerve lesions can cause sensory loss in the fifth finger and weakness of the remaining small muscles of the hands.

Answer to Question 11

B: radionuclide bone scan

In a patient with Paget's disease, focal bone pain can have numerous causes. It is important to exclude an osteosarcoma, so an X-ray of the right leg is entirely appropriate. However, although this will provide information about the cause of the pain it will not determine the extent of disease – for this a bone scan is most appropriate. The serum alkaline phosphatase also correlates with the extent of skeletal involvement.

Answer to Question 12

A: ectopia lentis

The Ghent nosology are used for the diagnosis of Marfan syndrome. Recent revisions place more emphasis on cardiovascular manifestations. The presence of aortic aneurysm and ectopia lentis is sufficient to establish the diagnosis. Although a high arched palate, pectus carinatum, scoliosis and skin striae are associated with Marfan syndrome, by themselves they are not sufficient to support a diagnosis.

Answer to Question 13

E: tryptase

The constellation of symptoms and their immediate relationship to the injection of contrast agent, coupled with the lack of a clear explanation for cardiovascular collapse at post-mortem, is suggestive of anaphylaxis. Of the biomarkers listed, only tryptase can be reliably assayed on post-mortem blood.

Answer to Question 14

C: mixed cryoglobulinaemia

The key clues to the diagnosis are a serum complement profile that shows classical pathway activation (reflected in a low C4) accompanied by a positive rheumatoid factor in the clinical context of purpura and dipstick haematuria. The only unifying explanation for this constellation of findings is mixed cryoglobulinaemia. All of the other diagnoses are associated with normocomplementaemia.

Answer to Question 15

C: inflammatory myositis

While interstitial lung disease has a broad differential diagnosis, the combination of an elevated creatine kinase (CK) and anti-Jo1 positivity is highly suggestive of inflammatory myositis. Because of the cytoplasmic distribution of Jo-1, anti-Jo-1 positivity is frequently detectable as cytoplasmic staining on HEp-2 cell substrates.

Answer to Question 16

E: total haemolytic complement activity

A history of two episodes of meningitis strongly suggests the possibility of underlying complement deficiency, particularly of terminal complement components underlying the importance of the C5b-9 complex in host defence against *Neisseria meningitidis*. Screening for the integrity of both classical and alternative pathways by assessing haemolytic complement activity is a rational first step to identifying complement component deficiency.

Answer to Question 17

D: negatively birefringent needle-shaped crystals

The feared cause of an acute monoarthritis is septic arthritis, but there is nothing in the history or examination to suggest infection. The most likely diagnosis is gout, given the possibility of alcohol intake (in a retired publican) and stage 3 chronic kidney disease, both of which increase serum urate levels. Pseudogout (pyrophosphate disease with brick-shaped positively birefringent crystals) is a possibility, but one would expect chondrocalcinosis on the X-ray.

Answer to Question 18

D: NSAIDs

The diagnosis is ankylosing spondylitis (AS), as evidenced by characteristic clinical and radiological features of spondyloarthritis, plus extra-spinal manifestations of iritis and tendinopathy. The treatment of choice is NSAIDs and physiotherapy (often hydrotherapy). Anti-TNF is indicated in disease that remains active despite an adequate trial of NSAIDs. Steroids / disease-modifying antirheumatic drugs (DMARDs) are not used in pure AS (although any additional peripheral disease such as hip/knee arthritis may respond).

Answer to Question 19

B: interstitial lung disease

This patient has features of pulmonary hypertension on a background of Scl70-positive diffuse scleroderma, making interstitial lung disease the most likely complication. Vasculopathy is associated with centromere positivity and would not produce crepitations; although an acute pulmonary embolism (PE) may produce right heart strain, the history is more insidious and there is no history of chest pain.

Answer to Question 20

D: renal biopsy

The presence of fluid overload, hypertension, oedema, proteinuria and haematuria is highly suggestive of renal lupus in this context, and a diagnostic renal biopsy should be sought, especially if there is any evidence of a rising creatinine (even if it is still within normal range). If renal lupus is confirmed on biopsy, therapeutic options would include steroids, cyclophosphamide or mycophenolate mofetil.

Answer to Question 21

D: tocilizumab

This patient meets standard (National Institute for Health and Care Excellence (NICE)) criteria for biologic therapy for rheumatoid arthritis. Since she is seronegative, she is not a candidate for rituximab, and TNF inhibition (adalimumab) is relatively contraindicated due to her recent previous malignancy. Cyclophosphamide is used primarily in vasculitis/connective tissue disease and not inflammatory joint disease. Ustekinumab (interleukin (IL)-12 / IL-23 inhibition) is not licensed for use in rheumatoid arthritis.

Answer to Question 22

D: rapid progression of symptoms

Rapid progression is a hallmark of anaphylaxis, which typically occurs immediately or within 30 minutes of contact with the allergen responsible.

Urticaria, although a feature of anaphylaxis, is often idiopathic.

ACE inhibitors are associated with non-allergic slow onset angio-oedema, which may potentially cause life-threatening airway obstruction that is resistant to conventional treatments.

Answer to Question 23

A: co-amoxiclav

Patients with antibody deficiency may require prolonged treatment of intercurrent infection. Initial antibiotics should be based on previous sputum isolates, or if unavailable, should cover common organisms until results of cultures are reported. Pneumocystis is not a common feature of antibody deficiency, but commonly occurs in T-cell or severe 'combined' immune deficiencies. The presentation is not suggestive of either cytomegalovirus (CMV) or fungal infection.

Answer to Question 24

A: chronic lymphocytic leukaemia

Primary immune deficiency such as common variable immunodeficiency can present at any age, but secondary antibody deficiency is more likely in an older person. In this case the high lymphocyte count suggests that chronic lymphocytic leukaemia, which is common in older people, is the cause of the antibody deficiency.

Answer to Question 25

B: Behçet's disease

This man does not satisfy all of the International Study Group (ISG) for Behçet's disease criteria, which require recurrent oral ulcers and at least two of uveitis, typical skin lesions, genital ulcers and pathergy, but it is still the most likely diagnosis. Anterior uveitis may not be visible on external inspection (or fundoscopy); detection requires slit-lamp examination.

Answer to Question 26

E: specific staining of biopsy tissue

The clinical context of retroperitoneal fibrosis associated with lymphoplasmacytic inflammation is highly suggestive of IgG4-related disease (IgG4-RD). Immunohistochemical staining of biopsy tissue for IgG4-expressing plasma cells would be critical in establishing the diagnosis. Serum IgG4 is of secondary importance, being elevated in only approximately 50% of cases.

Answer to Question 27

D: rituximab

As a therapeutic monoclonal antibody targeted against the CD20 antigen on B-cells, rituximab induces significant sustained hypogammaglobulinaemia accompanied by B-cell lymphopenia in a small minority of patients, some of whom will require immunoglobulin replacement. Adalimumab, infliximab and etanercept are targeted against the TNF pathway and do not affect serum immunoglobulin levels, and neither does tocilizumab (anti-IL-6 receptor).

Answer to Question 28

E: serum immunoglobulins

This patient's low total protein is a reflection of low total globulin levels (calculated by subtracting albumin from total protein). In this case this amounts to 13 g/L (normal range 17–24). Serum immunoglobulins are the major component of total globulins, hence it is very likely that this patient's immunoglobulin levels are low, which would explain his burden of infections.

Answer to Question 29

A: assessment of interferon-γ production by activated lymphocytes

Disseminated MAI infection in a young HIV-negative patient is highly suggestive of a defect in this patient's type I cytokine pathway (interleukin-12–interferon-γ axis). Assessment of interferon-γ production in response to lymphocyte activation is the key investigation to assess the integrity of this pathway.

Answer to Question 30

D: spondyloarthritis

He has features that are consistent with inflammatory back pain: it is worse in the morning, eases with use, involves the buttock and wakes him in the second half of the night. Pain in the buttocks suggests that he has sacroiliitis, which could be demonstrated with a FABER test. This involves the leg being Flexed at the hip, ABducted and Externally Rotated, which induces anterior ipsilateral pain in hip disease and posterior contralateral pain in sacroiliac disease. An MRI would be the investigation of choice to determine whether there is sacroiliitis.

Index

Note: page numbers in *italics* refer to figures, those in **bold** refer to tables.

non-rheumatoid pain and stiffness 40–2
  see also osteoarthritis (OA)
  see also rheumatoid arthritis (RA)
NSAIDs
  acute hot joints and 86
  gout and 120
  hypersensitivity 16–17, 17
  RA and 111
nuclear medicine 155–6
nut allergy 104, 105
  see also allergy

O

obstruction of major arteries 25
  see also Raynaud's phenomenon
ocular complications
  Behçet's disease and **73**, 74, 75, 138
  bilateral orbital masses in Wegener's
    granulomatosis 134
  Marfan syndrome and 67
  red eyes and oral ulcers 73–6
  Sjögren's syndrome and 125, 125,
    126
oedema, gout and 63
oesophageal dysmotility in scleroderma
  129
oligoarthritis 116
omalizumab for nut allergy 104, 105
opportunistic infection 82
oral allergy syndrome 104
organ damage analysis, Raynaud's
  phenomenon 26
osteoarthritis (OA)
  aetiology/pathophysiology/pathology
    108
  clinical presentation 108–9
  crepitus and 41
  hand 52–5, 109
  of hip and knee 109
  investigation 41–2
  involvement of particular joints in **41**
  joint changes in 108
  joint shape and 41

management 42
Paget's disease and 66
physical signs 109
psoriatic arthritis and 58
secondary causes of 109
osteoporosis 34, 86–8
  see also fractures, osteoporotic
oxygenation, septicaemia in asplenic
    patients and 77

P

Paget's disease of bone 65–6
palindromic RA 85
palpable purpura 18
palpitations, flushing and 13
PAN see polyarteritis nodosa (PAN)
pancreas, IgG4-RD and 130
panic attacks 81
paraesthesia 107
parotid enlargement, bilateral **28**
periodontal disease 4
peripheral perfusion 77
PET see positron emission tomography
    (PET)
phagocyte defect 149–50, 152
Phalen's test, carpal tunnel syndrome
    107
phenoxymethylpenicillin 7
photosensitivity 21
  see also arthralgia and photosensitive
    rash
plasma viscosity (PV) **144**, 145
platelet count in RA 111
PM see polymyositis (PM)
PMR see polymyalgia rheumatica (PMR)
Pneumocystis pneumonia 3, 134
Pneumovax 76
pollen-food syndrome 104
polyarteritis nodosa (PAN) 38–40
  aetiology/pathophysiology/pathology
    135
  clinical presentation 135
  complications 135

differential diagnosis 135
digital gangrene in 39
epidemiology 135
investigations 40, 135, 136
management 40
physical signs 135
prognosis 135
treatment 135
polyarthralgia 36, 41
polyarthritis 116
polymyalgia rheumatica (PMR) 29, 36
  giant cell arteritis and 131–3
polymyositis (PM) 29
positron emission tomography (PET),
    PAN and 40
pregnancy
  breathlessness and weakness 31
  C1 inhibitor deficiency and 9
primary antibody deficiency 89–92
  see also immunodeficiency
proximal myopathy 29–31
pseudogout 121
  see also gout
psoriatic arthritis 20, 56
  clinical presentation 115
  epidemiology 114
  hand examination 59
  osteoarthritis-like pattern 58
  prognosis 116
psoriatic arthropathy 52
psychosocial 'yellow flags 33–4
pulmonary complications
  in scleroderma 128
  in SLE 124
  in Wegener's granulomatosis 134
pulmonary function tests
  Sjögren's syndrome and 29
PV see plasma viscosity (PV)

R

RA see rheumatoid arthritis (RA)
radiograph/radiology
  ankylosing spondylitis and 65